Neurotransmitter Transporters

Contemporary Neuroscience

Neurotransmitter Transporters

Structure, Function, and Regulation

Edited by

Maarten E. A. Reith

College of Medicine, University of Illinois, Peoria, IL

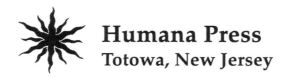

Humana Press
Totowa, New Jersey

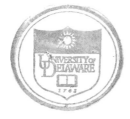

QP
364
.7
.N4757
1997

Cover illustration: Clearance of Extracellular Neurotransmitter by Presynaptic Neurotransmitter Transporters, courtesy of Randy D. Blakely, Vanderbilt Center for Molecular Neuroscience, Nashville, TN 37232-6600.

For additional copies, pricing for bulk purchases, and/or information about other Humana titles, contact Humana at the above address or at any of the following numbers: Tel.: 201-256-1699; Fax: 201-256-8314; E-mail: humana@interramp.com

Printed in the United States of America. 10 9 8 7 6 5 4 3 2 1

Library of Congress Cataloging in Publication Data

Main entry under title:

Neurotransmitter transporters: structure, function, and regulation / edited by Maarten E. A. Reith.
    p.   cm. — (Contemporary neuroscience)
    Includes index.
    ISBN 0-89603-372-4 (alk. paper)
    1. Neurotransmitters. 2. Carrier proteins.   I. Reith, Maarten E. A.
II. Series.
QP364.7.N4757   1997
612.8'22—dc20   96-36600
                                                        CIP

Preface

During neuronal activity a neurotransmitter is released into the synaptic cleft where it acts on various receptors positioned pre- and postsynaptically. Enormous progress has been made in characterizing neurotransmitter receptors and many books focus on the important advances in the receptor field. However, another vital aspect of synaptic transmission is the removal of transmitter from the synaptic cleft and the impact of relocated transmitter. A pivotal role in these processes is played by uptake of transmitter into neuronal or glial cells by specific transporter proteins that have been studied intensely over the last 25 years. Indeed, many advances have been made in the reuptake transporter area, but the information is scattered over a variety of publishing vehicles, making it difficult to conceptualize the different characteristics and physiological roles of these various transporters.

The primary aim of *Neurotransmitter Transporters: Structure, Function, and Regulation,* therefore, is to offer a comprehensive picture of the recent advances made in characterizing neurotransmitter transporters and understanding their biological roles. The current state of knowledge presents an optimal time for such a comprehensive focus on transmitter transporters because of the enormous progress made in cloning the genes coding for these different proteins. The information obtained from the application of molecular biological techniques builds on the results of the previous burst of findings with ligands that selectively target transporters, either as substrates or as blockers.

Interest in neurotransmitter transporters is steadily increasing, along with clearer understanding of their roles in the pathophysiology of schizophrenia, Tourette's syndrome, Parkinson's disease, neurotoxin accumulation and removal, brain ischemia, amyotrophic lateral sclerosis, or in the mechanisms of action of drugs of abuse, antidepressants, and antiepileptics. Thus, *Neurotransmitter Transporters: Structure, Function, and Regulation* will be of interest to scientists, graduate students, and advanced undergraduates who seek a comprehensive overview of this rapidly moving frontier in neuroscience. Selected chapters will also be of interest to physicians who are carrying out imaging and postmortem measurements of neurotransmitter transporters in the human brain.

Each chapter of *Neurotransmitter Transporters: Structure, Function, and Regulation* is not simply a review of the work carried out in the author's laboratory, but more importantly offers a critical survey and synthesis of achievements pertinent to the characterization, mechanism of action, regulation, and physiological relevance of each transporter. Chapters 1–7 focus on various neurotransmitter transporters located in neuronal or glial plasma membranes and in synaptic vesicles. The Na^+- and Cl^--dependent plasma membrane transporters are described for monoamines (Chapters 1–3) and for a number of compounds including amino acids (proline, glycine, GABA, taurine, betaine, creatine, choline) (Chapters 4,5). The separate family of Na^+-dependent glutamate transporters is discussed (Chapters 5,6) as well as the family of vesicular transporters for monoamines and acetylcholine (Chapter 7). Chapters 8–12 cover a variety of issues relevant to transporter structure and function. Chapter 8 describes posttranslational modifications with their important impact on the function of various transporters. Chapter 9 covers the wide variety of classes of recently developed blockers for the dopamine transporter, and Chapter 10 deals with the development of imaging techniques for neurotransmitter transporters to allow detection of changes in the living human brain. Characteristics of the dopamine transporter in human brain and alterations induced by cocaine use are described in Chapter 11, whereas the final chapter highlights the role of monoamine transporters in the action of monoamine uptake blockers both at the level of neuronal cell bodies and axon terminals.

The choice of authors for each neurotransmitter transporter reflects this editor's identification of investigators who have been instrumental in developing the field and are in the forefront of its ongoing elucidation. I thank the authors for their patience during the process of putting this book together and I am grateful for the excellent cooperation they have provided. I also appreciate the opportunity offered by Paul Dolgert, Tom Lanigan, and Tom Lanigan, Jr. at Humana Press for producing this book in recognition of the importance of neurotransmitter transporters in synaptic transmission.

Maarten E. A. Reith

Contents

Contributors

SUSAN G. AMARA • *Vollum Institute for Advanced Biomedical Research, Oregon Health Sciences University, Portland, OR*

RANDY D. BLAKELY • *Department of Pharmacology, Vanderbilt University Medical Center, Nashville, TN*

JOHN W. BOJA • *Department of Pharmacology, N.E. Ohio Universities College of Medicine, Rootstown, OH*

CHRISTOPHER C. BRADLEY • *Graduate Program in Neuroscience, Emory University School of Medicine, Atlanta, GA*

F. IVY CARROLL • *Department of Chemistry and Life Sciences, Research Triangle Institute, Research Triangle Park, NC*

NIAN-HANG CHEN • *Department of Pharmacology, Nanjing Medical University, Nanjing, Jiangsu, China*

BARBARA A. DOMIN • *Department of Neurobiology, Duke University Medical Center, Durham, NC*

ROBERT T. FREMEAU, JR. • *Department of Neurobiology, Duke University Medical Center, Durham, NC*

MATTHIAS A. HEDIGER • *Department of Medicine, Brigham and Women's Hospital, Harvard Medical School, Boston, MA*

YOSHIKATSU KANAI • *Department of Pharmacology, Kyorin University, Tokyo, Japan*

BARUCH I. KANNER • *Department of Biochemistry, Hadassah Medical School, The Hebrew University, Jerusalem, Israel*

DANIEL T. KLEVEN • *Department of Neurobiology, Duke University Medical Center, Durham, NC*

MICHAEL J. KUHAR • *Yerkes Regional Primate Research Center, Division of Neuroscience, Emory University, Atlanta, GA*

ANITA H. LEWIN • *Department of Chemistry and Life Sciences, Research Triangle Institute, Research Triangle Park, NC*

DEBORAH C. MASH • *Department of Neurology, University of Miami School of Medicine, Miami, FL*

JOSHUA W. MILLER • *Department of Neurobiology, Duke University Medical Center, Durham, NC*

STEPHAN NUSSBERGER • *Institut für Physiologische Chemie, Ludwig-Maximilians-Universität, Munich, Germany*

AMRAT P. PATEL • *Center for Drug Evaluation and Research, US Food and Drug Administration, Rockville, MD*

SUE L. POVLOCK • *Vollum Institute for Advanced Biomedical Research, Oregon Health Sciences University, Portland, OR*

YAN QIAN • *Graduate Program in Neuroscience, Emory University School of Medicine, Atlanta, GA*

SAMMANDA RAMAMOORTHY • *Department of Pharmacology, Vanderbilt University Medical Center, Nashville, TN*

MAARTEN E. A. REITH • *Department of Pharmacology, University of Illinois College of Medicine, Peoria, IL*

GARY RUDNICK • *Department of Pharmacology, Yale University School of Medicine, New Haven, CT*

URSULA SCHEFFEL • *Division of Nuclear Medicine, Department of Radiology, Johns Hopkins Medical Institute, Baltimore, MD*

SHIMON SCHULDINER • *Alexander Silberman Institute of Life Sciences, The Hebrew University, Jerusalem, Israel*

SALLY SCHROETER • *Department of Pharmacology, Vanderbilt University Medical Center, Nashville, TN*

JULIE K. STALEY • *Department of Molecular and Cellular Pharmacology, University of Miami School of Medicine, Miami, FL*

DAVIDE TROTTI • *Department of Medicine, Brigham and Women's Hospital, Harvard Medical School, Boston, MA*

DEAN F. WONG • *Division of Nuclear Medicine and Radiation Health Sciences, Johns Hopkins Medical Institute, Baltimore, MD*

CHAPTER 1

The Structure and Function of Norepinephrine, Dopamine, and Serotonin Transporters

Sue L. Povlock and Susan G. Amara

Introduction

Our first insights into the transport of monoamines came nearly 40 yrs ago when Axelrod et al. (7) injected [^{3}H]-epinephrine (EPI) into the femoral vein of anesthetized male rats in order to investigate the metabolism and physiological disposition of EPI and its metabolites. The data from this work demonstrated a selective, rapid accumulation of radiolabeled EPI in the adrenal gland, heart, and spleen (7). Shortly thereafter, similar results were obtained with [^{3}H]-norepinephrine (NE) (143) and the accumulation of both catecholamines was found to be dependent on intact sympathetic terminals (64,144) and associated with vesicles (147). These observations led to the proposal that the accumulation of the circulating catecholamines into specific tissues was responsible for their inactivation. Many drugs were known to affect the physiological actions of catecholamines and this prompted investigations into whether such compounds could act by blocking the accumulation of catecholamines. Indeed, transport of the catecholamines was inhibited by cocaine (144), reserpine, chloropromazine, imipramine, and amphetamine (8). Minimal amounts of the radiolabeled catecholamines were detected in the brain because they do not readily cross the blood–brain barrier (7,143), and thus, other investigators directly injected [^{3}H]-NE into the lateral ventricles and found that the radiolabeled compound selectively accumulated in catecholamine-rich areas (57). Further investigations into the fundamental properties of catecholamine transport were hindered by the

Neurotransmitter Transporters: Structure, Function, and Regulation
Ed. M. E. A. Reith Humana Press Inc., Totowa, NJ

lack of an in vitro system to study. Once methods to prepare synaptosomes were developed (*145*), experiments could be designed to explore the uptake of EPI and NE in brain tissues (*29,127*), thus allowing a more detailed investigation of the ion, pH, and temperature dependence of catecholamine transport (*62,68*).

Many years later, the field still draws great scientific and medical attention because the monoamine transporters are the primary sites of action for a wide spectrum of drugs which have both therapeutic and abuse potential. Inhibition of the dopamine transporter (DAT) has been closely linked to the euphoric and reinforcing properties of psychomotor stimulants, such as cocaine and amphetamines. The major classes of therapeutic antidepressants act by inhibiting the norepinephrine and/or serotonin transporters (NET and SERT), and many of these compounds have been proven clinically useful in treating an array of other behavioral syndromes, such as panic, stress, and obsessive compulsive disorders. The mechanism by which the transporter binds to and translocates its substrate across the plasma membrane is a fundamental issue for synaptic function, because reuptake along with diffusion can shape neurotransmission by limiting the extent, duration, and spacial domain of receptor activation. Progress in the monoamine transporter field had been impeded by the difficulties associated with purifying these membrane proteins which are relatively nonabundant in the central nervous system (CNS). However, the purification of a comparatively abundant γ-aminobutyric acid (GABA) transporter and the isolation of the corresponding cDNA clone, GAT-1, provided the first insight into the molecular details of neurotransmitter transporter structure (*61*). Shortly thereafter, a NET cDNA was isolated by a novel expression cloning technique and the sequence determined (*100*), thus allowing for the rapid cloning of the DAT and SERT. Elucidation of the basic function, structure–activity relationships, and regulation of the monoamine transporters are the current task at hand.

The monoamine transporters are members of a larger family of Na^+/Cl^--dependent transporters which also includes betaine, creatine, GABA, glycine, proline, and taurine carriers (*2,3,135*). The uptake process involves the translocation of substrate and cosubstrates Na^+ and Cl^- across the plasma membrane (*see* Fig. 1). Transport of substrate is energetically coupled to the transmembrane concentration gradient of Na^+, which is maintained by the activity of the Na^+/K^+-ATPase. Interestingly, when the ionic gradients are altered, such as when extracellular $[K^+]$ increases or extracellular

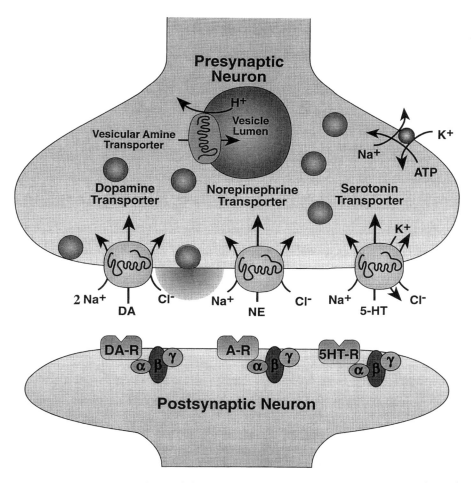

Fig. 1. The possible fates of the monoamine neurotransmitters once released from a vesicle into the synapse. DA, NE, and 5-HT diffuse across the synaptic cleft to bind to their respective receptors and alter the activity of the postsynaptic neurons. These neurotransmitters can be removed from the synapse by Na^+/Cl^--dependent monoamine transporters, thus limiting the stimulation of receptors. Once the neurotransmitter is transported into the cell, it can be taken up into vesicles by distinct carriers present on vesicular membranes.

[Na^+] and/or [Cl^-] decrease, transporters can function in reverse resulting in a net efflux of substrates and coupled ions out of a neuron (*36,42,87–89,125,131*). The recycling of SERT to an outwardly facing conformation requires K^+ (*98*), which may be replaced by H^+ or OH^- (*112*). There is no evidence that the other two monoamine transporters, NET and DAT, have such a requirement.

Isolation and Characterization of Transporter cDNAs

To circumvent the problems associated with the purification of low-abundance proteins in the brain, a novel expression cloning strategy was developed in order to isolate the NET cDNA from the human SK-N-SH cell line. This experimental approach involved expressing a library of SK-N-SH cDNAs in the COS-1 cell line (*100*). Individual cells expressing the NET were identified by autoradiography after incubation with [^{125}I]meta-iodobenzylguanidine, a catecholamine analog readily accumulated by NET. The sequence of NET contained many residues that were absolutely conserved with the GABA transporter (*61*), and thus defined a novel family of Na$^+$/Cl$^-$-dependent transporters (*see* Fig. 2, p. 6). Degenerate oligonucleotides, based on the conserved sequences between the GABA transporter and NET, were generated and employed either as probes for hybridization, or as primers for polymerase chain reactions to obtain DAT cDNA clones from various species: rat (*53,77,123*), bovine (*136*), and human (*55,105*). Similar strategies were used to clone the rat (*12,66*) human (*84,107*), and *Drosophila* (*28,35*) SERT cDNAs, and the bovine NET cDNA (*90*). The coding sequence for the transporters covers about 2 kb which corresponds to approx 617–630 amino acids, and the molecular weights of expressed proteins range from 60–97 kDa depending on the extent of glycosylation. A comparison of the primary sequences for the monoamine transporters demonstrates 80 and 69% homology between NET and DAT and DAT and SERT, respectively. Figure 2 highlights the conserved amino acids between the monoamine transporters and also the members of the Na$^+$/Cl$^-$-dependent neurotransmitter transporter family. The sequence is relatively more conserved in the putative transmembrane domains (TMs) and least conserved in the amino and carboxyl termini as well as the large extracellular loop between TMs 3 and 4. Preliminary structure–function analyses have provided some insights into which domains or specific amino acids are important to the binding of the antagonists, and this topic is discussed later.

Protein Sequence and Structure

Hydropathy analysis of the amino acid sequences predicted by the transporter clones suggests the presence of 12 putative TMs with a large extracellular loop between TMs 3 and 4, as shown in Fig. 3 (p. 8). Lack of a signal sequence followed by an even number of TMs implies that both the N- and C-termini reside within the cytoplasm, consistent with more recent data supporting this orientation. Some aspects of the general topology have been experimentally verified for NET and DAT. An indirect immunofluorescence study, employing antibodies raised against peptide sequences from the N- and C-termini and the large extracellular loop of NET, provided data to support the proposed orientation of these domains (*19*). For DAT, results from an electron microscopic immunochemical investigation provided support for the cytoplasmic location of the amino terminus (*99*). There are two cysteine residues located in the large extracellular loop which are conserved among all members of the family; these may form a disulfide bond thus maintaining a functional conformation of the transporter (*142*). A motif resembling a leucine zipper, which has been implicated in mediating protein–protein interactions, has been noted in TMs 2 and 9 (*3,52,65,100,119*), but there is no experimental evidence supporting the involvement of these leucines in possible subunit or membrane helix interactions of the transporters.

Consensus sites for glycosylation and phosphorylation are also present in the sequences encoded by the cDNAs. Sequence analysis of the human transporters predict three sites of N-linked glycosylation on the extracellular loop for NET and DAT, and two sites for SERT (*1,3,119*). Glycosylation has been shown to affect the surface expression and stability of the carriers (*95,133*). Neuraminidase treatment decreased the transport velocity of dopamine (DA) in striatal suspensions (*94*) and [^{3}H]-DA in synaptosomes (*149*) while having no affect on the affinity for substrates (*94,149*) or inhibitors. The influence of glycosylation on carrier structure and function will be reviewed in Chapter 8. Cytoplasmic consensus phosphorylation sites of protein kinase C, cAMP-dependent protein kinase, and Ca$^+$-calmodulin-dependent kinase are also inferred from the sequence (*3,52,65,134*), however as yet there is no experimental evidence to support a role for the direct phosphorylation of these residues in regulating the transporter function. The potential mechanisms for the direct or indirect regulation of carriers by phosporylation will be discussed in Chapters 2 and 8.

With much of the information on the structure of the monoamine transporters thus far derived from analysis of the primary sequence, attempts to elucidate the topology and subunit composition of these proteins have been limited. Two studies have attempted to estimate the size of the functionally active DAT by utilizing radiation inactivation analysis (*11,96*). However, the results of the studies are contradictory, predicting target sizes of 98 and 278 kDa, respectively.

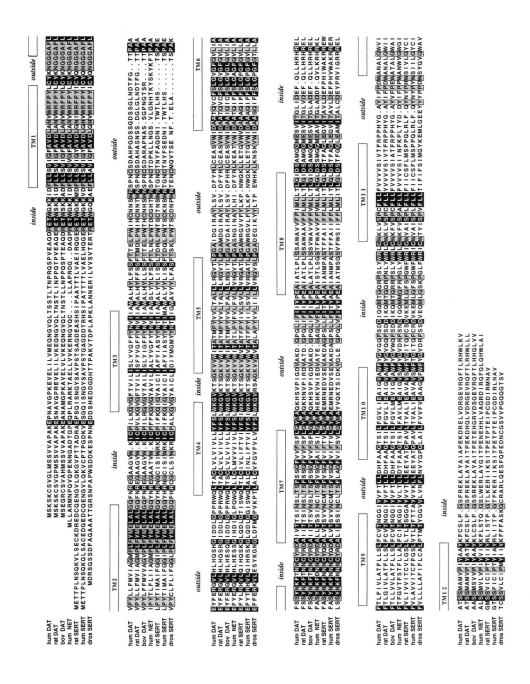

Molecular modeling techniques have been employed to simulate the tertiary structure of DAT using the primary sequence in conjunction with limited information from site-directed mutagenesis studies (*39*). The model predicts TMs that may be involved in the binding of DA and cocaine, however, no solid experimental evidence exists to corroborate this structural hypothesis for the transporter. The application of new experimental approaches for protein overexpression, topological and structural analyses, and determination of subunit composition will be required to address these issues.

Regional Distribution of Transporter mRNA and Protein

Investigations into the size and distribution of the mRNA of the monoamine transporters have employed techniques such as Northern blot analysis and *in situ* hybridization. Studies have shown that the expression of the mRNAs are localized to the cell bodies rather than to the neuronal terminals, are generally restricted to cells that synthesize the corresponding neurotransmitter, and thus are localized to distinct neuronal pathways of the brain. The regional expression pattern of the carrier mRNAs determines the substrates that they are likely to encounter and establishes which neuronal pathways will be influenced by the transporter activity. In contrast to the carriers for amino acid neurotransmitters for which glial expression is well documented, there is currently no indication that monoamine transporter mRNAs or proteins are expressed in glial cells. However several reports have noted monoamine transport activities in cultured glial cells (*33,78*). Additional studies will be required to resolve whether these activities correspond to known monoamine carriers expressed at levels below the sensitivity of detection by *in situ* hybridization and immunocytochemical methods.

DAT mRNA (approx 3.8 kb for rat and 3.0 kb for bovine) has been localized to the substantia nigra (SN) (*136*), the midbrain region (*92,124*), and the brain stem (*124*). *In situ* hybridization detected the highest expression of mRNA in the SN (*24,53,92,124*) and ventral

---

Fig. 2. An alignment of the protein sequences of the monoamine transporters. The amino acids shaded in gray represent residues common to all members of the Na^+/Cl^--dependent transporters including betaine, creatine, GABA, glycine, proline, and taurine carriers. Those residues conserved only between the monoamine transporters are denoted by white letters on a black background.

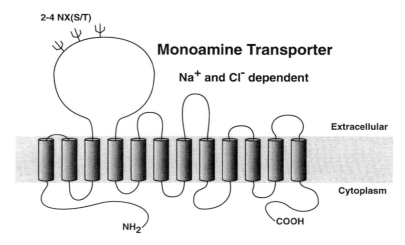

Fig. 3. The putative topology and structural features of the monoamine transporter proteins. As suggested by the primary sequence of the cDNAs, the proteins have 12 TMs with both the N- and C-termini oriented intracellularly. A large extracellular loop resides between TMs 3 and 4 and possesses anywhere from 2–4 consensus sites for glycosylation (AsnX[Ser/Tyr]).

tegmental area (VTA) (53,92,124), with the SN pars compacta (14,24,71,92,124) and the SN pars lateralis (92) having a more intense signals in comparison to that in the VTA (14,24,92,124). This evidence was further substantiated by demonstrating that the expression was localized to dopaminergic cell bodies using tyrosine hydroxylase immunostaining (5,14,92,136). Hybridization signals were also seen in the arcuate nucleus of the hypothalamus and glomerular layer of the olfactory bulb (24,92), zona incerta of the subthalamus (92), and cells of the inner nuclear layer of the retina (24). Developmental patterns of DAT expression also have been examined. Two independent investigations found that the DAT transcripts are detectable in the ventral mesencephalon of rats beginning on approximately embryonic d 15 (45,101). By embryonic d 18, expression of DAT mRNA in the VTA and SN resemble that found in adults (45). Information on the ontogeny of the DAT mRNA will enhance our understanding of the development of dopaminergic pathways and will aid in evaluating the impact of drugs of abuse at different developmental stages.

Various techniques and ligands have been used to assess the presence of DAT protein in regions of the brain receiving dopaminergic innervation (for a review *see* ref. *16* and Chapters 10 and 11). The production of transporter-specific antibodies (*140*) has led to the recent use of immunocytochemistry to determine the cellular localization of the transporter. Immunostaining has been detected in the SN (27,43,99), the dorsolateral striatum (27,43,99), medial forebrain bundle (27), arcuate nucleus and median eminence (113), certain nuclei of the VTA, nucleus accumbens, nigrostriatal bundle, lateral habenula, and olfactory tubercle (27,43). Using electron microscopic immunogold labeling, the transporter was detected in the plasma membranes of axons and dendrites in the SN, in the endoplasmic reticulum of dendrites in the SN, and in axon terminals of the striatum (99). The presence of DAT in dendrites suggests that the carrier may contribute to the dendritic release of DA by reverse transport and/or may influence local signaling mechanisms as a consequence of its ability to alter membrane potential (*see* section on Electrophysiological Properties). Both explanations warrant further investigation. This pattern of expression implies that DAT may influence pathways necessary for motor movements (30,59,132), motivation (15,31,72,73,126), and drug addiction (75,117).

The human NET probe selectively hybridized to two RNA species of approx 5.8 and 3.6 kb (92,100,108). The larger species was detected in the brainstem and in the adrenal gland, whereas the 3.6 kb species was expressed more widely at lower levels in other regions of the brain, as well as in the adrenal gland and placenta. Noradrenergic cells are highly restricted to the brainstem, and thus the 5.8 kb species most likely encodes the neuronal NET. Within the brainstem, the strongest labeling for NET mRNA was detected throughout the entire locus coeruleus complex in the dorsal pons, with the largest population of labeled cells localized in the nucleus locus coeruleus proper (40). Dopamine β-hydroxylase immunostaining together with *in situ* hybridization confirmed the localization of NET in the locus coeruleus and lateral tegmentum of the medulla and pons, regions encompassing most of the noradrenergic cell bodies in the CNS (92). The localization of NET mRNA in the locus coeruleus suggests that the transporter could influence many neuronal pathways because the noradrenergic terminals project widely to many different regions in the brain. Pathways involved in arousal, attention, autonomic and neuroendocrine regulation, as well as depression could be influenced by the modulation of NE transport activity.

Multiple species of SERT mRNA have also been noted. Northern blot analysis detected 8.2, 5.0, and 3.3 kb bands in the human brain (6) and 6.8, 4.9, and 3.0 kb bands in the human placenta (107). A single mRNA band (approx 3.8 kb) hybridized in the rat brainstem, midbrain, and adrenal gland (*12,84*). *In situ* hybridization detected strong labeling with a SERT probe in the dorsal and median raphe nuclear complex (*6,12,44*), and this general staining was further dissected and localized in the following raphe nuclei: raphe magnus nucleus, raphe pontis nuclei, raphe pallidus nucleus, and raphe obscurus nucleus (*44*). The cellular localization of the human SERT was determined using antibodies generated against the carboxyl terminal of human SERT (*106*). The immunoreactive fibers located in certain areas of the brain were consistent with those that exhibited high levels of antagonist binding (*32,47*), such as the cortex, the CA2–CA3 regions of the hippocampus, and the dorsal raphe nuclei (*26,38,70,130*). The serotonergic cell bodies present in the raphe nuclear com plex innervate many different regions of the brain and are involved various processes, including eating, sleeping, sexual behavior, circadian rhythmicity, neuroendocrine function, and mood disorders.

Organization of Transporter Genes

As noted in the previous section, multiple mRNA species have been found for NET (*92,100,108*) and SERT (*6,107*). However, there has been no indication of multiple subtypes with different primary sequences giving rise to structurally and functionally distinct carriers (*9*). A single mRNA species has been identified for DAT (*37,123,136*). As a result, the monoamine transporters appear to be encoded by three distinct genes that have been mapped to chromosomes 16q12–q21 (*20,50*), 5p15.3 (*55,137*), and 17q11.1–q12 (*51,107*) for the NET, DAT, and SERT, respectively. To date, these loci have not been linked to any established diseases, such as schizophrenia (*86*) or alcoholism (*97*).

The genes encoding the human SERT and NET have been identified and characterized (*83,103*). Both genes have a similar exon and intron structure and share the feature that each putative TM is encoded on a distinct exon. This is consistent with the structure of the GABA transporter gene (*82,91*), implying that this genomic organization may be conserved among the members of the Na^+/Cl^--dependent transporter family. One difference between the SERT and NET genes is that the NET gene has an additional exon encoding its C-terminus (*103*). Examination of the gene sequence for SERT revealed a number of putative binding sites for transcription factors that may influence the expression of the transporter gene. A TATA-like motif, an AP-1 binding site, and a cAMP response element are present in the sequence upstream from the initiator ATG codon (*83*).

Although the gene for DAT has not been characterized in its entirety, it is thought to span approx 70 kb of genomic DNA (*37*), a size roughly double that of SERT (31 kb) (*83*) and NET (45 kb) (*103*). As expected, the human DAT gene possesses a similar organization to the genes for other members of the family, but it appears to differ from SERT and NET in that it has only one exon encoding the region from TM 11 to the C-terminus. Sequence analysis of the upstream regions found it to contain a G-C rich domain and sequences with some similarity to the TATA and CAAT motifs (*37*), thus it is not yet understood whether the gene transcription of the DAT gene is driven by a classical TATA-box containing promoter or other sequence elements. The 3' untranslated region of the cDNA contains a novel repetitive (40 bp) element (*120,137,138*). The frequency of the 7-repeat allele has been reported to be higher in alcoholics with a mutant aldehyde dehydrogenase than in control subjects (*97*). A *Taq* I restriction fragment length polymorphism was also observed showing race-specific differences in the allelic frequencies (*138*).

Pharmacology of Monoamine Transport

Pharmacological characterization of the cloned monoamine transporters expressed in heterologous cell lines have confirmed the substrate specificities and inhibitor sensitivities of the transporters (*see* Table 1). NET transports both NE and DA very efficiently (*100*), whereas DAT mediates uptake of DA, but is an inefficient carrier of NE and other biogenic amines (*53,55,77,123,136*). Another substrate of DAT is the neurotoxin 1-methyl-4-phenylpyridinium (MPP$^+$) (*21,79,102*), a compound that causes a selective and irreversible loss of nigrostriatal dopaminergic neurons and provides the basis for an experimental model of Parkinson's disease (*17,128*). SERT shows a high selectivity for 5-HT but does not efficiently transport either NE or DA.

Drugs that block monoamine transport have powerful behavioral and physiological actions and have been the focus of extensive research into the development of useful therapeutic agents. The SERT is potently inhibited by many antidepressant drugs such as fluoxetine (Prozac™), sertraline, paroxetine, and citalopram (*see* ref. *46*). Other antidepressant drugs, such as the tricyclic antidepressant desipramine, are relatively selective inhibitors of NE uptake (*110,114*), and clinical studies of the actions of these drugs suggest that inhibition of NE reuptake also correlates with antidepressant activity (*114*). Tertiary amine tricyclic antidepressants, such as imipramine and

Table 1
Comparison of Various Inhibitors of the Transport of
Human Monoamine Clones

Inhibitors	K_i,nM DAT[a,b]	NET[c]	SERT[d,e]
Paroxetine		312	0.3
Citalopram		1000	5[e]
Fluoxetine			3[e]
Imipramine		65	5
Amitriptyline	3000[a]	100	15[d]
Mazindol	11, 60	1	98[e]
Cocaine	58, 743	140	611
Desipramine	13,000[a]	4	174
Nomifensine	17, 53	8	839
GBR12909	17, 14	133	
D-Amphetamine	2,260, 116	56	
L-Amphetamine	22,000[a]		
Nortriptyline	2300[a]	17	
DA	1220 (K_m), 1770	139	10,000
MPP+	10,000[a]		
NE	10,000, 8500	457 (K_m)	10,000
5-HT	10,000, 44,000	10,000	463 (K_m)

[a]The values of K_i were taken from Giros et al. (*55*) in Ltk⁻ cells.
[b]Values taken from Pristupa et al. (*105*) in COS-7 cells.
[c]Values taken from Pacholczyk et al. (*100*) in HeLa cells.
[d]Values taken from Ramamoorthy et al. (*107*) in HeLa cells.
[e]Values taken Demchyshyn et al. (*35*) in HeLa cells.

amytriptyline, have been found to be better inhibitors of SERT, whereas secondary tricyclic congeners, such as desipramine, antagonize NET to a greater extent (*100*). In contrast, psychomotor stimulants, such as cocaine and amphetamine, which nonselectively inhibit DAT, NET, and SERT, are poor antidepressants, despite the fact that they have stimulant and euphoric effects in some individuals.

Compounds that show greater potency as inhibitors of DAT than NET or SERT, include the diphenyl-piperazine derivatives, such as GBR12935, GBR12909, and LR1111 (*118*). Several reports have suggested that these agents demonstrate a nearly 400-fold greater selectivity for the inhibition of DA over NE uptake in synaptosomal preparations (*4*), but studies with the cloned carriers indicate a more limited 20-fold selectivity in their inhibition of DAT relative to NET

(22). These compounds also produce a spectrum of cocaine-like behavioral actions. For example, GBR12909 maintains iv self-administration in monkeys trained to self-administer cocaine (69), and supports increasing fixed-interval responding (69,76). In contrast, selective inhibitors of NE uptake (e.g., nisoxetine) or 5-HT transport (e.g., imipramine) do not maintain self-administration (67,148). Similarly, there are virtually no reports of abuse for mazindol, a more potent inhibitor of NET than DAT, that produces dysphoria in humans (25).

Cocaine is a moderately potent antagonist of all three monoamine transporters, but its actions on DAT have received the most attention because it appears to be the primary target for the addictive effects of cocaine (116). In these studies, the reinforcing effects have been attributed to inhibition of dopamine reuptake in the nucleus accumbens and related targets of the mesolimbic dopamine system. The effects of repeated cocaine, withdrawal from repeated cocaine, and withdrawal from self-administered cocaine on transport kinetics and DAT mRNA expression in both the striatum and nucleus accumbens have been reviewed (104). An exciting confirmation of the significance of DAT to the action of cocaine and amphetamines has come from the generation of a transgenic mouse line in which the dopamine transporter has been deleted by targeted disruption (54). The dramatic hyperactivity and neurochemical differences associated with the homozygote (DAT−/−) mouse strain are not altered by cocaine or amphetamine administration providing further support for the DAT as the obligatory target for the locomotor effects of these stimulant drugs of abuse. In addition to a markedly enhanced persistence of DA in the extracellular space, homozygotes display many neurochemical alterations in the nigrostriatal dopaminergic system, including diminished releasable pools of DA, reductions in number of D_2 autoreceptors, and decreases in the content of tyrosine hydroxylase, the rate-limiting enzyme in DA synthesis. Detailed examination of DA release and uptake in the nucleus accumbens has not been completed in homozygote mice, however, such studies are likely to provide further insight on the contribution of DAT to processes associated with addiction.

Probing Structure–Function Relationships

Preliminary investigations into the structure–function relationships of the monoamine transporters have employed many methodologies, including protein modification with residue-specific or photoaffinity reagents, as well as, more recently, the analysis of the pharmacological properties of chimeric or truncated proteins and site-directed mutants. Before the availability of cDNAs encoding the carriers, a variety of approaches employing chemical modification provided a glimpse into the relationships of the binding sites for different substrates and inhibitors and the existence of residues critical for activity. Both tyrosyl (49) and sulfhydryl (23,94) groups have been implicated to be involved in the basic functioning of the monoamine transporter proteins. In placental brush border membrane vesicles, a decrease has been reported in the V_{max} of [^{3}H]-5-HT transport in the presence of tyrosyl-specific reagents, n-acetylimidazole, 7-chloro-4-nitrobenzo-2-oxa-1,3-diazole, and tetranitromethane, whereas the K_m was uneffected. Similar effects on the velocity of DA transport have been obtained in both striatal suspensions (94) and striatal membranes (23) treated with the sulfhydryl reagent N-ethylmaleimide (NEM). Other sulfhydryl-specific reagents, such as mercuric chloride and 5,5′-dithiobis(2-nitrobenzoic acid) (DTNB), as well as NEM, have been found to inhibit the binding of antagonists of DAT, including [^{3}H]-cocaine (23,111,115), [^{3}H]-mazindol (111,115), [^{3}H]-CFT (111), and [^{3}H]-methylphenidate (121,122), without affecting the transporter density. The sensitivity to sulfhydryl modifying reagents suggests that cysteine residues may be involved in maintaining a protein conformation that allows binding of a ligand, or may actually reside within the binding site.

Sulfhydryl reagents have also been used to elucidate whether the binding sites for substrates and inhibitors are mutually exclusive, overlapping, or distinct. From the results of one study examining the relationship of the binding sites of mazindol, cocaine, DA, and amphetamine to DAT, cocaine, but not DA or amphetamine, could completely prevent the inhibition of [^{3}H]-mazindol binding by NEM. This suggested that part of the binding site shared by cocaine and mazindol is distinct from that of the substrates, DA and amphetamine (74). Evidence for a mutually exclusive site for both inhibitors and substrate was obtained using the more hydrophilic sulfhydryl reagent, DTNB. In this study, DTNB inhibited the binding of [^{3}H]-cocaine and [^{3}H]-GBR12783, but only the inhibition of [^{3}H]-cocaine binding could be reversed by mazindol and DA, implying that substrates and some nonsubstrate inhibitors bind to a similar site (109). Although these results may appear inconsistent, the use of compounds with varying capacities to interact with the hydrophobic membrane environment may result in the modification of distinct cysteine residues with different roles in determining the binding sites. Support for both mutually exclusive and overlapping binding sites for substrates and inhibitors has been presented in studies showing that the inhibition of [^{3}H]-paroxetine binding by NEM could be reversed by many inhibitors of SERT including fluoxetine, imipramine, cocaine, citalopram, as well as substrates tryptamine and 5-HT (58,146), however, not by p-chloroamphetamine and fenfluramine (146). Thus, there appears to be a common binding site on SERT for substrates and many, but not all, inhibitors of SERT.

Although strategies based on protein modification have provided some information on the possible residues involved in the transport activity and the binding of substrates and inhibitors to the transporter, they have not aided in elucidating specific regions of the protein responsible for these functions. Thus, as a general approach to study the superfamily of Na$^+$/Cl$^-$-dependent carriers, several laboratories have constructed and expressed functional chimeric transporters, in which similar sequence domains of closely related transporters are exchanged. These studies provide information on the domains that contribute to the unique properties of each carrier, such as its specificity for different substrates or its sensitivity to selective inhibitors. Unlike other conventional methods of mapping functional domains, such as analyses of site-directed or deletion mutants in which function is often compromised, chimeras can provide assayable phenotypes which allow delineation of functions associated with particular protein domains. For the monoamine transporters, chimeric proteins have been constructed from domains of DAT and NET (21,22,56) and human and rat SERT (10,13). The chimeric proteins were constructed using two basic experimental strategies: exchanging domains by exploiting unique restriction sites either already present in the sequence (10) or those engineered into the sequence by PCR (13,56), and using an in vivo method that generates chimeras within bacteria transformed with linear plasmid DNA containing a single copy of each parental cDNA in a tail-to-head configuration (21,22).

The structural domains of NET and DAT responsible for the substrate and inhibitor selectivity and substrate translocation have been localized to general areas of the transporter (21,22,56). The results of one study examining a series of highly functional chimeras between NET and DAT suggest that a region spanning TMs 5–8 is important for conferring inhibitor sensitivity to a variety of selective inhibitors, including the tricyclic antidepressant NET blocker desipramine and the DAT blocker GBR12935 (*22*). Furthermore, this region also appeared to be important for selective substrate translocation (V_{max}) (*21*). A second domain in NET spanning TMs 1–3 also contributed to the affinity of NET for antidepressants, whereas the corresponding region in DAT appeared to have a role in determining the affinity for the two GBR compounds. Interestingly, a recent report provides support for a direct interaction with this domain; [^{125}I]DEEP, a photoactive GBR derivative, appears to react with residues near TMs 1 and 2 of the DAT protein in the nucleus accumbens (*139*). Determinants responsible for the apparent affinities of catecholamine substrates are localized in the region spanning TMs 1–3 and residues that influence the affinity for MPP$^+$ appear to reside between TMs 11 and 12 (*21*).

A distinct set of chimeras between NET and DAT have been examined and although similar conclusions were obtained regarding the domain important for inhibitor interactions (TMs 5–8), some differences were apparent in regions contributing to substrate selectivity (*56*). In particular, Giros et al. (*56*) reported that TMs near the C-terminus, TMs 8–12, rather than TMs 1–3, have a more predominant influence on determining the apparent affinity and stereoselectivity for different substrates. Chimeras constructed between rat SERT and human SERT also have localized the determinants required for species-specific differences in binding of imipramine and D-amphetamine to TMs near the C-terminus (TM 11–12) (*10*). Although inconsistencies may arise from differences in chimera construction or the use of different expression systems, there is general agreement among the studies of chimeras (*21,56*) and truncations (*13*) that the determinants important for substrate affinity and translocation appear closely associated with TMs, and that the large extracellular loop and the intracellular portions of the N- and C-termini do not appear to be major determinants required for the selective substrate or inhibitor interactions with the monoamine carriers. As more information becomes available on the higher order structure of members of the family of sodium dependent transporters, precise interactions between residues and domains identified in these studies and their role in transport will become apparent.

Investigations employing site-directed mutagenesis with DAT have nicely complemented the more general overview of functional domains provided by the examination of the chimeric monoamine transporters. Replacement of an aspartate residue within TM 1 (D79) with alanine, glycine, or glutamate dramatically increased the K_d for binding of [^{3}H]-CFT, a cocaine analog, without affecting the B_{max}

(*80*). This mutation also resulted in a reduction in apparent affinity for [^{3}H]-DA and a markedly reduced V_{max} for transport of DA and other substrates (*80*), providing more evidence that determinants for substrate selectivity lie within the region containing TM 1–3. Mutations of serine residues in positions 356 and 359 in TM 7 had little effect on binding of [^{3}H]-CFT but resulted in a substantial reduction in the V_{max} for [^{3}H]-DA transport (*80*) again consistent with results implicating the involvement of TMs 5–7 in substrate translocation and V_{max}. Another study investigating the effects of mutations in TM 7 and TM 11 on the kinetics of MPP$^+$ transport obtained evidence that both domains contain determinants that influence substrate translocation and the affinity for the substrate MPP$^+$, respectively (*81*). Mutagenesis of cysteine residues may provide insight into the relationship of cysteine residues to drug and ion binding sites on the carrier and may in the future illuminate previous studies using sulfhydryl-specific modifying reagents. Alanine substitutions at four cysteines in DAT had no impact on the binding of a cocaine analog or dopamine binding, whereas, the mutation of two highly conserved cysteines residing in the extracellular loop resulted in a dramatic reduction in the surface expression of the transporter (*142*).

Electrophysiological Properties of Monoamine Transporters

Monoamine transport involves the cotransport of additional ions along with neurotransmitter, and depending on the net charge of substrates and ions, the process is potentially electrogenic. Estimates of the ionic stoichiometry of monoamine carriers have resulted predominantly from experiments measuring the ionic dependence of initial rates of substrate transport. These classical analyses have suggested that the carriers function in ways similar to enzymes, because the transport of substrate and cosubstrates follows Michaelis-Menten enzyme kinetics. NE and 5-HT are thought to be contransported with one sodium and one chloride ion, whereas DA appears to be transported with two sodium ions and one chloride ion, and hence transport processes would be predicted to be electrogenic. In constrast in mammals, 5-HT transport also appears to involve a countertransported potassium ion and has been thought to be electroneutral. Recent examination of cloned monoamine transporters have provided data generally consistent with these proposed stoichiometries (*60*).

Electrophysiological analyses of the currents associated with transport have provided additional insights into the electrical properties and the pathways of ion permeation of the carrier proteins (reviewed in ref. *85*). Although one might assume that the currents associated with these sodium-coupled cotransporters should reflect the net charge of substrates and ions transported, further electrophysiological investigation of neurotransmitter transporters demonstrates a much richer variety of electrical behaviors. Recent experiments clearly demonstrate that in addition to currents associated with substrate transport, members of the biogenic amine family of transporters can mediate macroscopic ionic currents that are not stoichiometrically linked to substrate movement. In the first series of experiments examining a mammalian monoamine carrier, several ionic currents were shown to be associated with the expression of the rat SERT in *Xenopus* oocytes (*93*). This study also suggested that rat SERT translocates 5–12 net charges/5-HT molecule, even though the transport-associated current displays an ionic dependence entirely consistent with an electroneutral stoichiometry as predicted from studies of the activation of transport activity. A discrepancy between charge movement and coupled transport has also been noted with the human NET in HEK cells, where a ratio of approx 200 charges/NE molecule has been observed (*48*) and also with the human DAT in oocytes where 2–15 net charges accompany each transported DA (*129*). The results of these studies support an emerging concept that transporters share more common properties with ionic channels than was previously thought (*34*).

A leak current associated with the carriers has also been noted for rat SERT (*93*), human NET (*48*) and human DAT (*129*). An interesting aspect of this finding is that application of nonsubstrate inhibitors such as cocaine, can generate a conductance change in the absence of substrates by blocking a leak conductance. Although we do not know what the consequence of this action might be, this result indicates that blockers can have effects on the cell that are distinct from their antagonist action on uptake.

Another intriguing consequence of the conductance changes associated with monoamine transporters is that the changes in membrane potential generated by a carrier could directly activate intracellular signaling mechanisms, much like an autoreceptor. The magnitude of the currents associated with the rat (*93*) and leech (*18*) 5-HT carriers, and NET (*48*) makes this a formal possibility. Recent examples have demonstrated that depolarization associated with glutamate (*141*) and GABA (*63*) transport is sufficient to activate voltage-gated calcium channels in some systems and it appears that some members of the glutamate carrier family may have evolved such that their ability to mediate transmembrane currents may be of greater physiological significance than their capacity to buffer extracellular glutamate concentrations (*41*). Taken together these studies support the hypothesis that transporter-mediated currents, generated either by cotransport or by the existence of thermodynamically uncoupled conductances, can alter membrane potential and suggest a greater diversity of roles for neurotransmitter transporter in regulating the action of neurotransmitters in the CNS.

Acknowledgements

The authors acknowledege support from NIDA, DA07595 (S. G. Amara), T32 DA07262 (S. L. Povlock), and the Howard Hughes Medical Institute.

References

1. Amara, S. G. Monoamine transporters: basic biology with clinical implications. *Neuroscientist* **1** (1995) 259–267.
2. Amara, S. G. and Arriza, J. L. Neurotransmitter transporters: three distinct gene families. *Curr. Op. Neurobiol.* **3** (1993) 337–344.
3. Amara, S. G. and Kuhar, M. Neurotransmitter transporters: recent progress. *Annu. Rev. Neurosci.* **16** (1993) 73–93.
4. Andersen, P. H. The dopamine uptake inhibitor GBR 12909: selectivity and molecular mechanisms of action. *Eur. J. Pharmacol.* **166** (1989) 493–504.
5. Augwood, S. J., Westmore, K., McKenna, P. J., and Emson, P. C. Co-expression of dopamine transporter mRNA and tyrosine hydroxylase mRNA in ventral mesencephalic neurons. *Mol. Brain Res.* **20** (1993) 328–334.
6. Austin, M. C., Bradley, C. C., Mann, J. J., and Blakely, R. D. Expression of serotonin transporter messenger RNA in the human brain. *J. Neurochem.* **62** (1994) 2362–2367.
7. Axelrod, J., Weil-Malherbe, H., and Tomchick, R. The physiological disposition of H^3-epinephrine and its metabolite metanephrine. *J. Pharmacol. Exp. Ther.* **127** (1959) 251–256.
8. Axelrod, J., Whitby, L. G., and Hertting, G. Effect of psychotropic drugs on the uptake of H^3-norepinephrine by tissues. *Science* **133** (1961) 383,384.
9. Barker, E. L. and Blakely, R. D. Norepinephrine and serotonin transporters. In Bloom, F. E. and Kupfer, D. J. (eds.), *Psychopharmacology: The Fourth Generation of Progress*, Raven, New York, 1995, pp. 321–333.
10. Barker, E. L., Kimmel, H. L., and Blakely, R. D. Chimeric human and rat serotonin transporters reveal domains involved in recognition of transporter ligands. *Mol. Pharmacol.* **46** (1994) 799–807.

11. Berger, S. P., Farrell, K., Conant, D., Kempner, E. S., and Paul, S. M. Radiation inactivation studies of the dopamine reuptake transporter protein. *Mol. Pharmacol.* **46** (1994) 726–731.

12. Blakely, R. D., Berson, H. E., Fremeau, R. T., Caron, M. G., Peek, M. M., Prince, H. K., and Bradley, C. C. Cloning and expression of a functional serotonin transporter from rat brain. *Nature* **354** (1991) 66–70.

13. Blakely, R. D., Moore, K. R., and Qian, Y. Tails of serotonin and norepinephrine transporters: deletions and chimeras retain function. In Reuss, L., Russell, J. M., Jr., and Jennings, M. L. (eds.), *Molecular Biology and Function of Carrier Proteins*, Rockefeller University Press, New York, 1993, pp. 284–300.

14. Blanchard, V., Raisman-Vozari, R., Vyas, S., Michel, P. P., Javoy-Agid, F., Uhl, G., and Agid, Y. Differential expression of tyrosine hydroxylase and membrane dopamine transporter genes in subpopulations of dopaminergic neurons of the rat mesencephalon. *Mol. Brain Res.* **22** (1994) 29–40.

15. Bloom, F. E., Schulman, J. A., and Koob, G. F. Catecholamines and behavior. In Trendelenburg, U. and Weiner, N. (eds.), *Handbook of Experimental Pharmacology*, Vol. 90. *Catecholamines II*, Springer-Verlag, Berlin, 1989, pp. 27–88.

16. Boja, J. W., Vaughan, R., Patel, A., Shaya, E. K., and Kuhar, M. J. The dopamine transporter. In Niznik, H. B. (ed.), *Dopamine Receptors and Transporter: Pharmacology, Structure and Function*, Dekker, New York, 1994, pp. 611–644.

17. Boyson, S. J. Parkinson's disease and the electron transport chain. *Ann. Neurol.* **30** (1991) 330,331.

18. Bruns, D., Engert, F., and Lux, H.-D. A fast activating presynaptic reuptake current during serotonergic transmission in identified neurons of Hirudo. *Neuron* **10** (1993) 559–572.

19. Brüss, M., Hammermann, R., Brimijoin, S., and Bönisch, H. Antipeptide antibodies confirm the topology of the human norepinephrine transporter. *J. Biol. Chem.* **270** (1995) 9197–9201.

20. Brüss, M., Kunz, J., Lingen, B., and Bonisch, H. Chromosomal mapping of the human gene for the tricyclic antidepressant-sensitive noradrenaline transporter. *Hum. Genet.* **91** (1993) 278–280.

21. Buck, K. J. and Amara, S. G. Chimeric dopamine norepinephrine transporters delineate structural domains influencing selectivity for catecholamines and 1-methyl-4-phenylpyridinium. *Proc. Natl. Acad. Sci. USA* **91** (1994) 12,584–12,588.

22. Buck, K. J. and Amara, S. G. Structural domains of catecholamine transporter chimeras involved in selective inhibition by antidepressants and psychomotor stimulants. *Mol. Pharmacol.* **48** (1995) 1030–1037.

23. Cao, C. J., Yound, M. M., Wong, J., Mahran, L. G., and Eldefrawi, M. E. Putative cocaine receptor in striatum is a glycoprotein with active thiol function. *Memb. Biochem.* **8** (1989) 207–220.

24. Cerruti, C., Walther, D. M., Kuhar, M. J., and Uhl, G. R. Dopamine transporter mRNA expression is intense in ratbrain neurons and modest outside midbrain. *Mol. Brain Res.* **18** (1993) 181–186.

25. Chait, L. D., Uhlenhuth, E. H., and Johanson, C. E. Reinforcing and subjective effects of several anorectics in normal human volunteers. *J. Pharmacol. Exp. Ther.* **242** (1987) 777–783.

26. Chen, H.-T., Clark, M., and Goldman, D. Quantitative autoradiolography of ^{3}H-paroxetine binding sites in rat brain. *J. Pharmacol. Toxicol. Methods* **27** (1992) 209–216.

27. Ciliax, B. J., Heilman, C., Demchyshyn, L. L., Pristupa, Z. B., Ince, E., Hersch, S. M., Niznik, H. B., and Levey, A. I. The dopamine transporter: immunochemical characterization and localization in brain. *J. Neurosci.* **15** (1995) 1714–1723.

28. Corey, J. L., Quick, M. W., Davidson, N., Lester, H. A., and Guastella, J. A cocaine-sensitive *Drosophila* serotonin transporter: cloning, expression, and electrophysiological characterization. *Proc. Natl. Acad. Sci. USA* **91** (1994) 1188–1192.

29. Coyle, J. T. and Snyder, S. H. Catecholamine uptake by synaptosomes in homogenates of rat brain: stereospecificity in different areas. *J. Pharmacol. Exp. Ther.* **170** (1969) 221–231.

30. Crossman, A. R. Primate model of dyskinesia: the experimental approach to the study of the basal gangla-related involuntary movement disorders. *Neuroscience* **21** (1987) 1–40.

31. Crow, T. J. The biology of schizophrenia. *Experientia* **38** (1982) 1275–1282.

32. D'Amato, R. J., Largent, B. L., Snowman, A. M., and Synder, S. H. Selective labeling of serotonin uptake sites in rat brain by [^{3}H] citalopram contrasted to labeling of multiple sites by [^{3}H] imipramine. *J. Pharmacol. Exp. Ther.* **242** (1987) 364–371.

33. Dave, V. and Kimelberg, H. K. Na$^+$-dependent, fluoxetine-sensitive serotonin uptake by astrocytes tissue-printed from rat cerebral cortex. *J. Neurosci.* **14** (1994) 4972–4986.

34. DeFelice, L. J. and Blakely, R. D. Pore models for transporters? *Biophys. J.* **70** (1996) 579,580.

35. Demchyshyn, L. L., Pristupa, Z. B., Sugamori, K. S., Barker, E. L., Blakely, R. D., Wolfgang, W. J., Forte, M. A., and Niznik, H. B. Cloning, and expression, and localization of a chloride-facilitated cocaine-sensitive serotonin transporter from *Drosophila melanogaster*. *Proc. Natl. Acad. Sci. USA* **91** (1994) 5158–5162.

36. Diliberto, P. A., Jeffs, R. A., and Cubeddu, L. X. Effects of low extracellular chloride on dopamine release and the dopamine transporter. *J. Pharmacol. Exp. Ther.* **248** (1989) 644–653.

37. Donovan, D. M., Vandenbergh, D. J., Perry, M. P., Bird, G. S., Ingersoll, R., Nanthakumar, E., and Uhl, G. R. Human and mouse dopamine transporter genes: conservation of 5'-flanking sequence elements and gene structures. *Mol. Brain Res.* **30** (1995) 327–335.

38. Duncan, G. E., Little, K. Y., Kirkman, J. A., Kaldas, R. S., Stumpf, W. E., and Bresse, G. R. Autoradiographic characterization of [^{3}H] imipramine and [^{3}H]citalopram binding in rat and human brain: species differences and relationships to serotonin innervation patterns. *Brain Res.* **591** (1992) 181–197.

39. Edvardsen, Ø. and Dahl, S. G. A putative model of the dopamine transporter. *Mol. Brain Res.* **27** (1994) 265–274.

40. Eymin, C., Charnay, Y., Greggio, B., and Bouras, C. Localization of noradrenaline transporter mRNA expression in the human locus coeruleus. *Neurosci. Lett.* **193** (1995) 41–44.

41. Fairman, W. A., Vandenberg, R. J., Arriza, J. L., Kavanaugh, M. P., and Amara, S. G. An excitatory amino-acid transporter with properties of a ligand-gated chloride channel. *Nature* **375** (1995) 599–603.

42. Fischer, J. F. and Cho, A. K. Chemical release of dopamine homogenates: evidence for an exchange diffusional model. *J. Pharmacol. Exp. Ther.* **208** (1979) 203–209.

43. Freed, C., Revay, R., Vaughan, R. A., Kriek, E., Grant, S., Uhl, G. R., and Kuhar, M. J. Dopamine transporter immunoreactivity in rat brain. *J. Comp. Neurol.* **359** (1995) 340–349.

44. Fujita, M., Shimada, S., Maeno, H., Nishimura, T., and Tohyama, M. Cellular localization of serotonin transporter mRNA in the rat brain. *Neurosci. Lett.* **162** (1993) 59–62.

45. Fujita, M., Shimada, S., Nishimura, T., Uhl, G. R., and Tohyama, M., Ontogeny of dopamine transporter mRNA expression in the rat brain. *Mol. Brain Res.* **19** (1993) 222–226.

46. Fuller, R. W. Minireview: uptake inhibitors increase extracellular serotonin concentration measured by brain microdialysis. *Life Sci.* **55** (1994) 163–167.

47. Fuxe, K., Calza, L., Benfenati, F., Zini, I., and Agnati, L. F. Quantitative autoradiographic localization of [^{3}H] imipramine binding sites in the brain of the rat: relationship to ascending 5-hydroxytryptamine neurons systems. *Proc. Natl. Acad. Sci. USA* **80** (1983) 3836–3840.

48. Galli, A., DeFelice, L. J., Duke, B.-J., Moore, K. R., and Blakely, R. D., Sodium-dependent norepinephrine-induced currents in norepinephrine-transporter-transfected HEK-293 cells blocked by cocaine and antidepressants. *J. Exp. Biol.* **198** (1995) 2197–2212.

49. Ganapathy, V., Kulanthaivel, P., Tiruppathi, C., Mahesh, V. B., and Leibach, F. H. Inactivation of the human placental serotonin transporter by tyrosyl group-specific reagents. *J. Pharmacol. Exp. Ther.* **251** (1989) 9–15.

50. Gelernter, J., Kruger, S., Pakstis, A. J., Pacholczyk, T., Sparkes, R. S., Kidd, K. K., and Amara, S. G. Assignment for the norepinephrine transporter protein (NET1) locus to chromosome 16. *Genomics* **18** (1993) 690–692.

51. Gelernter, J., Pakstis, A. J., and Kidd, K. K. Linkage mapping of serotonin transporter protein gene SLC6A4 on chromosome 17. *Hum. Genet.* **95** (1995) 677–680.

52. Giros, B. and Caron, M. G. Molecular characterization of the dopamine transporter. *Trends Pharmacol. Sci.* **14** (1993) 43–49.

53. Giros, B., El Mestikawy, S., Bertrand, L., and Caron, M. G. Cloning and functional characterization of a cocaine-sensitive dopamine transporter. *FEBS Lett.* **295** (1991) 149–154.

54. Giros, B., Jaber, M., Jones, S. R., Wightman, R. M., and Caron, M. G. Hyperlocomotion and indifference to cocaine and amphetamine in mice lacking the dopamine transporter. *Nature* **379** (1996) 606–612.

55. Giros, B., Mestikawy, S. E., Godinot, N., Zheng, K., Han, H., Yang-Feng, T., and Caron, M. G. Cloning, pharmacological characterization, and chromosome assignment of the human dopamine transporter. *Mol. Pharmacol.* **42** (1992) 383–390.

56. Giros, B., Wang, Y.-M., Suter, S., McLeskey, S. B., Pifl, C., and Caron, M. G. Delineation of discrete domains for substrate, cocaine, and tricyclic antidepressant interactions using chimeric dopamine-norepinephrine transporters. *J. Biol. Chem.* **269** (1994) 15,985–15,988.

57. Glowinski, J., Kopin, I. J., and Axelrod, J. Metabolism of [^{3}H]norepinephrine in the rat brain. *J. Neurochem.* **12** (1965) 25–30.

58. Graham, D., Esnaud, H., Habert, E., and Langer, S. Z. A common binding site for tricyclic and nontricyclic 5-hydroxytryptamine uptake inhibitors at the substrate recognition site of the neuronal sodium-dependent 5-hydroxytryptamine transporter. *Biochem. Pharmacol.* **38** (1989) 3819–3826.

59. Graybiel, A. M. Neurotransmitters and neuromodulators in the basal ganglia. *TiNS* **13** (1990) 244–254.

60. Gu, H., Wall, S. C., and Rudnick, G. Stable expression of biogenic amine transporters reveals differences in inhibitor sensitivity, kinetics, and ion dependence. *J. Biol. Chem.* **269** (1994) 7124–7130.

61. Guastella, J., Nelson, N., Nelson, H., Czyzk, L., Keynan, S., Miedel, M., Davidson, N., Lester, H., and Kanner, B. Cloning and expression of a rat brain GABA transporter. *Science* **249** (1990) 1303–1306.

62. Harris, J. E. and Baldessarini, R. J. The uptake of [³H]dopamine by homogenates of rat corpus striatum: effects of cations. *Life Sci.* **13** (1973) 303–312.

63. Haugh-Scheidt, L., Malchow, R. P., and Ripps, H. GABA transport and calcium dynamics in horizontal cells from the skate retina. *J. Physiol.* **488** (1995) 565–576.

64. Herttig, G., Axelrod, J., Kopin, I. J., and Whitby, L. G. Lack of uptake of catecholamines after chronic denervation of sympathetic nerves. *Nature* **189** (1961) 66.

65. Hoffman, B. J. Molecular biology of dopamine transporters. In Niznik, H. B. (ed.), *Dopamine Receptors and Transporter: Pharmacology, Structure, and Function*, Dekker, New York, 1994, pp. 645–668.

66. Hoffman, B. J., Mezby, E., and Brownstein, M. J. Cloning of a serotonin transporter affected by antidepressants. *Science* **254** (1991) 79,80.

67. Hoffmeister, F. and Goldberg, S. R. A comparison of chlorpromazine, imipramine, morphine and D-amphetamine self-administration in cocaine-dependent rhesus monkeys. *J. Pharmacol. Exp. Ther.* **187** (1973) 8–14.

68. Holz, R. W. and Coyle, J. T. The effects of various salts, temperature, and the alkaloids veratridine and Batrachotoxin on the uptake of [³H] dopamine into synaptosomes from rat striatum. *Mol. Pharmacol.* **10** (1974) 746–758.

69. Howell, L. L. and Byrd, L. D. Characterization of the effects of cocaine and GBR 12909, a dopamine uptake inhibitor, on behavior in the squirrel monkey. *J. Pharmacol. Exp. Ther.* **258** (1991) 178–185.

70. Hrdina, P. D., Foy, B., Hepner, A., and Summers, R. J. Antidepressant binding sites in brain: autoradiographic comparison of [³H] paroxetine and [³H] imipramine localization and relationship to serotonin transporter. *J. Pharmacol. Exp. Ther.* **252** (1990) 410–418.

71. Hurd, Y. L., Pristupa, Z. B., Herman, M. M., Niznik, H. B. and Kleinman, J. E. The dopamine transporter and dopamine D_2 receptor messenger RNAs are differentially expressed in limbic- and motor-related subpopulations of human mesencephalic neurons. *Neuroscience* **63** (1994) 357–362.

72. Iversen, L. L. Monoamines in the mammalian central nervous system and the actions of antidepressant drugs. *Biochem. Soc. Spec. Publ.* **1** (1973) 81–96.

73. Iversen, L. L. Uptake processes for biogenic amines. In Iversen, C., Iversen, S. D., and Snyder, S. H. (eds.), *Handbook of Psychopharmacology*, Plenum, New York, 1977, pp. 381–442.

74. Johnson, K. M., Bergmann, J. S., and Kozilowski, A. P. Cocaine and dopamine differentially protect [^{3}H]-mazindol binding sites from alkylation by N-ethylmaleimide. *Eur. J. Pharmacol.* **227** (1992) 411–415.

75. Kalivas, P. W. and Stewart, J. Dopamine transmission in the initiation and expression of drug- and stress-induced sensitization of motor activity. *Brain Res. Rev.* **16** (1991) 223–244.

76. Kelly, A. E. and Lang, C. G. Effects of GBR 12909, a selective dopamine uptake inhibitor, on motor activity and operant behavior in the rat. *Eur. J. Pharmacol.* **167** (1989) 385–395.

77. Kilty, J., Lorang, D., and Amara, S. G. Cloning and expression of a cocaine-sensitive dopamine transporter. *Science* **254** (1991) 578,579.

78. Kimelberg, H. K. and Katz, D. M. Regional differences in 5-hydroxytryptamine and catecholamine uptake in primary astrocytic cultures. *J. Neurochem.* **47** (1986) 1647–1652.

79. Kitayama, S., Shimada, S., and Uhl, G. R. Parkinsonism-inducing neurotoxin MPP$^+$: uptake and toxicity in nonneuronal COS cells expressing dopamine transporter cDNA. *Ann. Neurol.* **32** (1992) 109–111.

80. Kitayama, S., Shimada, S., Xu, H., Markham, L., Donovan, D. M., and Uhl, G. R. Dopamine transporter site-directed mutations differentially alter substrate transport and cocaine binding. *Proc. Natl. Acad. Sci. USA* **89** (1992) 7782–7785.

81. Kitayama, S., Wang, J. B., and Uhl, G. R. Dopamine transporter mutants selectively enhance MPP$^+$ transport. *Synapse* **15** (1993) 58–62.

82. Lam, D. M.-K., Fei, J., Zhang, X.-Y., Tam, A. C. W., Zhu, L.-H., Huang, F., King, S. C., and Guo, L.-H. Molecular cloning and structure of the human (GABATHG) GABA transporter gene. *Mol. Brain Res.* **19** (1993) 227–232.

83. Lesch, K.-P., Balling, U., Gross, J., Strauss, K., Wolozin, B. L., Murphy, D. L., and Riederer, P. Organization of the human serotonin transporter gene. *J. Neural Transm. Gen. Sect.* **95** (1994) 157–162.

84. Lesch, K.-P., Wolozin, B. L., Estler, H. C., Murphy, D. L., and Riederer, P. Isolation of a cDNA encoding the human brain serotonin transporter. *J. Neural Transm. Gen. Sect.* **91** (1993) 67–72.

85. Lester, H. A., Mager, S., Quick, M. W., and Corey, J. L. Permeation properties of neurotransmitter transporters. *Annu. Rev. Pharmacol. Toxicol.* **34** (1994) 219–249.

86. Li, T., Yang, L., Wiese, C., Xu, C. T., Zeng, Z., Giros, B., Caron, M. G., Moises, H. W., and Liu, X. No association between alleles or genotypes at the dopamine transporter gene and schizophrenia. *Psychiatry Res.* **52** (1994) 17–23.

87. Liang, N. Y. Comparison of the release of [^{3}H]dopamine from isolated corpus striatum by amphetamine, fenfluramine, and unlabelled dopamine. *Biochem. Pharmacol.* **31** (1982) 983–992.

88. Liang, N. Y. and Rudledge, C. O. Evidence for carrier mediated efflux of dopamine from corpus striatum. *Biochem. Pharmacol.* **31** (1982) 2479–2484.

89. Liang, N. Y. and Rutledge, C. O. Calcium-independent release of [^{3}H]dopamine by veratridine in pargyline- and reserpine-treated corpus striatum. *Eur. J. Pharmacol.* **89** (1983) 153–155.

90. Lingen, B., Brüss, M., and Bönisch, H. Cloning and expression of the bovine sodium- and chloride-dependent noradrenaline transporter. *FEBS Lett.* **342** (1994) 235–238.

91. Liu, Q.-R., Mandiyan, S., Nelson, H., and Nelson, N. A family of genes encoding neurotransmitter transporters. *Proc. Natl. Acad. Sci. USA* **89** (1992) 6639–6643.

92. Lorang, D., Amara, S. G., and Simerly, R. Cell-type specific expression of catecholamine transporters in the rat brain. *J. Neurosci.* **14** (1994) 4903–4914.

93. Mager, S., Min, C., Henry, D. J., Chavkin, C., Hoffman, B. J., Davidson, N., and Lester, H. A. Conducting states of mammalian serotonin transporter. *Neuron* **12** (1994) 845–859.

94. Meiergerd, S. M. and Schenk, J. O. Striatal transporter for dopamine: catechol structure–activity studies and susceptibility modification. *J. Neurochem.* **62** (1994) 998–1008.

95. Melikian, H. E., McDonald, J. K., Gu, H., Rudnick, G., Moore, K. R., and Blakely, R. D. Human norepinephrine transporter. Biosynthetic studies using a site-directed polyclonal antibody. *J. Biol. Chem.* **269** (1994) 12,290–12,297.

96. Milner, H. E., Béliveau, R., and Jarvis, S. M. The in situ size of dopamine transporter is a tetramer as estimated by radiation inactivation. *Biochim. Biophys. Acta* **1190** (1994) 185–187.

97. Muramatsu, T. and Higuchi, S. Dopamine transporter gene polymorphism and alcoholism. *Biochem. Biophys. Res. Commun.* **211** (1995) 28–32.

98. Nelson, P. J. and Rudnick, G. Coupling between platelet 5-hydroxytryptamine and potassium transport. *J. Biol. Chem.* **254** (1979) 10,084–10,089.

99. Nirenberg, M. J., Vaughen, R. A., Uhl, G. R., Kuhar, M. J., and Pickel, V. M. The dopamine transporter is localized to dendritic and axonal plasma membranes of nigrostriatal dopaminergic neurons. *J. Neurosci.* **16** (1996) 436–447.

100. Pacholczyk, T., Blakely, R. D., and Amara, S. G. Expression cloning of a cocaine- and antidepressant-sensitive human noradrenaline transporter. *Nature* **350** (1991) 320–353.

101. Perrone-Capano, C. Target cells modulate dopamine transporter gene expression during brain development. *NeuroReport* **5** (1994) 1145–1148.

102. Pifl, C., Giros, B., and Caron, M. Dopamine transporter expression confers cytotoxicity to low doses of the parkinsonism-inducing neurotoxin 1-methyl-4-phenylpyridinium. *J. Neurosci.* **13** (1993) 4246–4253.

103. Pörzgen, P., Bönisch, H., and Brüss, M. Molecular cloning and organization of the coding region of the human norepinephrine transporter gene. *Biochem. Biophys. Res. Commun.* **215** (1995) 1145–1150.

104. Povlock, S. L., Meiergerd, S. M., and Schenk, J. Kinetic mechanisms of the dopamine transporter: a comparison with biogenic amine transporters. In Stone, T. W. (ed.), *CNS Neurotransmitters and Neuromodulators: Dopamine*, CRC Press, Boca Raton, FL, 1996, pp. 21–39.

105. Pristupa, Z. B., Wilson, J. M., Hoffman, B. J., Kish, S. J., and Niznik, H. B. Pharmacological heterogeneity of the cloned and native human dopamine transporter: dissociation of [^{3}H]WIN 35,428 and [^{3}H]GBR 12,935 binding. *Mol. Pharmacol.* **45** (1994) 125–135.

106. Qian, Y., Melikian, H. E., Rye, D. B., Levey, A. I., and Blakely, R. D. Identification and characterization of antidepressant-sensitive serotonin transporter proteins using site-specific antibodies. *J. Neurosci.* **15** (1995) 1261–1274.

107. Ramamoorthy, S., Bauman, A. L., Moore, K. R., Han, H., Yang-Feng, T., Chang, A. S., Ganapathy, V., and Blakely, R. D. Antidepressant- and cocaine-sensitive

human serotonin transporter: molecular cloning, expression, and chromosomal localization. *Proc. Natl. Acad. Sci. USA* **90** (1993) 2542–2546.

108. Ramamoorthy, S., Prasad, P. D., Kulanthaivel, P., Leibach, F. H., Blakely, R. D. and Ganapathy, V. Expression of a cocaine-sensitive norepinephrine transporter in the human placental syncytiotrophoblast. *Biochemistry* **32** (1993) 1346–1353.

109. Refahi-Lyamani, F., Saadouni, S., Costentin, J., and Bonnet, J. J. Interaction of two sulfhydryl reagents with a cation recognition site on the neuronal dopamine carrier evidences small differences between [H-3]GBR 12783 and [H-3] cocaine binding sites. *Naunyn-Schmiedeberg's Arch. Pharmacol.* **351** (1995) 136–145.

110. Rehavi, M., Skolnick, P., Hulihan, B., and Paul, S. M. High affinity binding of [^{3}H]desipramine to rat cerebral cortex: relationship to tricyclic antidepressant-induced inhibition of norepinephrine uptake. *Eur. J. Pharmacol.* **70** (1981) 597–599.

111. Reith, M. E. A. and Selmeci, G. Radiolabeling of dopamine uptake sites in mouse striatum: comparison of binding sites for cocaine, mazindol, and GBR 12935. *Naunyn-Schmiedeberg's Arch. Pharmacol.* **345** (1992) 309–318.

112. Reith, M. E. A., Zimanyi, I., and O'Reilly, C. A. Role of ions and membrane potential in uptake of serotonin into plasma membrane vesicles from mouse brain. *Biochem. Pharmacol.* **38** (1989) 2091–2097.

113. Revay, R., Vaughan, R., Grant, S., and Kuhar, M. J. Dopamine transporter immunohistochemistry in median eminence, amygdala, and other areas of the rat brain. *Synapse* **22** (1996) 93–99.

114. Richelson, E. and Pfenning, M. Blockade by antidepressants and related compounds of biogenic amine uptake into rat brain synaptosomes: most antidepressants selectively block norepinephrine uptake. *Eur. J. Pharmacol.* **104** (1984) 277–286.

115. Richfield, E. K. Zinc modulation of drug binding, cocaine affinity states, and dopamine uptake on the dopamine uptake complex. *Mol. Pharmacol.* **43** (1993) 100–108.

116. Ritz, M. C., Lamb, R. J., Goldberg, S. R., and Kuhar, M. J. Cocaine receptors on dopamine transporters are related to self-administration of cocaine. *Science* **237** (1987) 1219–1223.

117. Roberts, D. C. S., Koob, G. F., Klonoff, P., and Fibiger, H. C. Extinction and recovery of cocaine self-administration following 6-hydroxydopamine lesions of the nucleus accumbens. *Pharmacol. Biochem. Behav.* **12** (1980) 781–787.

118. Rothman, R. B., Lewis, B., Dersch, C., Xu, H., Radesca, L., Decotsa, B. R., Rice, K. C., Kilburn, R. B., Akunne, H. C., and Pert, A. Identification of a GBR12935 homolog, LR1111, which is over 4,000 fold selective for the dopamine transporter, relative to serotonin and norepinephrine transporters. *Synapse* **14** (1993) 34–39.

119. Rudnick, G. and Clark, K. From synapse to vesicle: the reuptake and storage of biogenic amine neurotransmitters. *Biochim. Biophys. Acta* **1144** (1993) 249–263.

120. Sano, A., Kondoh, K., Kakimoto, Y., and Kondon, I. A 40-nucleotide repeat polymorphism in the human dopamine transporter gene. *Hum. Genet.* **91** (1993) 405,406.

121. Schweri, M. M. N-ethylmaleimide irreversibly inhibits the binding of [^{3}H]threo-(±)-methylphenidate to the stimulant recognition site. *Neuropharmacology* **29** (1990) 901–908.

122. Schweri, M. M. Mercuric chloride and *p*-chloromercuriphenylsulfonate exert a biphasic effect on the binding of the stimulant [^{3}H]methylphenidate to the dopamine transporter. *Synapse* **16** (1994) 188–194.

123. Shimada, S., Kitayama, S., Lin, C.-L., Patel, A., Nanthakumar, E., Gregor, P., Kuhar, M., and Uhl, G. Cloning and expression of a cocaine-sensitive dopamine transporter complementary DNA. *Science* **254** (1991) 576–578.

124. Shimada, S., Kitayama, S., Walther, D., and Uhl, G. Dopamine transporter mRNA: dense expression in ventral midbrain neurons. *Mol. Brain Res.* **13** (1992) 359–362.

125. Sitges, M., Reyes, A., and Chiu, L. M. Dopamine transporter mediated release of dopamine: role of chloride. *J. Neurosci. Res.* **39** (1994) 11–22.

126. Snyder, S. H. Amphetamine psychosis: a "model" of schizophrenia mediated by catecholamines. *Am. J. Psych.* **130** (1973) 61–67.

127. Snyder, S. H. and Coyle, J. T. Regional differences in H^3-norepinephrine and H^3-dopamine uptake into rat brain homogenates. *J. Pharmacol. Exp. Ther.* **165** (1969) 78–86.

128. Snyder, S. H. and D'Amato, R. J. MPTP: a neurotoxin relevant to the pathophysiology of Parkinson's disease. *Neurology* **36** (1986) 250–258.

129. Sonders, M. S. Characterization of two steady-state conductances mediated by the electrogenic human dopamine transporter. *Biophys. J.* **70** (1996) A98.

130. Souza, E. B. D. and Kuyatt, B. L. Autoradiographic localization of ^{3}H-paroxetine-labeled serotonin uptake sites in rat brain. *Synapse* **1** (1987) 488–496.

131. Sulzer, D., Chen, T.-K., Lau, Y. Y., Kristensen, H., Rayport, S., and Ewing, A. Amphetamine redistributes dopamine from synaptic vesicles to the cytosol and promotes reverse transport. *J. Neurosci.* **15** (1995) 4102–4108.

132. Swanson, L. W. The projections of the ventral tegmental area and adjacent regions: a combined fluorescent retrograde tracer and immunofluorescence study in the rat. *Brain Res. Bull.* **9** (1982) 321–353.

133. Tate, C. G. and Blakely, R. D. The effect of N-linked glycosylation on activity of the Na$^+$- and Cl$^-$-dependent serotonin transporter expressed using recombinant Baculovirus in insect cells. *J. Biol. Chem.* **269** (1994) 26,303–26,310.

134. Uchikawa, T., Kiuchi, Y., Yura, A., Nakachi, N., Yamazaki, Y., Yokomizo, C., and Oguchi, K. Ca^{2+}-dependent enhancement of [^{3}H]dopamine uptake in rat striatum: possible involvement of calmodulin-dependent kinases. *J. Neurochem.* **65** (1995) 2065–2071.

135. Uhl, G. R. and Johnson, P. S. Neurotransmitter transporters: three important gene families for neuronal function. *J. Exp. Biol.* **196** (1994) 229–236.

136. Usdin, T. B., Mezey, E., Chen, C., Brownstein, M. J., and Hoffman, B. J. Cloning of the cocaine-sensitive bovine dopamine transporter. *Proc. Natl. Acad. Sci. USA* **88** (1991) 11,168–11,171.

137. Vandenbergh, D. J., Persico, A. M., Hawkins, A. L., Griffin, C.A., Li, X., Jabs, E. W., and Uhl, G. R. Human dopamine transporter gene (DAT1) maps to chromosome 5p15.3 and displays a VNTR. *Genomics* **14** (1992) 1104–1106.

138. Vandenbergh, D. J., Persico, A. M., and Uhl, G. R. A human dopamine transporter cDNA predicts reduced glycosylation, displays a novel repetitive element and provides racially-dimorphic *Taq I* RFLPs. *Mol. Brain Res.* **15** (1992) 161–166.

139. Vaughan, R. A. Photoffinity-labeled ligand binding domains on dopamine transporters identified by peptide mapping. *Mol. Pharmacol.* **47** (1995) 956–964.

140. Vaughan, R. A., Uhl, G., and Kuhar, M. J. Recognition of dopamine transporters by antipeptide antibodies. *Mol. Cell. Neurosci.* **4** (1992) 209–215.
141. Villalobos, C. and García-Sancho, J. Glutamate increases cytosolic calcium in GH₃ pituitary cells acting via a high-affinity glutamate transporter. *FASEB J.* **9** (1995) 815–819.
142. Wang, J. B., Moriwaki, A., and Uhl, G. R. Dopamine transporter cysteine mutants: second extracellular loop cysteines are required for transporter expression. *J. Neurochem.* **64** (1995) 1416–1419.
143. Whitby, L. G., Axelrod, J., and Weil-Malherbe, H. The fate of H³-norepinephrine in animals. *J. Pharmacol. Exp. Ther.* **132** (1961) 193–201.
144. Whitby, L. G., Hertting, G., and Axelrod, J. Effect of cocaine on the disposition of noradrenaline labelled with tritium. *Nature* **187** (1960) 604,605.
145. Whittaker, V. P. Catecholamine storage particles in the central nervous system. *Pharmacol. Rev.* **18** (1966) 401–412.
146. Wolf, W. A. and Kuhn, D. M. Role of essential sulfhydryl groups in drug interactions at the neuronal 5-HT transporter. *J. Biol. Chem.* **267** (1992) 20,820–20,825.
147. Wolfe, D. E., Potter, L. T., Richardson, K. C., and Axelrod, J. Localizing tritiated norepinephrine in sympathetic axons by electron microscopic autoradiography. *Science* **138** (1962) 440–442.
148. Woolverton, W. L. Evaluation of the role of norepinephrine in the reinforcing effects of psychomotor stimulands in rhesus monkeys. *Pharmacol. Biochem. Behav.* **26** (1987) 835–839.
149. Zaleska, M. M. and Erecinska, M. Involvement of sialic acid in high-affinity uptake of dopamine by synaptosomes from rat brain. *Neurosci. Lett.* **82** (1987) 107–112.

CHAPTER 2

Regulation of Antidepressant-Sensitive Serotonin Transporters

Randy D. Blakely, Sammanda Ramamoorthy,
Yan Qian, Sally Schroeter, and
Christopher C. Bradley

Introduction

The indoleamine serotonin (5-hydroxytryptamine [5HT]) plays an important role as a chemical messenger in the adult central nervous system (CNS) and periphery, regulating a host of diverse processes, including mood, sleep, sexual drive, gastrointestinal motility, thyroid function, and vasoconstriction (38,55). Though more than a half dozen distinct 5HT receptor subtypes exist to confer the specific actions of 5HT on target cells (45), a single gene product (11,51,71,102) encoding the serotonin transporter (SERT), appears to be exclusively responsible for the inactivation of extracellular 5HT. SERTs are members of a large gene family of Na^+ and Cl^- coupled, plasma membrane transporters (1,10), most closely related in sequence to the 1-norepinephrine (NE) transporter (NET) (73,96) and the dopamine (DA) transporter (DAT) (44,60,113,119). SERT expression in the adult CNS appears to be predominantly, if not exclusively, neuronal (5,11,20,100), restricted to serotonergic neurons of the raphe complex and their projections. Clearance of synaptic and extrasynaptic 5HT appears to be the principal role for SERTs; however, certain cells, notably platelets (100,116), utilize SERTs to acquire 5HT from the environment for subsequent release, since they lack the essential biosynthetic machinery for 5HT synthesis. SERTs have also been identified in intestinal crypt epithelia (121), adrenal chromaffin cells (13,118), mast cells (51), medullary thyroid carcinoma cells (21), thyroid follicular cells (117), and placenta (8).

Neurotransmitter Transporters: Structure, Function, and Regulation
Ed. M. E. A. Reith Humana Press Inc., Totowa, NJ

In the placenta, SERTs are enriched in apical, brush-border membranes, where they are poised to provide a pathway for transplacental transfer of maternal 5HT in embryonic development (*112*), and/or a mechanism for maintenance of appropriate placental perfusion by limiting 5HT-induced constriction of placental blood vessels. Together, these sites of SERT gene and protein expression constitute small populations of highly specialized cells whose capacity to clear extracellular 5HT constrains the amine's action in time and space.

SERT antagonists, including antidepressants and cocaine, limit clearance of extracellular 5HT to the level achieved either by simple diffusion or lower affinity transport pathways, significantly elevating 5HT concentrations at receptors. Since prolonged receptor action leads to adaptive target responses, the question arises as to how SERT expressing cells establish the appropriate abundance of surface transporters to quantitatively attain the appropriate efficiency of 5HT clearance. Are SERT expression levels or catalytic transport rates modulated to effect changes in 5HT signaling? What are the rate-limiting steps in 5HT translocation that might be targets for rapid modulation of transport? Does 5HT itself, acting through 5HT receptors, provide an important signal to establish the appropriate level of SERT expression? Is SERT gene expression linked to 5HT production or growth factors promoting cell survival and differentiation? Are changes in SERT gene expression or regulation predisposing factors in mental illness?

Changes in SERT activity or expression reviewed herein suggest a role for both transcriptional and postranscriptional mechanisms for appropriate SERT regulation. The present chapter seeks to organize published findings, to highlight opportunities for mechanistic insight into regulation at the gene and protein level. In many cases, insights have been gained not from neurons but from more tractable peripheral cell model systems. Since SERT antagonists are efficacious in a wide spectrum of neuropsychiatric disturbances (*39,87*) and SERT activity or density has been reported to be affected in mental illness, particularly in depression (*80,95*), a clearer understanding of the mechanisms by which SERT gene expression and transport activity are regulated may provide additional diagnostic criteria and therapeutic strategies.

SERT Regulation: General Models

Cells that are specialized to accumulate 5HT via expression of SERT might do so constitutively, allowing variations in release and response to influence 5HT signaling. However, environmental factors and pharmacologic agents have been reported to influence 5HT uptake, radioligand binding, and/or SERT gene expression (Tables 1 and 2), suggesting the presence of endogenous regulatory mechanisms. Depending on whether changes in SERT activity or expression are rapid (seconds to minutes) or delayed (hours or days), we label such regulation acute or long-term, respectively. Conceivably, immediate effects may lead to, or occur in parallel with, long-term changes, although present data suggests distinct pathways for modulation. Given that several hours are required to translate elevated transporter mRNA into processed, surface-resident transporter proteins (78) and even longer periods would be required to affect transporter protein levels in the distant terminals of serotonin neurons, alterations in gene expression are unlikely to contribute to acute regulation. Acute changes in 5HT uptake are thus most likely to arise from local alterations in substrate gradients, cell surface distribution of SERT proteins, reversible interactions of SERT proteins with regulatory proteins or reversible posttranslational modifications in SERT proteins already inserted in the presynaptic membrane. Evidence now exists to support several of these possibilities that, in concert with alterations in SERT gene expression, establish appropriate levels of 5HT clearance.

Acute Modulation of SERT Activity

Mechanistic Considerations for Rapid Transporter Regulation

Observations of acute changes in SERT activity (Table 1) could reflect a number of direct and indirect mechanisms, altering the cell's capacity to accumulate 5HT. To carry out clearance of extracellular 5HT, SERTs must be inserted in the plasma membrane in an active form. This may require targeting the carrier to certain plasma membrane domains but not to others. For example, in the CNS, SERTs should be positioned near sites of 5HT release in varicosities or terminals. Electron microscopic (EM) studies localizing the homologous rat DAT reveal that this carrier is enriched in the plasma membrane of varicosities, terminals, and dendritic spines, but is reduced or absent in surface membranes of axonal intervaricose segments and the cell body region (91). Light microscopic studies with SERT antibodies demonstrate labeling of axons and dendrites as well (100), with preliminary EM studies from our lab consistent with DAT observations (Schroeter, unpublished). In the periphery, antidepres-

Table 1
Acute Regulation of Serotonin Transport[a]

Preparation	Agent[a]	Condition	Change	Refs.
In vivo studies				
Perfused lung (rabbit)	β-PMA	80 nM	Decrease clearance (V_{max}/K_m)	90
	β-PMA	30 µg/kg	Decrease clearance (V_{max}/K_m)	106
Hippocampal dialysis (rat)	TIA	ip 10 mg/kg	Reduce 5HT overflow	126
Hippocampal voltammetry (rat)	TIA	ip 10 mg/kg	Increase 5HIAA efflux	28
Synaptosome (rat)	TIA	ip 10 mg/kg, 1 h prior to assay	Increase uptake	82
	TIA	ip 10 mg/kg twice over 2 h period	Increase uptake	35
Brain slice (rat)	novel environment, cat odor	5 min exposure 5–30 min prior to sacrifice	Biphasic change in uptake	36
In vitro studies				
Endothelial cells (cow)	β-PMA	0.1 nM to 1 µM, 0–120 min	Decrease uptake	89
	4β-PDBu	0.1 nM to 1 µM, 30 min	Decrease uptake	
	Mezerein	0.1 nM to 1 µM, 30 min	Decrease uptake	
Platelet (rabbit)	ConA	.2–.5 mg/mL	Decrease uptake	93
	ConA	.135 mg/mL	Decrease uptake	57

Cell type	Compound	Concentration, time	Effect	Ref.
Platelet (human)	β-PMA	1 pM to 10 µM, 1–30 min	Decrease uptake (V_{max})	2
	Mezerein	0.1 nM to 1 µM, 5 or 20 min	Decrease uptake	
	Histamine	10 nM to 0.25 µM, 0–15 min	Increase uptake (V_{max})	66
	Impromidine	0.25–3 µM, 0–10 min	Increase uptake	
	Dimaprit	1–100 nM, 5 min	Increase uptake	
	PEA	0.01–10 µM, 5 min	Increase uptake	
	SNP	0.1 µM, 5 min	Increase uptake	
	EGTA	1 mM, 0–60 min	Decrease uptake	92
	Thapsigargin	0.1 µM, 0–45 min	Decrease uptake	
	Genistein	0.1–100 nM, 1–30 min	Decrease uptake	50
	MHC	0.1–100 nM, 1–30 min	Decrease uptake	
RBL–2H3 cells	β-PMA	0.1 µM, 0–24 h	Decrease uptake (V_{max})	84
	NECA	1 µM, 10–60 min	Increase uptake (V_{max}, K_m)	
	N6-CPA	10 µM, 15 min	Increase uptake	
	8-Br-cGMP	10 µM, 15 min	Increase uptake	
	SNAP	100 µM, 1–15 min	Increase uptake	
	Hydroxylamine	100 µM, 1–15 min	Increase uptake	
	Calmidazolium	10 µM, 30 min	Decrease uptake	
	LY-83583	10 µM, 30 min	Decrease uptake	
	Methylene blue	10 µM, 20 min	Decrease uptake	
JAR cells	β-PMA	1 µM, 2 h	Decrease uptake	101
	CGS9343B	0–100 µM, 0–60 min	Decrease uptake (V_{max}, K_m)	56
			Decrease Na and Cl dep.	

(continued)

33

Table 1 (*continued*)

Preparation	Agent[a]	Condition	Change	Refs.
BeWo cells	CGS9343B	75 μM, 1 h	Decrease uptake	56
Raphe culture (rat)	β-PMA	0.01 μM, 10–12 min	Decrease uptake	3
Brain slice (hip)	DOI	EC$_{50}$ 6 nM, 15 min	Decrease uptake	85
Brain slice (ctx)	DOI	EC$_{50}$ 40 nM, 15 min	Decrease uptake	
SERT (rat)-Transfected COS cells	β-PMA	Dose-dependent	Decrease uptake	52
SERT (rat)-Transfected COS cells	Interferon-α	Dose-dependent	Decrease uptake (V_{max})	109
SERT (human) Transfected HEK-293 cells	β-PMA	Dose-dependent	Decrease uptake (V_{max})	99

[a]Abbreviations: ConA, concanavalin A; DOI, 2,5-dimethoxy-4-iodoamphetamine; 8-Br-cAMP, 8-bromo cyclic adenosine monophosphate; EGTA, ethyleneglycol bis(β-aminoethylester)-N,N,N′,N′-tetraacetate; MHC, methyl 2,5-dihydroxycinnamate; NECA, 5′-N-ethylcarboxamidoadenosine; PDBu, phorbol12,13-dibutyrate; PEA, 2-(2-pyridylethyl)amine; PMA, phorbol 12-myristate 13-acetate; SNAP, S-nitroso-N-acetylpenicillamine; SNP, sodium nitroprusside; TIA, tianeptine.

Table 2
Long-term Regulation of Serotonin Transport[a]

Measure	Change	Treatment	Preparation	Refs.
In vivo studies				
5HT uptake	Increase	Darkness	SCN slice (rat)	83
	Increase	Darkness	Hypothal. slice (rat)	14
	Increase (V_{max})	Long day	Hypothal. slice (rat)	107
	Increase	Progesterone	Septal slice (rat)	127
	Increase	Estradiol	Synaptosome (rat)	19
	Increase (V_{max})	IMI, DMI	Synaptosome (rat)	9
	Decrease (V_{max})	FLX	Synaptosome (rat)	53
	Decrease	CMI	Platelet	59
	Decrease	PAR	Hipp/raphe slice	97
	Increase (V_{max})	TIA	Synaptosome (rat)	82
	Increase	TIA	Synaptosome (rat)	86
	Increase	TIA	Platelet (rat)	86
	Increase	TIA	Platelet	59
	Increase	TIA	Synaptosome (rat)	35
	Increase	TIA	Brain dialysis (rat)	126
	Biphasic change	Prenatal ACTH, NIC	Synaptosome (rat)	61
IMI binding	Decrease	DMI	Cortical memb. (rat)	100a
	Decrease (B_{max})	IMI	Hypothal. memb. (cat)	4
	Decrease (B_{max})	IMI	Platelet memb. (cat)	4
	Decrease	IMI	Cortical memb. (rat)	61a
	Decrease (B_{max})	IMI	Brain and platelet (cat)	16a

(*continued*)

Table 2 *(continued)*

Measure	Change	Treatment	Preparation	Refs.
	Decrease (B_{max})	IMI, DMI	Hipp. memb. (rat)	9
	Decrease	DEP	Cortical homog.	130
	Decrease (K_D)	FLX, NRT, MAP, PHEN	Cortical memb. (rat)	53
	Increase (B_{max})	Long day	Hypothal. slice (rat)	107
PAR binding	Decrease	LIT	Whole brain memb.	98
	Decrease	Estradiol benzoate	Hipp. sections *in situ*	81
	Decrease	TIA, IMI	Hipp. CTX *in situ*	122
	Decrease	TIA	Dorsal raphe *in situ*	64
	Decrease (B_{max})	PAR	Cort./hipp. memb.	97
CYN binding	Increase	DEP, PHEN	Rat brain *in situ*	62
	Decrease	SER	Rat brain *in situ*	62
5HT response	Delayed recovery	PAR	Hippocamp. in vivo	97
SERT mRNA	Decrease	IMI, DMI, CMI, FLX	Raphe nuclei (rat)	67
	Decrease	TIA	Dorsal raphe (rat)	64
	Increase	CMI, IMI	Raphe *in situ*	76
	Decrease	PCPA, IMI	Raphe nuclei (rat)	74
	Decrease	PCPA	Raphe nuclei (rat)	129
	Increase	Age	Raphe *in situ* (rat)	77a
In vitro studies				
Primary cultures				
5HT uptake	Increase	ACTH	Raphe neuron (rat)	6
	Increase	Glial cond. media	Raphe neuron (rat)	123
	Increase	S100β	Raphe neuron (rat)	7
	Biphasic change	dbcAMP, (Rp)-cAMPS, 8-Br-cAMP, forskolin	Raphe neuron (rat)	37
	Increase	FGF-5	Raphe neuron (rat)	72

	Effect	Treatment	Cell line	Ref
	Increase (V_{max})	hypoxia	Endothel. cell (pig)	10b
SERT mRNA	Increase	NGF	Thyroid C-cells (rat)	21
	Increase	NGF	Thyroid C-cell (rat)	21

In vitro studies

Transformed cell lines

	Effect	Treatment	Cell line	Ref
5HT uptake	Induce	dbcAMP, cyclohexane-carboxylate	IC11 (mouse terat.)	16b
	Increase (V_{max})	CTX, forskolin dbcAMP, BMX	JAR	22
	Increase (V_{max})	CTX, forskolin, IBMX	JAR	61
	Increase (V_{max})	Staurosporine	JAR	101
	Increase (V_{max})	Interleukin-1β	JAR	105
	Increase	Staurosporine	BeWo	101
	Decrease (complex)	CTX, forskolin, IBMX	PC12	61
	Increase	ACTH4-10, forskolin, dbcAMP, S100β	RN46A	32
RTI-55 binding	Increase (B_{max})	CTX, forskolin	JAR	104
	Increase (B_{max})	Staurosporine	JAR	101
	Increase (B_{max})	Interleukin-1β	JAR	105
SERT mRNA	Increase	CTX	JAR	104
	Increase	Staurosporine	JAR	101
	Increase	Interleukin-1β	JAR	105

[a]Abbreviations: ACTH, adrenocorticotrophic hormone; CMI, clomipramine; CTX, cholera toxin; CYN, cyanoimipramine; dbcAMP, dibutyryl cyclic adenosine monophosphate; DEP, deprenyl; DMI, desmethylimipramine; FGF, fibroblast growth factor; FLX, fluoxetine; IBMX, isobutylmethylxanthine; IMI, imipramine; LIT, lithium; MAP, maprotiline; NGF, nerve growth factor; NIC, nicotine; NRT, nortriptyline; PAR, paroxetine; PCPA, paeacholophenylalanine; PHEN, phenelzine; (Rp)-cAMPs, (Rp) adenosine 3'5'-cydic phosphorothioate; SCN, suprachiasmatic nucleus; SER, sertraline; TIA, tianeptine.

sant-sensitive 5HT uptake is enriched in placental apical brush-border membranes (*8*). Recently, Gu et al. (*48*) found SERT expression to be polarized in basolateral membranes of transfected Madine-Darby Canine Kidney (MDCK) cells, whereas DAT expression was predominantly apical. These data suggest active mechanisms to insert or exclude SERT and homologs from discrete plasma membrane domains. Might membrane retrieval and insertion be a mechanism for acute SERT regulation? Perhaps the best-studied example of hormone-activated transporter regulation, involving insulin-activated glucose transport, involves selective redistribution of a specific glucose transporter (GLUT4) isoform (*58,115*). Regarding the SERT gene family, studies by Corey et al. (*23*), with a homologous GABA transporter (GAT1) expressed in *Xenopus laevis* oocytes, indicate that protein kinase C (PKC)-mediated upregulation of GAT activity arises through rapid redistribution of surface carriers.

In addition to a loss of SERTs from the plasma membrane, the catalytic efficiency of a fixed population of carriers could change, so that transport rates are altered. To understand the possible control points for regulating catalytic efficiency, we need to understand the basic mechanism of ion-coupled 5HT translocation. This is discussed in detail in Chapter 3, but it is briefly covered here, to provide continuity with the presentation of regulatory mechanisms. 5HT is believed to be transported as a cation (Fig. 1). Ion dependence and equilibrium studies suggest that single Na^+ and Cl^- ions move in parallel with 5HT down their concentration gradients to provide the energy required for amine uptake against its concentration gradient. Once unloaded in the cytoplasm, 5HT in neurons, platelets, and endocrine cells is further sequestered into secretory vesicles by a vesicular monoamine transporter (VMAT) (*33*). A single K^+ ion is believed to be countertransported in a step in the transport cycle after 5HT release, and may contribute energy for reorientation of the unloaded carrier for subsequent rounds of uptake.

Stable decreases in 5HT affinity would be predicted to reduce transport rates and at low substrate concentrations could be discernible as an alteration in transport K_m. Because the transport of 5HT is gradient driven, however, changes in ion or 5HT gradients will also influence levels and rates of 5HT accumulation without a requirement for a physical change in SERT proteins. Thus indirect effects on other plasma membrane ion pumps, or in the activity of VMATs, might read out as a change in maximal 5HT transport capacity or V_{max}. The extracellular release of 5HT through vesicular fusion could elevate extracel-

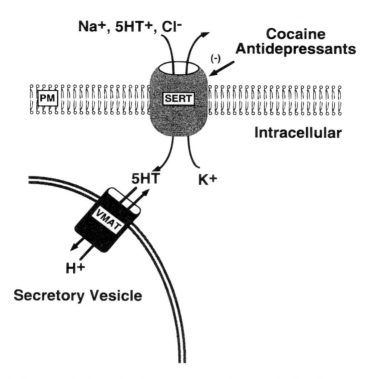

Fig. 1. Ion-coupled serotonin transport and sequestration in neurons and platelets. Serotonin is shown transported as the charged cation, $5HT^+$, across the plasma membrane (PM) via the antidepressant- and cocaine-sensitive SERT. Single Na^+, Cl^-, and K^+ ions move down their electrochemical gradients in a coupled fashion to drive $5HT^+$ influx. The neutral form of 5HT is shown preferentially accumulated by a secretory VMAT, using an antiport mechanism with coupled efflux of intravesicular H^+.

lular 5HT. The latter effect would be equivalent to adding an unlabeled, competitive inhibitor to flux assays and would reduce the apparent 5HT K_m, but would not reflect an intrinsic change in SERT proteins. However, changes in SERT's affinity for coupling ions, or in its ability to shift protein conformation as a consequence of ion binding, could alter rates of flux. For example, K^+-assisted reorientation has been identified as a rate-limiting step in 5HT transport and, thus, modulation of intracellular K^+ recognition or its actions may contribute to acute regulation. Thus, a reduction in available internal K^+ could lead to a decrease in apparent K_m because of saturation at lower substrate levels. Such explanations become attractive in the absence of a change in surface density and when proper controls reveal no influence of other ion and 5HT flux pathways. Other membrane channels and pumps achieve modulation in intrinsic activity via reversible post-translational modifications, such as phosphorylation, or through direct interactions with second messengers and accessory proteins. Recently, uncoupled ion flow, apparently through a transiently open ion pore, has been discovered in GAT, NET, and SERT (*12,18,40,77*). The significance of this ion flow for the transport mechanism is unclear but must be considered in the future as a potential target for modulatory influences. Mammalian SERT (but not *Drosophila* SERT [*24*]) appears to conduct voltage-insensitive 5HT accumulation (*77*). This suggests that acute regulation noted below cannot be explained simply as an indirect result of membrane potential perturbation; more likely, changes arise from the impact of altered substrate gradients or alterations in SERT surface density, and/or modulation of intrinsic catalytic efficiency of 5HT translocation.

Acute SERT Regulation In Vivo

Because of constraints and complexities in being able to provide a stimulus and then monitor the consequences for SERT activity in vivo minutes later, much of our understanding of acute SERT regulation arises from more tractable in vitro preparations, such as harvested platelets, cultured cell lines, brain slices, and synaptosomes. Gillis and coworkers (*42,43*) noted efficient clearance of 5HT from the lung through an antidepressant-sensitive mechanism presumed to reflect SERT activity. Meyers and Pitt (*90*) used the perfused lung preparation to test the effects of PKC activation of 5HT clearance in vivo. These investigators noted that addition of the PKC activator phorbol myristate acetate (PMA) to perfusates (25 min) significantly reduced 5HT extraction. Additional studies (*106*) revealed that this reduced clearance was not an indirect effect of pulmonary edema, since catalase reduced the edema produced, but not the reduction in 5HT clearance, suggesting that a PKC-modulated pathway exists in lung for 5HT clearance.

Acute upregulation of SERT activity has been noted following ip administration of the atypical antidepressant tianeptine (*59,86*). Most antidepressants are inhibitors of 5HT uptake, but tianeptine, given to animals, results in an elevation in 5HT transport from synaptosomes harvested 1 h later (*35,82*), with no effect on antagonist site density ([^{3}H]imipramine) or evoked 5HT release. Supporting evidence for acute effects on neuronal 5HT clearance arises from in vivo dialysis

(*126*) and voltammetry studies (*28*), in which monitoring of 5HT or metabolite spillover can be monitored prior to and after tianeptine administration. Since tianeptine does not elevate 5HT transport when applied in vitro to synaptosomes, its actions appear to require an intact serotonin neuron, target cell, or animal. Because of the compound's antidepressant utility, it will be interesting to determine whether other clinically efficacious agents can be found that upregulate SERT expression. Finally, File et al. (*36*) reported alterations in 5HT uptake in hippocampal and cortical brain slices, when slices were taken from rats given a brief (5 min) exposure to a novel environment or cat odor. As noted, the complexity of these preparations raises more questions than answers, although they do suggest important in vivo regulatory phenomena that may utilize one or more of the SERT regulatory pathways traced in vitro.

Regulatory Pathways for Acute Modulation of SERT Activity: Ca^{2+} and Calmodulin

Release of 5HT, like many other neurotransmitters and hormones, is mediated by a rise in intracytoplasmic Ca^{2+}. It seems reasonable then, to consider whether elevated cytoplasmic Ca^{2+} affects 5HT transport. Studies by Nishio and Segawa (*93*) found that brief (minutes) treatment of rabbit platelets with concanavalin A (ConA) significantly reduces 5HT uptake. ConA elevates influx of Ca^{2+}, an effect blocked by $LaCl_3$, an inorganic Ca^{2+} entry blocker (*57*). ConA also elevated Ca^{2+}-dependent protein kinase activity in platelets (*57*). Notably, staurosporine and K-252a, inhibitors of PKC, but not KT5720 (a PKA inhibitor), blocked the ConA-mediated reduction in 5HT uptake and induced platelet phosphorylation, suggesting an involvement of activated PKC (*see* next section) in Ca^{2+}-modulated SERT activity (*57*). Kinase inhibitors themselves had no inhibitory effects on 5HT uptake, precluding SERT-targeted nonspecific effects.

These studies led Nishio and colleagues (*92*) to subsequently examine the role of intracellular Ca^{2+} on platelet SERT expression. Extracellular Ca^{2+} chelation with EGTA was found to rapidly deplete intracellular Ca^{2+} and led to a time-dependent decrease in 5HT uptake. The effect of EGTA on 5HT uptake could be enhanced (90% decrease vs 40% decrease) by the addition of 10 μM BAPTA-AM, an intracellular Ca^{2+} chelator, or by 0.1 μM thapsigargin, an endoplasmic Ca^{2+}-ATPase inhibitor reported to cause depletion of intracellular Ca^{2+} stores. However, BAPTA-AM itself did not have obvious effect on 5HT uptake; thapsigargin only slightly decreased 5HT uptake (10%

decrease). These results suggest that the basal intracellular level of Ca^{2+} maintained by influx of extracellular Ca^{2+} and/or Ca^{2+} released through ER is required to maintain resting levels of platelet 5HT uptake activity. Since Ba^{2+}, but not Sr^{2+}, can substitute for extracellular Ca^{2+}, whereas both ions substitute for PKC-mediated thrombin effects, a site independent of PKC activation may be involved in basal Ca^{2+} modulation.

One of the major mediators of Ca^{2+} effects in cells is the soluble Ca^{2+} binding protein calmodulin, which can complex and regulate numerous proteins, including kinases, phosphatases, nitric oxide synthase (NOS), and membrane transporters. Jayanthi et al. (56) reported that treatment of SERT-expressing JAR cells (derived from the human placenta), with the selective calmodulin antagonist CGS 9343B, rapidly (minutes) inhibits 5HT uptake in a time- and dose-dependent manner, with a 85% decrease in activity evident after 1 h incubation. Kinetic analysis suggested that the effect of CGS was mainly caused by a decrease in transport V_{max}. A slight increase in K_m (0.25–0.11 µM) as well as a significant decrease in the apparent affinity to Cl^- (K_m: 11.3–22.7 mM) and Na^+ (K_m: 33–42 mM) were also observed. Treatment with another calmodulin antagonist, W7 (10 µM), for 1 h also decreased 5HT uptake to 50% in JAR cells. However, 20 µM calmidazolium, another calmodulin antagonist, failed to decrease 5HT uptake within 1 h incubation. None of these three calmodulin compounds had obvious effects on Na^+-dependent alanine uptake and in fact stimulated Na^+-independent leucine uptake, suggesting that their inhibitory effect was SERT-specific. The inhibitory effect of CGS on 5HT uptake also could be observed in membrane vesicles harvested from CGS-treated JAR cells, indicating that the effect is unrelated to a change in ion gradients and can be long lasting. Similar findings were obtained with BeWo cells, another placental choriocarcinoma cell line. CGS treatment did not affect the density or affinity of antagonist binding (RTI-55) or SERT mRNA levels; however, surface density of SERT was not directly assessed and could explain the findings, if binding sites for the lipophilic ligand used are sequestered but not eliminated. Placental cells lack VMATs (Ganapathy, V. personal communication), suggesting that a vesicular storage process is probably not involved in changes in 5HT uptake. Further studies are warranted to determine whether calmodulin itself, or a calmodulin-dependent protein, affects SERT activity in JAR cells. Thus, studies have yet to link the effects of calmodulin antagonists to changes in cellular Ca^{2+} dynamics or to the involvement of calmodulin itself in regulatory events. Recently, Miller and Hoffman (*84*) also demonstrated a reduction in 5HT transport in RBL2H3 cells following calmodulin antagonist treatment (calmidazolium), suggesting that calmodulin may play a role in SERT regulation in a number of cell types.

Regulatory Pathways for Acute Modulation of SERT Activity: PKC

As noted, studies with Ca^{2+} depletion and mobilization implicate PKC as a regulator of SERT activity. Activators of PKC, such as PMA, have been shown in a number of systems to rapidly reduce 5HT transport. For example, PMA reduces 5HT transport in cultured bovine pulmonary artery endothelial cells (*89*), human platelets (*2*), rat basophilic leukemia (RBL2H3) cells (*84*), and JAR cells (*101*). The inhibitory effect by PMA can be observed as early as a few minutes and may last for several hours. In human platelets (*2*), a 5-min pretreatment with PMA lowered the rate of 5HT uptake, largely as a decrease in transport capacity (V_{max}) with little change for the apparent affinity to 5HT (K_m). Time-course analysis of the effects of 1 μM PMA shows maximal reduction (48%) of 5HT uptake observed at 20 min. Similar changes in transport V_{max} were noted in PMA studies with RBL cells. Anderson and coworkers (*3*) recently reported acute downregulation of 5HT uptake by PKC activators in primary neuronal cultures from the embryonic (E13.5) rat brainstem, suggesting that nonneuronal and neuronal SERTs are sensitive to PKC activation.

Various control experiments have been performed to confirm the specificity of PMA's effect on activation of PKC. First, the effects of PMA are found to be stereospecific (*2*). β-PMA, the active PKC activator, reduces 5HT uptake, but α-PMA, the inactive isomer, lacks effects. Second, other PKC activators, such as mezerein or phorbol dibutyrate, have been found to reduce 5HT uptake (*2,89*). Third, the effect of PMA is paralleled by an activation and translocation of PKC (*2*) and can be blocked by PKC inhibitors, such as staurosporine (*2*). Finally, PMA effects appear specific for SERT. Consequently, PMA treatment has negligible effects on Na^+-dependent alanine uptake and stimulates Na^+-independent leucine uptake in RBL2H3 cells (*84*), reducing concern for a generalized effect on membrane permeability. Inhibitory effects of PMA also can be observed in plasma membrane vesicle preparations where artificial ion gradients are imposed (*84*).

Some of the effects of PMA might be mediated indirectly via effects on 5HT release. Indeed, PMA does induce release of 5HT from platelets (2), but to a much smaller extent than found for reductions in uptake. Importantly, SERT regulation by PMA has recently been reported in transfected cells devoid of vesicular storage pathways. Hoffman and Miller (52) reported that PMA reduced 5HT transport capacity in COS cells transiently transfected with the rat SERT cDNA. Saito and coworkers (109) noted that similarly transfected COS cells exhibit SERT downregulation by interferon-α, although it is unclear whether activation of PKC is linked to this effect. We (99) reproduced PMA effects in human SERT stably transfected HEK-293 cells. Kinetic analysis in HEK-SERT cells shows that PMA (1 μM) treatment for 20 min causes a 46% decrease in transport V_{max} with little or no change in 5HT K_m (Fig. 2). Significant effects can be seen with as little as 10 nM PMA. As with platelet preparations, the α isomer is ineffective. The effect of 1 μM PMA on 5HT uptake can be blocked by cotreatment with staurosporine, but staurosporine alone does not acutely affect 5HT uptake. In addition, we found that PMA also reduces SERT-mediated, 5HT-gated currents in whole-cell patch-clamp studies, effects reversed by staurosporine (Quian et al., submitted). The opportunity to rapidly regulate 5HT uptake in transfected cells and record transport activity, using sensitive patch-clamp techniques, provides a new paradigm to dissect mechanisms responsible for PKC-mediated SERT regulation.

Regulatory Pathways for Acute Modulation of SERT Activity: NO and PKG

In addition to a PKC-mediated pathway for acute SERT downregulation, receptor-mediated signaling through the NOS-cGMP pathway has been reported to activate SERT in platelets (66), and RBL2H3 cells (84). In human platelets, histamine pretreatment for 5 min increased 5HT uptake to 236% of control. Kinetic analysis showed that this effect was through an increase of transport capacity (V_{max}) with no obvious changes in apparent 5HT affinity (K_m). Histamine was also shown to rapidly (5 min) elevate cGMP levels. In addition, the cGMP-inducing agent sodium nitroprusside (0.1 μM) also increased 5HT uptake (to 230% of control). The stimulatory effect of histamine on 5HT uptake could be blocked by the guanylate cyclase inhibitor LY-83588 or the NOS inhibitor NMMA, but LY-83588 and NMMA alone did not have any effect on 5HT uptake. These data suggest that downstream targets of NO and cGMP, such as protein kinase G (PKG) can activate SERT.

In RBL2H3 cells (84), treatment with the adenosine receptor agonist NECA increased 5HT uptake. The effect is primarily caused by an

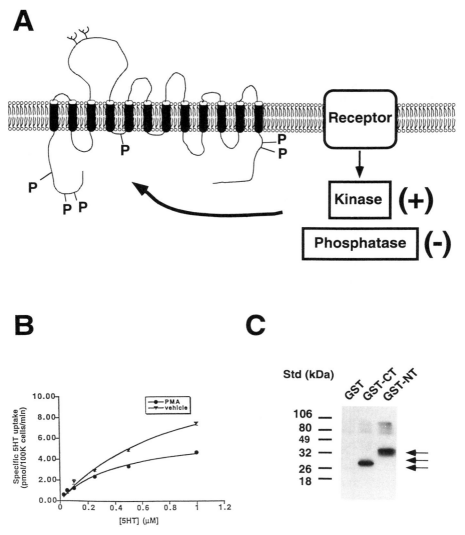

Fig. 2. Possibilities for protein phosphorylation in the acute regulation of SERT. **(A)** Hydrophobicity-based model of SERT protein structure showing 12 putative transmembrane domains (TMDs), a large N-glycosylated extracellular loop between TMDs 3 and 4, and multiple canonical sites for Ser/Thr protein phosphorylation in cytoplasmic domains. *See* text for evidence that kinase-activated pathways acutely modulate SERT catalytic activity or surface expression. **(B)** SERT activity in HEK-293 cells stably transfected with human SERT cDNA is downregulated by treatment of cells with the PKC activator PMA. Kinetic studies reveal a significant reduction in transport capacity (V_{max}) as observed in native preparations (*see text*). **(C)** SERT amino (NT) and carboxy termini (CT) can be phosphorylated in vitro by PKC. Fusion proteins with each termini were produced with glutathione-S-transferase (GST) to yield GST-NT and GST-CT. Arrows indicate the position of fusion proteins visualized by in vitro phosphorylation by PKC. Note GST is only lightly labeled, but prominent labeling is observed for GST-NT and GST-CT.

increase in V_{max}. A slight increase of 5HT K_m (0.2–0.6 μM) was also observed. The maximal effect of NECA could be reached within 10 min and was followed by a gradual return toward basal rates. Pretreatment of the cells with the NOS inhibitor L-NAME (100 μM) or L-NMMA (100 μM) could block the effect of 1 μM NECA. The NO donor SNAP (100 μM) and hydroxylamine (100 μM) also stimulated 5HT uptake, with maximal effect reached within 10 min and a time-course of action similar to NECA. SNAP and NECA were both found to elevate cellular cGMP levels; 10 μM 8-Br-cGMP also stimulated 5HT uptake. Together, these data suggest that the effect of NECA on 5HT uptake may be mediated by a NO-activated guanylate cyclase, as suggested in the platelet studies. Calmidazolium and methylene blue, a scavenger of NO, and the guanylate cyclase inhibitor LY82583, inhibit 5HT uptake when added alone, suggesting tonic activation of the NO-cGMP pathway may regulate the activity of the 5HT transporter under basal condition. However, NOS inhibitors have no effect on basal 5HT uptake, suggesting greater complexities than a simple linear path from NO to PKG. It will be interesting to determine whether the tonic modulation exerted by Ca^{2+} and calmodulin and the NOS/cGMP pathway are part of similar or distinct SERT regulatory pathways.

Recently, Miller and coworkers (*85*) reported similar involvement of a cGMP/NO pathway in rat brain synaptosomes, triggered by 5HT receptors. The $5HT_2$ receptor agonist DOI was found to elevate 5HT uptake in hippocampal synaptosomes. In the same preparation, a 117% increase in cGMP level and 41% increase in nitrite level were also observed. Qualitatively similar observations were found in cortical synaptosomes. In both preparations, the effect of DOI could be blocked by LY82583, although LY82583 itself did not have obvious effect on 5HT uptake. These results suggest that activation of pre- and/or postsynaptic $5HT_2$ receptors, coupled to a NOS-cGMP pathway, may regulate SERT in presynaptic neuronal terminals.

At present, a mechanistic basis for the regulation of 5HT uptake through NOS-cGMP pathway is undefined. In RBL2H3 cells, the stimulatory effect of SNAP and 8-Br-cGMP was specific, since similar treatments did not have any effects on the Na^+-dependent alanine uptake and inhibited Na^+-independent leucine uptake. The stimulatory effect of SNAP and 8-Br-cGMP could also be observed in a plasma membrane vesicle preparation with established ion gradients, suggesting effects are unrelated to changes in membrane permeability. Histamine and NECA treatment fail to alter SERT protein levels as assessed by radioligand binding of intact platelets or RBL cells.

However, these ligands are relatively lipophilic and may bind to sequestered, inactive transporters. In RBL2H3 cells, the stimulatory effect of 1 μ*M* NECA could be blocked by pretreatment of the cells with 10 μ*M* H8, a relatively selective cyclic-nucleotide dependent protein kinase inhibitor. H8 itself did not affect 5HT uptake, suggesting a phosphorylation process may mediate the effect of NECA on the transporter protein. Whether the target is SERT itself remains to be clarified (*see* Structural Basis for Acute SERT Regulation). Reconstituted cGMP/NO activated SERT regulation in transfected cells has yet to be reported.

Regulatory Pathways for Acute Modulation of SERT Activity: Tyrosine-Kinase

Although we have emphasized biochemical cascades that might influence Ser and Thr protein kinases (PKC, PKG), many membrane proteins, including growth factor receptors, receptors, and ion channels are modified by reversible tyrosine phorphorylation. Recently, Helmeste and Tang (*50*) reported that structurally distinct inhibitors of tyrosine kinases (genistein, herbimycin A, and methyl 2,5-dihydroxycinnamate) induce rapid and dramatic reductions in 5HT uptake in human platelets. Genistein treatment (100 n*M*) for 1 min caused a 34% decrease of 5HT uptake. Maximal effects (~90% decrease) could be observed within 5 min and remained after 30-min treatment. Methyl 2,5-dihydroxycinnamate 100 n*M* caused a 46% decrease of 5HT uptake after 5-min treatment. However, because the compound is unstable in solution, it was less effective after 10-min treatment (only 30% decrease) and became ineffective after 30-min treatment. The effects of genistein, herbimycin A, and methyl 2,5-dihydroxycinnamate on 5HT uptake were dose-dependent. Consistent decrease of 5HT uptake could be observed at concentrations >1 n*M*. At concentrations up to 10 μ*M*, neither genistein nor methyl 2,5-dihydroxycinnamate inhibited [^{3}H]imipramine binding, suggesting that the effect of these agents on 5HT uptake was not caused by the direct binding of these drugs to the transporter (*49*). Genistein is known to decrease intracellular Ca^{2+} levels in platelets and, as noted, reductions in cytoplasmic Ca^{2+} levels have been associated with decreased 5HT uptake. However, genistein (100 n*M*) caused only a 28% decrease in intracellular Ca^{2+} level, but affected a decrease in 5HT uptake of 86%; thus, either SERT is highly sensitive to small changes in intracellular Ca^{2+} or additional Ca^{2+}-independent pathways are involved.

Structural Basis for Acute SERT Regulation

Although significant data has accumulated to suggest that SERT activity in platelets, mast cells, placenta, and brain neurons can be acutely regulated by second messengers and protein kinases, the physical basis for SERT regulation is unclear. SERT contains multiple consensus sites for Ser/Thr phosphorylation, with most of these sites found in the presumed cytoplasmic NH_2 and COOH termini (10,84). Tyrosine phosphorylation sites have not been described.

Hoffman and Miller (52) noted that 5HT uptake in COS cells transfected with a rat SERT bearing an N-terminal truncation partially blunted the downregulation of 5HT uptake induced by PMA. Largely because of the low abundance of the transporter protein in native tissues and cell lines and, until recently, an absence of SERT antibodies (100), no in vivo or in vitro phosphorylation of SERT has been reported. In preliminary studies, we (99) found that fusion proteins that contain either the NH_2 or COOH terminal tail of rat SERT can be phosphorylated in vitro (Fig. 2). Phosphoaminoacid analyses show labeling of both serine and threonine residues. However, site-directed mutagenesis studies demonstrate the phosphorylation is not at canonical sites for PKC. Cautious extrapolation from these data for functional significance is warranted, since PKA also phosphorylates these tail domains in vitro and yet no data implicates PKA in SERT regulation. One possibility is that PKA phosphorylation might only yield functional consequences in the presence of additional modifications, requiring more elaborate functional paradigms to dissect a hierarchical network of regulatory events. Potential phosphorylation sites for PKG exist on cytoplasmic SERT domains, yet fusion proteins of the NH_2-terminal or COOH-terminal domains are not phosphorylated by PKG in vitro. If phosphorylation of SERT by cGMP-dependent protein kinase mediates the effect of NECA or histamine on 5HT uptake, a canonical PKG phosphorylation site (rat SERT Ser 277) in the intracellular domain between transmembrane domains 4 and 5 might also be important for this process. As mentioned, GABA transporters expressed in *Xenopus laveis* oocytes (23) also respond to PMA, even with canonical PKC sites mutated; here, the regulation of GABA transport activity appears to best correlate with surface redistribution. Although PMA treatments do not change [³H]imipramine or [³H]paroxetine binding to intact platelets or RBL2H3 cells, and have been used to investigate change in SERT density, the ligands may cross the membrane to label intracellular pools of transporter. Recently, we have combined membrane impermeant biotinylation with immunoprecipitation by transporter-specific antibodies to reveal changes in surface density following PMA treatment (Qian et al., submitted). These studies, along with further efforts to identify potential phosphorylation sites on SERT in vivo, should allow us to determine whether second-messenger and kinase pathways converge to affect SERT surface trafficking or catalytic efficiency, or both.

Long-Term Modulation of SERT Activity

Evidence for Long-Term SERT Regulation In Vivo

Changes in antidepressant-sensitive 5HT uptake or SERT-associated antidepressant binding site density have been found in a number of paradigms employing environmental perturbations or pharmacologic challenges (Table 2). Meyer and Quay (*83*) noted ultradian and circadian changes in 5HT uptake capacity in hypothalamus and suprachiasmatic nucleus (SCN) of male and proestrous female rats, respectively. Interestingly, the peak in 5HT uptake in the SCN just preceded the luteinizing hormone (LH) surge of proestrous females. In addition, [^{3}H]imipramine binding density as a measure of SERT expression has been reported to vary with a circadian pattern in the SCN (*107*). Rovescalli and colleagues (*107*) reported that entrainment on different photoperiods (long dark or long light), to mimic seasonal variations in sunlight, also leads to significant alterations in 5HT uptake capacity (V_{max}) and [^{3}H]imipramine binding density (B_{max}) in hypothalamus, but cortex uptake and binding sites were found to be unaltered. Although concurring in detection of variations in 5HT uptake across a standard 12:12 light–dark cycle, Blier and coworkers (*14*) could find no change in SERT antagonist-mediated 5HT overflow or fenfluramine-induced release of 5HT from hypothalamic slices, measures that might detect changes in plasma membrane SERT expression. Alternative explanations for the discrepancy between the studies are that SERT expression in the entire hypothalamus may not respond to light/dark cycle variations like the SCN, or that changes in uptake and binding may reflect altered storage, release, or radioligand sites not associated with 5HT terminals.

Conceivably, changes in 5HT uptake observed in circadian and seasonal paradigms may reflect a sensitivity of SERT expression to light-modulated hormonal rhythms. Ovarian steroids (estradiol and progesterone) have been reported to acutely diminish the capacity of hypothalamic slices to accumulate 5HT, with significant effects for estradiol observed at subnanomolar concentrations (*34*). Chronic administration of either agent to ovariectomized rats was without effect on uptake. However, others (*19,127*) have found region-specific elevations in 5HT uptake after administration of estradiol or progesterone to ovariectomized rats. Mendelson and coworkers (*81*) reported estradiol-induced reductions in [³H]paroxetine binding, a more specific ligand for 5HT uptake sites than imipramine, in hippocampal subfields. In vivo studies also suggest that corticosteroids may influence SERT expression, particularly during ontogeny. ACTH and nicotine (which releases ACTH), administered at birth to rats, have been reported to significantly increase levels of synaptosomal 5HT uptake in the neonate, although prenatal administration of these agents reduced expression (*61*). However, in the adult rat, 14 d restraint stress with attendant elevations in plasma cortisol appear not to affect SERT antagonist sites in cortex, septum, or hippocampus, as labeled by [³H]paroxetine (*122*). In addition, adrenalectomy failed to alter SERT mRNA levels in the adult rat (*63*). These latter data suggest that if the effects of ACTH on 5HT uptake are indirectly mediated by secretion of cortisol, a critical period of sensitivity during development for SERT regulation may be present. In addition, studies reviewed below suggest that ACTH has direct effects on differentiation of raphe neurons and SERT expression, independent of its actions on the adrenal gland.

Regulation of SERT Expression In Vivo After Chronic Antidepressant Administration

Changes in 5HT uptake and/or radioligand binding have been noted in human brain and platelets in depression and suicide (*80,95*). To date, a structural basis for these changes has not been established (*69*); indeed, the more prevalent suggestion of alterations in transport capacity and site density, rather than substrate or antagonist affinity, suggests an inappropriately low level of SERT gene and/or protein expression, rather than a heritable defect in SERT proteins. Since antagonist blockade of SERT (and NET) occurs immediately, yet antidepressant effects require chronic administration, therapeutic benefits are presumably derived from compensatory changes following increased occupancy of pre- and postsynaptic 5HT receptors.

One compensatory effect evaluated has been the level of SERT expression itself. SERT antagonist binding sites as a measure of SERT protein levels have been found to be altered (generally decreased) following chronic antidepressant treatment, although there is by no means a consensus in the literature on this issue. In early studies,

Arbilla and coworkers (4) noted that cat brain and platelet sites labeled by [^{3}H]imipramine exhibited a reduced density after chronic (two injections/d, 21 d treatment) administration of imipramine with no change in ligand affinity. However, Barbacia and colleagues (9) noted increased rat hippocampal 5HT uptake in parallel with decreased imipramine binding (B_{max}) binding following chronic desipramine or imipramine treatments. It is unlikely that residual imipramine was responsible for the latter effect, because there was a sufficiently long in vivo wash-out time of 3 d, the preparation consisted of washed membranes, and such a phenomenon would have elevated the imipramine binding K_d (which it did not). Rather, the results suggest a change in the expression of the site labeled by the SERT antagonist; the speculated endogenous inhibitor, postulated to explain the opposite binding and uptake effects (9), has not been identified. The issue of residual drug effects was again noted by Hrdina (53), who observed changes in [^{3}H]imipramine affinity following chronic treatment with a number of SERT antagonists, although the investigator also found changes in rat brain synaptosomal 5HT uptake capacity. Other studies have found either reduced density of [^{3}H]imipramine binding sites (Table 2) or no change following antidepressant treatments.

Although these changes in transport or binding suggest a responsiveness of SERT activity or protein expression to environment, hormones, and drugs, changes in uptake must always be cautiously interpreted, since parallel changes in vesicular storage, release, or ion gradients may contribute to the alterations in transport observed. In addition, many have noted the problems associated with use of [^{3}H]imipramine as a SERT-specific marker (26), and recent studies with more specific SERT radioligands, such as [^{3}H]cyanoimipramine, [^{3}H]paroxetine, or [^{3}H]citalopram, have often suggested fairly subtle or no influence of chronic antidepressant administration on SERT expression. Thus, Graham and coworkers (46) found no changes in 5HT uptake or [^{3}H]paroxetine in rat cortex or hippocampus following either acute or chronic treatment (ip, once/d, 18 d) of rats with clorgyline, deprenyl, chlomipramine, or citalopram. Using quantitative autoradiographic techniques, Kovachich and colleagues (62) found elevations in [^{3}H]cyanoimipramine binding following chronic treatment with monoamine oxidase (MAO) inhibitors and reductions following sertraline treatment, though the changes were restricted to small regions of the CNS, and no changes were found after citalopram, protriptyline, or mianserin administration. Watanabe and coworkers (*122*) reported significant, region-specific reductions in cortex and hippocampal [^{3}H]paroxetine binding following chronic (ip, twice daily, 14 d treatment) imipramine treatment. Clearly, dosage, delivery, duration, and quantitation variables exist in these studies and deserve greater attention before firm conclusions can be drawn as to SERT responsiveness to antidepressant administration. In this regard, the non-SERT-directed antidepressant lithium (5 mo treatment, ip injections) has also been reported to cause a reduction in [^{3}H]paroxetine binding in rat brain, but the effect is not seen if lithium levels are elevated through dietary administration (*98*), a delivery route that elevates plasma levels with a more stable profile. In elegant recent studies, Piñeyro et al. (*97*) utilized in vivo electrophysiologic techniques, along with measures of uptake and binding, to establish a downregulation of SERT-mediated clearance following 2 or 21 d paroxetine treatment. These investigators utilized the recovery time of firing activity after microiontophoretic application of 5HT in the rat dorsal hippocampus as an indication of changes in vivo 5HT clearance. Paroxetine administration led to a sustained increase in the duration of recovery from effects of applied 5HT, an effect paralleled (though not exactly matched) by reductions in 5HT uptake measured in slices and [^{3}H]paroxetine binding capacity (B_{max}). The authors of the latter study suggested the presence of spare transporters, so that reductions in density need to be significant to achieve a functional modulation in clearance.

As noted, the atypical tricyclic antidepressant tianeptine, a compound itself ineffective at blocking 5HT uptake in vitro, has been reported to have the paradoxical ability to elevate 5HT uptake in acute or chronically-treated rats and humans (*86*). Platelet and brain uptake of 5HT was found to exhibit an elevated transport capacity with no change in K_m. Although the uptake-enhancing effects of tianeptine have been validated in a number of labs, at least one group has found a reduction in SERT density ([^{3}H]paroxetine binding) following chronic treatment (*122*). A change in SERT density might bring tianeptine in line with other antidepressant agents, but its low potency in vitro and its ability to upregulate expression are puzzling pieces in an enigma yet to be solved.

Several recent studies have reported significant changes in SERT gene expression in the raphe nuclei of rats treated with antidepressants, effects that may lead to long-term alterations in SERT activity and density. Lesch et al. (*67*), using RNA-PCR techniques, reported significant reductions in SERT mRNA following chronic treatment of rats with nonselective and selective SERT antagonists, including imipramine, desipramine, clomipramine, and fluoxetine. The MAO inhibitor clorgyline did not alter SERT mRNA levels, although it should increase synaptic 5HT by elevation of cytoplasmic pools. No effects were observed following treatment with a nonselective 5HT receptor agonist (mCPP) or with selective $5HT_{1a}$ (8-OHDPAT), $5HT_{1c/2}$ (DOI), receptor agonists. The authors suggested that loss of SERT expression may not reflect events subsequent to transport blockade, but rather may indicate a direct effect on the SERT gene. One problem with this hypothesis is that the tricyclics have a structure distinct from fluoxetine, requiring that potential transcriptional regulators share pharmacologic characteristics with SERT. As with studies measuring changes in SERT antagonist density, other groups using different drug treatment protocols come to different conclusions regarding the sensitivity of SERT gene expression to antidepressant administration. Burnet and coworkers (17) found chronic imipramine treatment to have no effects on SERT gene expression measured autoradiographically in three different strains of rats. To complete the spectrum. López et al. (76) found significant elevations in SERT gene expression following chronic ip injections of imipramine and clorgyline. Tianeptine has been reported to reduce SERT mRNA levels in dorsal but not median raphe nuclei, consistent with changes observed in [^{3}H]paroxetine binding (64), but not with reports of enhanced uptake. As with radioligand binding studies, further analyses of the dose and treatment variables required to modulate SERT gene expression in vivo by SERT antagonists and other antidepressants are needed.

If SERT antagonists affect SERT gene expression through alterations in 5HT receptor signaling, 5HT itself (or a lack thereof) might be expected to influence SERT expression. Yu et al. (129) and Linnet et al. (74) both recently reported that SERT mRNA is significantly reduced in rats by depletion of 5HT with p-chlorophenylalanine (PCPA). Since the magnitude of CNS 5HT reduction was not reported and peripheral 5HT synthesis also might be affected, the results described should be cautiously interpreted, although they suggest that compensatory changes in 5HT synthesis and release that follow antidepressant treatment (88) also may contribute to changes in SERT expression. In an earlier study with the same depletion paradigm, [^{3}H]paroxetine binding was not found to be reduced (30), and Yu et al. (129) were also unable to detect changes in [^{3}H]cyanoimipramine binding, suggesting that changes in SERT mRNA require considerably longer periods to affect a change in transporter protein in terminals. Finally, significantly elevated SERT mRNA has been reported in studies with aged rats. Although the proximal causes and consequences of elevated expression are unknown, it is tempting to speculate that elevated SERT gene expression may be an important compensatory response to achieve greater 5HT clearance and reduced 5HT effects in older animals.

In summary, evidence suggests that SERT levels may be modulated by hormones and pharmacologic agents, although in most cases the link between agent and target is tenuous and methodological issues continue to cloud the picture, particularly with in vivo studies. These findings have led investigators to consider regulatory mechanisms in more defined in vitro preparations, when the direct influences of trophic factors, hormones, and second messengers on SERT gene and protein expression can be directly evaluated. Here, consistent effects are emerging for brain and peripheral control mechanisms for long-term SERT regulation. In addition, since some of the preparations are of human origin (JAR cells), experimental paradigms arise that would be difficult, if not possible, to achieve in vivo. Nonetheless, the hope is that information from cell culture studies can be used to frame hypotheses directly relevant to the function of intact tissues and organisms.

Regulation of SERT Expression in Cultured 5HT Neurons and Neuronal Cell Lines

The restricted nature of CNS SERT expression in raphe neurons has been well established in multiple vertebrate species, including humans (5,100), and must depict precise mechanisms for cell-specific gene expression possibly shared with other serotonergic genes, including those that encode the biosynthetic enzyme tryptophan hydroxylase (TpH), the vesicular amine transporters, VMATs, and raphe and platelet 5HT receptors. 5HT appears to be a trophic/differentiation factor for the development of serotonergic neurons (29,124). Pronounced morphological abnormalities have been noted in mouse embryos cultured in the presence of SERT antagonists (114,128), although sites of action for these agents have not been established. In the developing rat CNS, blockade of 5HT synthesis with PCPA delays the onset of neuronal differentiation (65). This raises the possibility that precocious SERT expression may assist in the maintenance of appropriate extracellular 5HT levels required for proper neuronal development.

In the mouse CNS, SERT expression appears to be among the earliest characteristics of serotonergic neurons evident. SERT mRNAs can be detected as early as d 10 (where EØ = day of vaginal plug) in developing neurons that will migrate toward the midline to give rise to midbrain and brainstem raphe nuclei (*111,112*). SERT radioligands and SERT antibodies detect murine SERT protein expression in raphe cell bodies and processes soon thereafter, consistent with reports of 5HT uptake expression in embryonic raphe neurons and growth cones prior to target innervation (*54*). Cloning of the murine SERT gene (Bauman et al., 1996) offers the opportunity to manipulate SERT gene expression nonpharmacologically in transgenic animals to evaluate the role of SERT expression in the early embryo.

Like the mouse embryo, RN46A cells (*31,125*), a transformed line of embryonic rat raphe neuroblasts, demonstrate a precocious expression of SERT activity. Undifferentiated, but neuronally committed, RN64A cells express Na^+-dependent, antidepressant-sensitive 5HT uptake (*31*) but little or no 5HT synthesis, while dividing under the control of a temperature-sensitive SV40 T-antigen. Undifferentiated RN64A cells also express $5HT_{1a}$ receptors, implicated in somatodendritic regulation of neuronal electrical activity in the adult (*31*). A shift of culture temperature to inactivate T-antigen results in morphological differentiation, maintenance of 5HT uptake, and induction of TpH and $5HT_{1a}$ receptors. Further differentiation conditions, including treatment with brain-derived neurotrophic factor (BDNF) and partial depolarizing conditions, which do not affect 5HT uptake expression, are required to establish significant 5HT synthesis and storage. Thus, the transcription factors that first establish SERT expression in the CNS may be responsive to the earliest signals triggering development of a serotonergic phenotype, with distinct controls evident for essential proteins characteristic of the serotonergic phenotype. Differential, tissue-specific control of serotonergic gene expression is clearly evident in nonneural sites of SERT expression, such as platelet and placenta, where TpH is not expressed. In these tissues, vesicular transport proteins are also either absent (placenta) (Ganapathy, V., personal communication) or derived from a VMAT gene product distinct from that found in CNS neurons (platelets). Recently, Clark et al. (*21*) established that cultured thyroid C-cells can be differentiated to a serotonergic neuronal phenotype, with the resultant expression of SERT mRNA. This differentiation can be enhanced by NGF, with the consequent induction of 5HT uptake and SERT gene expression. In C-cells, dexamethasone and retinoic acid repress neuronal characteristics (*108*); it will be interesting to determine whether SERT expression is downregulated in parallel with other neuronal characteristics, and whether these agents identify important negative regulatory pathways for SERT gene expression nonneuronal cells and nonserotonergic neurons. In C-cells, SERT mRNA is elevated by NGF, along with $5HT_{1b}$ receptor mRNA, yet TpH mRNA levels appear unchanged, again revealing distinct pathways mediating regulation of serotonergic genes.

Once established in developing neurons, 5HT uptake can be modulated by multiple factors thought to act endogenously to support serotonergic differentiation, or by drugs, presumably affecting one or more intracellular pathways controlling SERT expression. Vesicular 5HT release may be constitutive during raphe neuron development (*31*), with the released amine acting on glial 5HT receptors to trigger secondary release of other substances affecting serotonergic differentiation. Serotonergic neurons develop and migrate along transient, radial glial processes immunoreactive for S-100β (*120*). 5HT, acting through $5HT_{1a}$ receptors, releases S-100β from astroglial cultures in vitro (*123,124*). In turn, chronic, but not acute, administration of S-100β enhances morphological differentiation of 5HT neurons and elevates 5HT uptake independent of cell survival (*75,124*). Subcellular mechanisms transducing the effect of S-100β on SERT expression have not been identified, although availability of the protein in the raphe appears to be transient, suggesting a critical period of response or the involvement of additional supportive factors later in development.

In primary cultures of raphe neurons, ACTH peptides (particularly $ACTH_{4-10}$) elevate 5HT uptake (*6*). This effect is replicated in RN46A cells, where chronic administration of $ACTH_{4-10}$ can upregulate 5HT uptake as much as sevenfold (*32*). Importantly, $ACTH_{4-10}$-mediated upregulation of 5HT uptake is not simply accounted for by increased survival of serotonergic neurons, since the survival-promoting effects of ACTH appear to require further treatment of cells under partial depolarizing conditions. $ACTH_{4-10}$ elevates cAMP levels in RN46A cells and exogenous treatments with either an adenylyl cyclase activator (forskolin) or the cAMP analog dibutyryl cAMP also elevates levels of 5HT uptake, as it can in primary cultures (*37*). In RN46A cells, basal and $ACTH_{4-10}$-induced 5HT uptake are reduced by chronic administration of the Ca^{2+} channel antagonist nifedipine, suggesting the involvement of Ca^{2+}-regulated processes in SERT induction. Partial depolarizing conditions are required to affect maximal ACTH-mediated effects on TpH activity, 5HT levels, and 5HT1a receptor expression in these cells, but depolarizing conditions fail to further affect expression of 5HT uptake. Since coculture of raphe neurons with hippocampal neurons has been reported to both induce 5HT uptake and to eliminate the effects of ACTH peptides (6), $ACTH_{4-10}$ and other target-derived factors may activate a common intracellular pathway (perhaps cAMP) in support of the molecular differentiation of serotonergic neurons.

Fibroblast growth factor-5 (FGF-5), synthesized and secreted by many CNS regions that receive a serotonergic innervation, has been suggested to enhance differentiation of raphe neurons, upregulating 5HT uptake capacity (72). Specific intracellular pathways supporting SERT expression have not been identified. FGF receptors may trigger kinase-activated signaling pathways that parallel, or interact with, cAMP-mediated signaling to coordinate appropriate levels of SERT expression during differentiation in the CNS. Target-derived support of SERT gene expression would require the retrograde transport of signals to activate the SERT gene in the nuclei of raphe neurons. NGF, BDNF, or neurotrophin-3 do not significantly affect 5HT uptake, although BDNF itself appears trophic for survival of serotonergic neurons (7,31). Since 5HT uptake and mRNA are induced by NGF in C-cells as part of a generalized induction to a neuronal phenotype, absence of effects of NGF in RN46A cells suggests cell-specificity in NGF-mediated SERT regulation (serotonin neurons from C-cells are presumably neural crest progeny, but RN46A neurons derive from the CNS). Finally, it is worth noting that studies on cultured raphe neurons and RN46A cells have relied exclusively on measurements of $[^{3}H]5HT$ uptake and are not explicitly indicative of altered gene expression. However, the rather slow induction of uptake in vitro is most consistent with changes in SERT transcription. Morphological differentiation itself must dictate elevated SERT protein levels to keep pace with an increased number of varicosities and 5HT release sites.

A plausible working model for regulated SERT gene expression in support of neural development is one in which SERT is first activated at commitment of neuroblasts to a serotonergic phenotype, followed by subsequent amplification of expression sustained by extracellular trophic molecules. Extracellular differentiating molecules sustain SERT expression through cAMP and tyrosine-kinase mediated signaling pathways. One economical aspect of a model of second messenger-mediated amplification of SERT gene expression is that it does not involve serotonin neuron-specific proteins or pathways, since many agents might elevate SERT expression at different stages of development, using common second-messenger pathways. If SERT gene induction and level of expression are set through independent mechanisms, studies with peripheral cell models might provide important insights for quantitative regulation of SERT gene expression in the brain, particularly if common or linked promoters drive SERT expression in different tissues. Chromosomal mapping studies reveal that SERTs derive from a single genomic locus (*see* next section) in humans (*103*) and a single syntenic position in mouse (*47*). Recent studies in human placental JAR cells echo and extend findings from studies with raphe preparations, and have provided the first direct evidence for independent subcellular mechanisms in control of SERT gene expression.

SERT Gene Expression in Placental JAR Cells

JAR cells are a choriocarcinoma cell line derived from human placenta (*8*). Balkovetz et al. (*8*) first demonstrated that JAR cells exhibit antidepressant-sensitive 5HT transport and SERT antagonist binding, activity that can be increased by activators of $G\alpha s$ (cholera toxin, CTX) or adenylyl cyclase (forskolin), phosphodiesterase inhibition (IBMX), and the membrane-permeant cAMP analog dbcAMP (*22,104*). 5HT uptake elevations are blocked by inhibitors of cAMP-dependent protein kinase, require chronic stimulation, and are dependent on sustained RNA and protein synthesis (*22*). Indeed, CTX and forskolin elevate cAMP levels maximally within 2 h, but changes in transporter activity are only observed after approx 8 h of treatment, suggesting multiple steps are involved from activated PKA to changes in cell-surface SERT expression. Kinetically, transport capacity (V_{max}) is markedly elevated by 100 ng/mL CTX, with little or no change in 5HT concentration dependence (K_m). This effect is paralleled by a corresponding increase in membrane binding capacity (B_{max}) for the SERT antagonist RTI-55 (*104*), consistent with elevated levels of SERT protein in treated cells. Under these conditions, steady state SERT mRNA levels in JAR cells are elevated nearly 10-fold, despite no changes in mRNA half-life (*16*). Together, these findings suggest that activation of PKA activates SERT gene expression, with the time delay in elevated activity caused by time required for translocation of PKA, activation of cAMP-response element binding protein (CREB), and the subsequent delays imposed by transcription, mRNA processing, and transporter protein processing. Pulse-chase analysis of NET biosynthesis in transfected LLC-PK1 cells (*78*) and cell-surface biotinylation experiments (*79*) demonstrate that homologous NET proteins take several hours to reach the mature state of glycosylation displayed by surface transporters.

Although elevated SERT expression by activation of cAMP-dependent pathways appears to be similar in placental cells and raphe neurons, PC12 cells, an adrenal chromaffin cell tumor line of neural crest origin, have been reported to exhibit reduced 5HT uptake in response to CTX. Because of the low level of 5HT uptake measured in these cells, the nonselective antagonist (imipramine) used to define specific transport, and an absence of data with specific gene or protein probes, these effects may reflect an alteration in PC12 NE transporter gene expression rather than alterations in SERT expression. The recent demonstration of high-level SERT gene expression in rodent adrenal glands (*13*), and the finding that neural crest derivatives in the thyroid transdifferentiate to a serotonergic neuronal phenotype, suggests interesting aspects of SERT gene expression might be identified by further studies with cultured adrenal chromaffin cells.

Additional studies with JAR cells have provided further insight into cAMP-mediated SERT expression and suggest additional kinase-linked pathways involved in SERT gene expression. Staurosporine, a microbial alkaloid antagonist of PKC, PKG, and PKA, induces a similar activation of 5HT uptake and increase in SERT mRNA levels as CTX, yet with no alteration in cAMP levels (*101*). Presuming that staurosporine is acting through kinase inhibition (it has no effects directly on SERT), these findings indicate the presence of a pathway to negatively regulate SERT gene expression. Since CTX-mediated SERT activation is not additive with staurosporine-induced effects, however, this kinase is likely to be poised downstream of PKA, either in a linear sequence, or the two kinases may share a common regulatory target. SERT is not upregulated by other PKA, PKC, and PKG, and tyrosine kinase antagonists, and so these traditional pathways are not likely to be responsible for staurosporine's effects. Equivalent effects have yet to be reported in cultured neurons; comparative studies would be useful in exploring the generality of these effects and their relationship to the effects of CNS trophic factors.

Recently, Ramamoorthy et al. (*105*) found that the cytokine interleukin-1β (IL-1β) elevates SERT gene expression in JAR cells. Like CTX and staurosporine effects, sustained mRNA synthesis is required for IL-1β-induced activation of 5HT uptake and elevation of SERT mRNA levels, consistent with activation of SERT transcription. Like staurosporine, IL-1β does not alter JAR cell cAMP or cGMP levels. Unlike staurosporine, however, IL-1β's effects on uptake are additive with CTX. IL-1 signaling is thought to be mediated through recruitment and oligomerization of nonreceptor kinases (*94*). Receptors for IL-1β are found on serotonergic neurons (*25*), although no data is available to implicate the cytokine in regulation of neuronal SERT gene expression. IL-1 itself is synthesized by neurons and glial cells, although raphe neurons may also respond to IL-1 delivered by white blood cells penetrating endothelial barriers (diapedesis) during inflammation (*25*). Thus, studies with SERT gene expression in placental JAR cells may reflect regulatory pathways at work as well in CNS neurons. Since ACTH-regulated expression of 5HT uptake in raphe neurons and cell lines appears to correspond to the cAMP-coupled pathway first identified in JAR cells, it will be useful to examine whether other inducers of serotonergic differentiation and 5HT uptake, such as S100β and FGF, utilize cAMP-independent pathways for SERT gene activation identified in JAR cells.

Structural Analysis of Regulatory Elements in the SERT Gene

SERT cDNAs have been identified from rat (*11,51*), mouse (*20*), human (*70,71,103*), and *Drosophila* (*24,27*). The existence of a homologous *Drosophila melanogaster* transporter with the substrate specificity of SERT, and partially overlapping sensitivity to antagonists (*24,27*), suggests that a single gene for 5HT clearance evolved prior to the separation of invertebrate and vertebrate lineages. Although originally reported with divergent sequences, rat brain and mast cell SERTs appear to be identical proteins of 630 amino acids. Consistent with these data, identical human SERT cDNAs have been identified from placenta (*103*), brain, and platelets (*70,71*). A single SERT genomic locus has been identified on human chromosome 17q11.2 (Fig. 3) by Southern analysis, somatic cell hybrid analysis, and *in situ* hybridization (*103*) and this has been recently confirmed by linkage mapping (*41*). An initial report of the intron/exon structure of the human SERT gene (*68*) suggests the presence of at least 14 exons spanning more than 30 kb of genomic DNA, findings we have recently confirmed and extended (Fig. 4). The start site for transcription, as determined by primer extension and 5'RACE reactions on brain RNA, was reported to fall 207 bp upstream of the initiator ATG codon (*68*). In addition, we have noted that multiple SERT mRNAs are found in human brain (*5*) and placenta (*103*) and preliminary data suggests some of these mRNAs may initiate from distinct promoters (Fig. 4). A large initial intron (3–6 kb) appears to separate

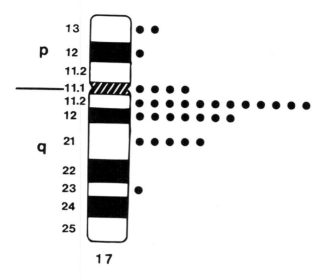

Fig. 3. Localization of the human SERT gene on chromosome 17. Somatic cell hybrid studies (not shown) and *in situ* hybridization of spread and banded chromosomes reveal significant labeling of human chromosome 17, centered at 17q11.2. Dots indicate relative abundance of silver grains deposited after labeling with human SERT cDNA probes. No other chromosomal locus labeled above background. Figure reproduced with permission from Ramamoorthy et al. (*102*).

transcription start sites from the first coding exon (exon 2). Tissue-specific initiation and promoter usage has been described for glycine transporters (*15*), homologous members of the GAT1 gene family. Distinct promoters may serve to provide additional flexibility in the coordination of SERT expression in different tissues, since both glycine transporters exhibit distinct patterns of distribution in the CNS and periphery. In the human SERT gene, 10 copies of a 17 bp polymorphism (GGCT-GYGACCY[R]GRRTG) have been found upstream of a putative AP1 site in intron 2 (*68*), although the significance of this element for regulation of SERT transcription is unclear. Upstream of the distal SERT transcription start site observed in human brain, binding sites for transcription factors, including a TATA-like motif, an AP1 site, and an element for CREB binding (CRE), have been described (*68*). Similar sequences are found upstream of the mouse SERT (mSERT) promoter (*110*) and have been reported to direct elevated reporter gene expression in transfected COS cells in the presence of cAMP elevating agents. In addition, the putative promoter region for mSERT contains motifs reminiscent of

Genomic Organization for the Human Serotonin Transporter

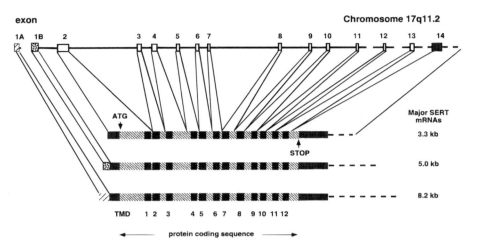

Fig. 4. Genomic organization of the human SERT gene. Shown are at least 14 exons that encode SERT mRNA noncoding and coding sequences. Gaps in the genomic structure indicate unresolved distances between exons. Dotted lines in the genomic and mRNA structures indicate suspected, but as yet unidentified, noncoding exons contribution to mRNA heterogeneity. Multiple transcription initiation sites have been identified, resulting in mRNA beginning at exons 1a, 1b, or 2. Three SERT mRNA sizes are produced with varying representation in different tissues (placenta 3.3 > 5.0 > 8.2; brain 3.3 = 8.2 > 5.0, from Ramamoorthy et al. [*102*] and Austin et al. [*5*]). Regions of mRNAs with diagonal hatching are hydrophilic, and regions in black indicate 12 hydrophobic regions presumed to be TMDs. Note that all but TMD 11 is uninterrupted by intron/exon boundaries, placing these TMDs in a separate exon.

AP-2, α-INF, γ-IRE, NF-IL6, NF-κB, and SP1 sites, some of which may be responsible for cAMP-independent pathways of SERT gene regulation. Indeed, IL-1 has been shown to activate or induce (among other things) *jun, fos*, NF-IL6, and NF-κB (*94*). Together, these studies suggest structural bases for elevated SERT gene expression by cAMP-depedent and independent pathways. Along with information delineating biochemical pathways for acute SERT regulation, this initial framework (Fig. 5) suggests opportunities for significant progress in the coming years on mechanisms of how cells regulate their ability to clear 5HT and how we might manipulate these pathways for therapeutic benefit.

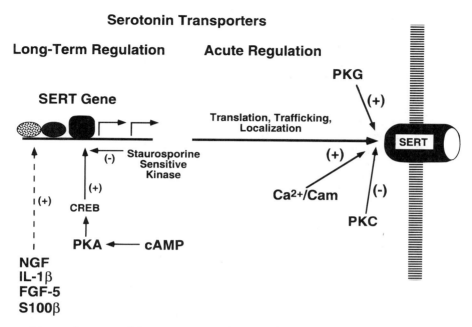

Fig. 5. Acute and long-term regulation of serotonin transport: an initial roadmap. The SERT gene is shown bound by constitutive and regulated transcription factors driving transcription at multiple promoters (arrows). SERT gene expression is suggested to be positively regulated by hormones, such as ACTH, elevating cAMP and activating PKA and presumably CREB. A staurosporine-sensitive inhibitory pathway, perhaps mediated by an unidentified kinase, can inhibit gene activation through the PKA pathway. In parallel with the PKA pathways are other as yet unidentified pathways transducing upregulation of SERT expression noted for NGF, IL-1β, FGF-5, and S100β. Following transcription, SERTs are translated and transported to their membrane sites of expression in cells. Ca^{2+}, calmodulin (Cam), PKG, and PKC have been implicated in acute regulation of expressed SERT, with the mechanism of regulation and potential for interaction of multiple effectors awaiting clarification. The diagram serves to organize regulatory influences suggested to occur at either the gene or protein level, but should not be taken to imply that all pathways are operational in any one cell type.

Acknowledgments

The authors acknowledge the support of the National Institute on Drug Abuse and the National Association for Research in Schizophrenia and Affective Disorders (R. Blakely) and the PhRMA Foundation (S. Schroeter) and Maarten Reith for his patience and encouragement.

References

1. Amara, S. G. and Kuhar, M. J. Neurotransmitter transporters: recent progress. *Annu. Rev. Neurosci.* **16** (1993) 73–93.
2. Anderson, G. M. and Horne, W. C. Activators of protein kinase C decrease serotonin transport in human platelets. *Biochim. Biophys. Acta* **1137** (1992) 331–337.
3. Anderson, G. M., Vaccadino, F. M., and Hall, L. M. Short-term regulation of glial and neuronal serotonin uptake. *Soc. Neurosci. Abstr.* **21** (1995) 344.16.
4. Arbilla, S., Briley, M., Cathala, F., Langer, S. Z., Pornin, C., and Raisman, R. Parallel changes in [^{3}H]-imipramine binding sites in cat brain and platelets following chronic treatment with imipramine. *Proc. BPS.* **1** (1980) 154P,155P.
5. Austin, M. C., Bradley, C., Blakely, R. D., and Mann, J. Expression of 5HT transporter gene in the human brainstem. *J. Neurochem.* **62** (1994) 2362–2367.
6. Azmitia, E. C. and de Kloet, E. R. ACTH neuropeptide stimulation of serotonergic neuronal maturation in tissue culture: modulation by hippocampal cells. *Prog. Brain Res.* **72** (1987) 311–318.
7. Azmitia, E. C., Dolan, K., and Whitaker-Azmitia, P. M. S100β but not NGF, EGF, insulin or calmodulin is a CNS serotonergic growth factor. *Brain Res.* **516** (1990) 354–356.
8. Balkovetz, D. F., Tiruppathi, C., Leibach, F. H., Mahesh, V. B., and Ganapathy, V. Evidence for an imipramine-sensitive serotonin transporter in human placental brush-border membranes. *J. Biol. Chem.* **264** (1989) 2195–2198.
9. Barbaccia, M. L., Gandolfi, O., Chuang, D., and Costa, E. Modulation of neuronal serotonin uptake by a putative endogenous ligand of imipramine recognition sites. *Proc. Natl. Acad. Sci. USA* **80** (1983) 5134–5138.
10. Barker, E. L. and Blakely, R. D. Norepinephrine and serotonin transporters: molecular targets of antidepressant drugs. In Bloom, F. E. and Kupfer, D. J. (eds.), *Psychopharmacology: The Fourth Generation of Progress*, Raven, New York, 1995, pp. 321–333.
10a. Bauman, A. L., Flattem, N., Malone, M. D., Fritz, J. D., and Blakely, R. D. Molecular cloning of the murine serotonin transporter gene and identification of brain transcription initiation sites. *Soc. Neurosci. Abstr.* **22** (1996) in press.
10b. Bhat, G. B. and Block, E. R. Hypoxia directly increases serotonin transport by porcine pulmonary artery endothelial cell-plasma membrane vesicles. *Am. J. Respir. Cell Mol. Biol.* **3** (1990) 363–367.
11. Blakely, R. D., Berson, H. E., Fremeau, R. T., Jr., Caron, M. G., Peek, M. M., Prince, H. K., and Bradley, C. C. Molecular cloning and functional expression of a rat brain serotonin transporter. *Nature* **354** (1991) 66–70.
12. Blakely, R. D., DeFelice, L. J., and Hartzell, H. C. Molecular physiology of norepinephrine and serotonin transporters. *J. Exp. Biol.* **196** (1994) 263–281.
13. Blakely, R. D., Wise, K. R., and Schroeter, S. Localization of the serotonin transporter to rodent adrenal chromaffin cells: support for a role of 5HT in adrenal physiology. *Soc. Neurosci. Abstr.* **21** (1995) 316.1.
14. Blier, P., Galzin, A., and Langer, S. Z. Diurnal variation in the function of serotonin terminals in the rat hypothalamus. *J. Neurochem.* **52** (1989) 453–459.
15. Borowsky, B., Mezey, E., and Hoffman, B. J. Two glycine transporter variants with distinct localization in the CNS and peripheral tissues are encoded by a common gene. *Neuron.* **10** (1993) 851–863.

16. Bradley, C. C. and Blakely, R. D. Transcriptional regulation and message hetero-geneity of the human serotonin transporter. *Soc. Neurosci. Abstr.* **21** (1995) 344.8.

16a. Briley, M., Raisman, R., Arbilla, S., Casadamont, M., and Langer, S. Z. Concomitant decrease in [3H] imipramine binding in cat brain and platelets after chronic treatment with imipramine. *Eur. J. Pharmacol.* **81** (1982) 309–314.

16b. Buc-Caron, M. H., Launay, J. M., Lamblin, D., and Kellermann, O. Serotonin uptake, storage, and synthesis in an immortalized committed cell line derived from mouse teratocarcinoma. *Proc. Natl. Acad. Sci USA* **87** (1990) 1922–1926.

17. Burnet, P. W. J., Michelson, D., Smith, M. A., Gold, P. W., and Sternberg, E. M. The effect of chronic imipramine administration on the densities of 5HT1A and 5HT2 receptors and the abundancies of 5HT receptor and transporter mRNA in the cortex, hippocampus, and dorsal raphe of three strains of rat. *Brain Res.* **638** (1994) 311–324.

18. Cammack, J. N., Rakhilin, S. V., and Schwartz, E. A. A GABA transporter oper-ates asymmetrically with variable stoichiometry. *Neuron* **13** (1994) 949–960.

19. Cardinali, D. P. and Gomez, E. Changes in hypothalamic noradrenaline, dopamine, and serotonin uptake after oestradiol administration to rats. *J. Endocrinol.* **73** (1977) 181,182.

20. Chang, A. S., Chang, S. M., Starnes, D. M., Schroeter, S., and Blakely, R. D. Molecular cloning and expression of the mouse serotonin transporter. *Mol. Brain Res.* (1996), in press.

21. Clark, M. S., Lanigan, T. M., Page, N. M., and Russo, A. F. Induction of a sero-tonergic and neuronal phenotype in thyroid C-cells. *J. Neurosci.* **15** (1995) 6167–6178.

22. Cool, D. R., Leibach, F. H., Bhalla, V. K., Mabesh, V. B., and Ganapathy, V. Expression and cyclic AMP-dependent regulation of a high affinity serotonin transporter in the human placental choriocarcinoma cell line (JAR). *J. Biol. Chem.* **266** (1991) 15,750–15,757.

23. Corey, J. L., Davidson, N., Lester, H. A., Brecha, N., and Quick, M. W. Protein kinase c modulates the activity of a cloned γ-aminobutyric acid transporter expressed in *Xenopus* oocytes via regulated subcellular redistribution of the transporter. *J. Biol. Chem.* **269** (1994) 14,759–14,767.

24. Corey, J. L., Quick, M. W., Davidson, N., Lester, H. A., and Guastella, J. A cocaine-sensitive *drosophila* serotonin transporter: cloning, expression, and electrophysiological characterization. *Proc. Natl. Acad. Sci. USA* **91** (1994) 1188–1192.

25. Cunningham, E. T. and de Souza, E. B. Interleukin 1 receptors in the brain and endocrine tissues. *Immunol. Today* **14** (1996) 171–176.

26. D'Amato, R. J., Largent, B. L., Snowman, A. M., and Snyder, S. H. Selective label-ing of serotonin uptake sites in rat brain by [^{3}H]citalopram contrasted to label-ing of multiple sites by [^{3}H]imipramine. *J. Pharmacol. Exp. Ther.* **242** (1987) 364–371.

27. Demchyshyn, L. L., Pristupa, Z. B., Sugamori, K. S., Barker, E. L., Blakely, R. D., Wolfgang, W. J., Forte, M. A., and Niznik, H. B. Cloning, expression, and local-ization of a chloride-facilitated, cocaine-sensitive serotonin transporter from *Drosophila melanogaster*. *Proc. Natl. Acad. Sci. USA* **91** (1994) 5158–5162.

28. De Simoni, M. G., De Luigi, A., Clavenna, A., and Manfridi, A. In vivo studies on the enhancement of serotonin reuptake by tianeptine. *Brain Res.* **574** (1992) 93–97.

29. De Vitry, F., Hamon, M., Catelon, J., Dubois, M., and Thibault, J. Serotonin initiates and autoamplifies its own synthesis during mouse central nervous system development. *Proc. Natl. Acad. Sci. USA.* **83** (1986) 8629–8633.

30. Dewar, K. M., Grondin, L., Carli, M., Lima, L., and Reader, T. A. [³H]Paroxetine binding and serotonin content of rat cortical areas, hippocampus, neostriatum, ventral mesencephalic tegmentum, and midbrain raphe nuclei region following p-chlorophenylalanine and p-chloroamphetamine treatment. *J. Neurochem.* **58** (1992) 250–257.

31. Eaton, M. J., Staley, J. K., Globus, M. Y., and Whittemore, S. R. Developmental regulation of early serotonergic neuronal differentiation: the role of brain derived neurotrophic factor and membrane depolarization. *Dev. Biol.* **170** (1995) 169–182.

32. Eaton, M. J. and Whittemore, S. R. Adrenocorticotropic hormone activation of adenylate cyclase in raphe neurons: multiple regulatory pathways control serotonergic neuronal differentiation. *J. Neurobiol.* **28** (1995) 465–481.

33. Edwards, R. H. The transport of neurotransmitters into synaptic vesicles. *Curr. Opinion Neurobiol.* **2** (1992) 594–596.

34. Endersby, C. A. and Wilson, C. A. The effect of ovarian steroids on the accumulation of ³H-labelled monoamines by hypothalamic tissue in vitro. *Brain Res.* **73** (1974) 321–331.

35. Fattaccini, C. M., Bolaños-Jimenez, F., Gozlan, H., and Hamon, M. Tianeptine stimulates uptake of 5-hydroxytryptamine in vivo in the rat brain. *Neuropharmacology* **29** (1990) 1–8.

36. File, S. E., Zangrossi, H., and Andrews, N. Novel environment and cat odor change GABA and 5-HT release and uptake in the rat. *Pharmacol. Biochem. Behav.* **45** (1993) 931–934.

37. Foguet, M., Hartikka, J. A., Schmuck, K., and Lubbert, H. Long-term regulation of serotonergic activity in the rat brain via activation of protein kinase A. *EMBO J.* **12** (1993) 903–910.

38. Fozard, J. (ed.) *Peripheral Actions of 5-Hydroxytryptamine*, Oxford University Press, New York, 1989.

39. Fuller, R. W. and Wong, D. T. Serotonin uptake and serotonin uptake inhibition. *Ann. NY Acad. Sci.* **600** (1990) 68–78.

40. Galli, A., DeFelice, L. J., Duke, B. J., Moore, K. R., and Blakely, R. D. Sodium-dependent norepinephrine-induced currents in norepinephrine transporter transfected HEK-293 cells blocked by cocaine and antidepressants. *J. Exp. Biol.* (1995), 2197–2212.

41. Gelernter, J., Pakstis, A. J., and Kidd, K. K. Linkage mapping of serotonin transporter protein gene SLC6A4 on chromosome 17. *Hum. Genet.* **95** (1995) 677–680.

42. Gillis, C. N. Peripheral metabolism of serotonin. In Vanhoutte, P. M. (ed.), *Serotonin and the Cardiovascular System*, Raven, New York, 1985, pp. 27–36.

43. Gillis, C. N. and Pitt, B. R. The fate of circulation amines within the pulmonary circulation. *Annu. Rev. Neurosci.* **44** (1982) 269–281.

44. Giros, B., Mestikawy, S. E., Bertrand, L., and Caron, M. G. Cloning and functional characterization of a cocaine-sensitive dopamine transporter. *FEBS Lett.* **295** (1991) 149–154.

45. Glennon, R. A. and Dukat, M. Serotonin receptor subtypes. In Bloom, F. E. and Kupfer, D. J. (eds.), *Psychopharmacology: The Fourth Generation of Progress*, Raven, New York, 1995, pp. 415–429.

46. Graham, D., Tahraoui, L., and Langer, S. Z. Effect of chronic treatment with selective monoamine oxidase inhibitors and specific 5-hydroxytryptamine uptake inhibitors on [³H]paroxetine binding to cerebral cortical membranes of the rat. *Neuropharmacology* **26** (1987) 1087–1092.

47. Gregor, P., Patel, A., Shimada, S., Lin, C., Rochelle, J. M., Kitayama, S., Seiden, M. F., and Uhl, G. R. Murine serotonin transporter: sequence and localization of chromosome 11. *Mammal. Genome* **4** (1993) 283,284.

48. Gu, H. H., Ahn, J., Caplan, M. J., Blakely, R. D., Levey, A. I., and Rudnick, G. Sorting of biogenic amine transporters expressed in epithelial cells. *J. Biol. Chem. (1996)*, in press.

49. Helmeste, D. M. and Tang, S. W. Kinase inhibitors complete with imipramine for binding and inhibition of serotonin transport. *Eur. J. Pharmacol.* **267** (1994) 239–242.

50. Helmeste, D. M. and Tang, S. W. Possible regulation of platelet serotonin uptake by tyrosine kinase. *Soc. Neurosci. Abstr.* **21** (1995) 345.12.

51. Hoffman, B. J., Mezey, E., and Brownstein, M. J. Cloning of a serotonin transporter affected by antidepressants. *Science* **254** (1991) 579,580.

52. Hoffman, B. J. and Miller, K. J. The N-terminal domain of the 5HT transporter partially mediates the regulation of uptake by protein kinase C (PKC). *Soc. Neurosci. Abstr.* **20** (1994) 267.4.

53. Hrdina, P. D. Regulation of high- and low-affinity [³H]imipramine recognition sites in rat brain by chronic treatment with antidepressants. *Eur. J. Pharmacol.* **138** (1987) 159–168.

54. Ivgy-May, N., Tamir, H., and Gershon, M. D. Synaptic properties of serotonergic growth cones in developing rat brain. *J. Neurosci.* **14** (1994) 1011–1029.

55. Jacobs, B. and Azmitia, E. C. Structure and function of the brain serotonin system. *Physiol. Rev.* **72** (1992) 165–229.

56. Jayanthi, L. D., Ramamoorthy, S., Mahesh, V. B., Leibach, F. H., and Ganapathy, V. Calmodulin-dependent regulation of the catalytic function of the human serotonin transporter in placental choriocarcinoma cells. *J. Biol. Chem.* **269** (1994) 14,424–14,429.

57. Jikoh, Y., Nishio, H., Okugawa, K., and Segawa, T. Effect of concanavalin A on serotonin transport into blood platelets: possible involvement of protein kinase C. *Jpn. J. Pharmacol.* **53** (1990) 403–410.

58. Kasanicki, M. A. and Pilch, P. F. Regulation of glucose-transporter function. *Diabetes Care* **13** (1990) 219–227.

59. Kato, G. and Weitsch, A. F. Neurochemical profile of tianeptine, a new antidepressant drug. *Clin. Neuropharmacol.* **11(Suppl. 2)** (1988) S43–S50.

60. Kilty, J. E., Lorang, D., and Amara, S. G. Cloning and expression of a cocaine-sensitive rat dopamine transporter. *Science* **254** (1991) 578–580.

61. King, J. A., Davila-Garcia, M., Azmitia, E. C., and Strand, F. L. Differential effects of prenatal and postnatal ACTH or nicotine exposure on 5-HT high affinity uptake in the neonatal rat brain. *Int. J. Dev. Neurosci.* **9** (1991) 281–286.

61a. Kinnier, W. J., Chuang, D., and Costa, E. Down regulation of dihydroalprenolol and imipramine binding sites in brain of rats repeatedly treated with imipramine. *Eur. J. Pharmacol.* **67** (1980) 289–294.

62. Kovachich, G. B., Aronson, C. E., and Brunswick, D. J. Effect of repeated administration of antidepressants on serotonin uptake sites in limbic and neocortical

structures of rat brain determined by quantitative autoradiography. *Neuropsychopharmacology* **7** (1992) 317–324.

63. Kuroda, Y., Watanabe, Y., Albeck, D. S., Hastings, N. B., and McEwen, B. S. Effects of adrenalectomy and type I or type II glucocorticoid activation on 5HT1A and 5HT2 receptor binding and 5HT transporter mRNA expression in rat brain. *Brain Res.* **648** (1994) 157–161.

64. Kuroda, Y., Watanabe, Y., and McEwen, B. S. Tianeptine decreases both serotonin transporter RNA and binding sites in rat brain. *Eur. J. Pharmacol.* **268** (1994) R3–R5.

65. Lauder, J. M. and Krebs, H. Effects of p-chlorophenylalanine on time of neuronal origin during embryogenesis in the rat. *Brain Res.* **107** (1976) 638–644.

66. Launay, J., Bondoux, D., Oset-Gasque, M., Emami, S., Mutel, V., Haimart, M., and Gespach, C. Increase of human platelet serotonin uptake by atypical histamine receptors. *Am. J. Physiol.* **266** (1994) 526–536.

67. Lesch, K. P., Aulakh, C. S., Wolozin, B. L., Tolliver, T. J., Hill, J. L., and Murphy, D. L. Regional brain expression of serotonin transporter mRNA and its regulation by reuptake inhibiting antidepressants. *Mol. Brain Res.* **17** (1993) 31–35.

68. Lesch, K. P., Balling, U., Gross, J., Strass, K., Wolozin, B. L., Murphy, D. L., and Riederer, P. Organization of the human serotonin transporter gene. *J. Neural Transm.* **95** (1994) 157–162.

69. Lesch, K. P., Gross, J., Franzek, E., Wolozin, B. L., Riederer, P., and Murphy, D. L. Primary structure of the serotonin transporter in unipolar depression and bipolar disorder. *Biol. Psychiatry* **37** (1995) 215–223.

70. Lesch, K. P., Wolozin, B. L., Estler, H. C., Murphy, D. L., and Riederer, P. Isolation of a cDNA encoding the human brain serotonin transporter. *J. Neural Transm.* **91** (1993) 67–72.

71. Lesch, K. P., Wolozin, B. L., Murphy, D. L., and Riederer, P. Primary structure of the human platelet serotonin uptake site: identity with the brain serotonin transporter. *J. Neurochem.* **60** (1993) 2319–2322.

72. Lindholm, D., Hartikka, J., Berghazui, M. D., Castren, E., Tzimagiorgis, G., Hughes, R. A., and Thoene, H. Fibroblast growth factor-5 promotes differentiation of cultured rat septal cholinergic and raphe serotonergic neurons: comparison with the effects of neurotrophins. *Eur. J. of Neurosci.* **6** (1994) 244–252.

73. Lingen, B., Bruss, M., and Bonisch, H. Cloning and expression of the bovine sodium- and chloride-dependent noradrenaline transporter. *FEBS Lett.* **342** (1994) 235–238.

74. Linnet, K., Koed, K., Wiborg, O., and Gregersen, N. Serotonin depletion decreases serotonin transporter mRNA levels in rat brain. *Brain Res.* **697** (1995) 251–253.

75. Liu, J. P. and Lauder, J. M. S-100β and insulin-like growth factor-II differentially regulate growth of developing serotonin and dopamine neurons in vitro. *J. Neurosci. Res.* **33** (1992) 248–256.

76. López, J. F., Chalmers, D. T., Vazquez, D. M., Watson, S. J., and Akil, H. Serotonin transporter mRNA in rat brain is regulated by classical antidepressants. *Biol. Psychiatry* **35** (1994) 287–290.

77. Mager, S., Min, C., Henry, D. H., Chavkin, C., Hoffman, B. J., Davidson, N., and Lester, H. A. Conducting states of a mammalian serotonin transporter. *Neuron* **12** (1994) 845–859.

77a. Meister, B., Johnson, H., and Ulfhake, B. Increased expression of serotonin transporter messenger RNA in raphe neurons of the aged rat. *Mol. Brain Res.* **33** (1995) 87–96.

78. Melikian, H. E., McDonald, J. K., Gu, H., Rudnick, G., Moore, K. R., and Blakely, R. D. Human norepinephrine transporter: biosynthetic studies using a site-directed polyclonal antibody. *J. Biol. Chem.* **269** (1994) 12,290–12,297.

79. Melikian, H. E., Ramamoorthy, S., Tate, C. G., and Blakely, R. D. N-glycosylation deficient human norepinephrine transporter: transport deficits arise from a combination of decreased protein stability, reduced surface abundance, and compromised amine translocation independent of ligand recognition. *Mol. Pharmacol.* **50(2)** (1996), in press.

80. Meltzer, H. Y. Role of serotonin in depression. *Ann. N. Y. Acad. Sci.* **600** (1990) 486–499.

81. Mendelson, S. D., McKittrick, C. R., and McEwen, B. S. Autoradiographic analyses of the effects of estradiol benzoate on [^{3}H]paroxetine binding in the cerebral cortex and dorsal hippocampus of gonadectomized male and female rats. *Brain Res.* **601** (1993) 299–302.

82. Mennini, T., Mocaer, E., and Garattini, S. Tianeptine, a selective enhancer of serotonin uptake in rat brain. *Naunyn-Schmiedebergs Arch. Pharmacol.* **336** (1987) 478–482.

83. Meyer, D. C. and Quay, W. B. Hypothalamic and suprachiasmatic uptake of serotonin in vitro: twenty-four-hour changes in male and proestrous female rats. *Endocrinology* **98** (1976) 1160–1165.

84. Miller, K. J. and Hoffman, B. J. Adenosine A$_3$ receptors regulate serotonin transport via nitric oxide and cGMP. *J. Biol. Chem.* **269** (1994) 27351–27356.

85. Miller, K. J. and Hoffman, B. J. 5HT2 receptors increase 5HT transport via nitric oxide and cGMP *Soc. Neurosci. Abstr.* **21** (1995) 344.4.

86. Mocaër, E., Rettori, M. C., and Kamoun, A. Pharmacological antidepressive effects and tianeptine-induced 5-HT uptake increase. *Clin. Neuropharmacol.* **11(Suppl. 2)** (1988) S32–S42.

87. Montgomery, S. A. Selective serotonin reuptake inhibitors in the acute treatment of depression. In Bloom, F. E. and Kupfer, D. J. (eds.), *Psychopharmacology: The Fourth Generation*, Raven, New York, 1995, pp. 1043–1051.

88. Moret, C. and Briley, M. Effect of antidepressant drugs on monoamine synthesis in brain in vivo. *Neuropharmacology* **31** (1992) 679–684.

89. Myers, C. L., Lazo, J. S., and Pitt, B. R. Translocation of protein kinase C is associated with inhibition of 5-HT uptake by cultured endothelial cells. *Am. J. Physiol.* **257** (1989) L253–L258.

90. Myers, C. L. and Pitt, B. R. Selective effect of phorbol ester on serotonin removal and ACE activity in rabbit lungs. *J. Appl. Physiol.* **65** (1988) 377–384.

91. Nirenberg, M. J., Vaughan, R. A., Uhl, G. R., Kuhar, M. J., and Pickel, V. M. The dopamine transporter is localized to dendritic and axonal plasma membranes of nigrostriatal dopaminergic neurons. *J. Neurosci.* **16** (1996) 436–447.

92. Nishio, H., Nezasa, K., and Nakata, Y. Role of calcium ion in platelet serotonin uptake regulation. *Eur. J. Pharmacol.* **288** (1995) 149–155.

93. Nishio, H. and Segawa, T. Effect of concanavalin A on 3H-5-hydroxytryptamine uptake in rabbit blood platelets: interaction with adenylate cyclase activity. *Jpn. J. Pharmacol.* **33** (1983) 79–84.

94. O'Neill, L. A. J. Towards an understanding of the signal transduction pathways for interleukin 1. *Biochim. Biophys. Acta* **1266** (1995) 31–44.

95. Owens, M. J. and Nemeroff, C. B. Role of serotonin in the pathophysiology of depression: focus on the serotonin transporter. *Clin. Chem.* **40** (1994) 288–295.

96. Pacholczyk, T., Blakely, R. D., and Amara, S. G. Expression cloning of a cocaine- and antidepressant-sensitive human noradrenaline transporter. *Nature* **350** (1991) 350–354.

97. Piñeyro, G., Blier, P., Dennis, T., and de Montigny, C. Desensitization of the neuronal 5HT carrier following long-term blockade. *J. Neurosci.* **14** (1994) 3036–3047.

98. Plenge, P., Mellerup, E. T., and Jorgensen, O. S. Lithium treatment regimens induce different changes in [^{3}H]paroxetine binding protein and other rat brain proteins. *Psychopharmacology* **106** (1992) 131–135.

99. Qian, Y., Melikian, H. E., Moore, K. R., Duke, B. J., and Blakely, R. D. Phosphorylation of serotonin transporter domains and ther role of phosphorylation in acute transporter regulation. *Soc. Neurosci. Abstr.* **21** (1995) 344.7.

100. Qian, Y., Melikian, H. E., Rye, D. B., Levey, A. I., and Blakely, R. D. Identification and characterization of antidepressant-sensitive serotonin transporter proteins using site-specific antibodies. *J. Neurosci.* **15** (1995) 1261–1274.

100a. Raisman, R., Briley, M. S., and Langer, S. Z. Specific tricyclic antidepressant binding sites in rat brain characterized by high-affinity 3-H imipramine binding. *Eur. J. Pharmacol.* **61** (1980) 373–380.

101. Ramamoorthy, J. D., Ramamoorthy, S., Papapetropoulos, A., Catravas, J. D., Leibach, F. H., and Ganapathy, V. Cyclic AMP-independent up-regulation of the human serotonin transporter by staurosporine in choriocarcinoma cells. *J. Biol. Chem.* **270** (1995) 17,189–17,195.

102. Ramamoorthy, S., Bauman, A. L., Moore, K. R., Han, H., Yang-Feng, T., Chang, A. S., Ganapathy, V., and Blakely, R. D. Antidepressant- and cocaine-sensitive human serotonin transporter: molecular cloning, expression, and chromosomal localization. *Proc. Natl. Acad. Sci. USA* **90** (1993) 2542–2546.

103. Ramamoorthy, S., Bradley, C. C., Bauman, A. L., Leibach, F. H., Ganapathy, V., and Blakely, R. D. Human serotonin transporter: molecular cloning, genomic organization, and mRNA regulation. *Soc. Neurosci. Abstr.* **19** (1993) 7.5.

104. Ramamoorthy, S., Cool, D. R., Mahesh, V. B., Leibach, F. H., Melikian, H., Blakely, R. D., and Ganapathy, V. Regulation of the human serotonin transporter: cholera toxin-induced stimulation of serotonin uptake in human placental choriocarcinoma cells is accompanied by increased serotonin transporter mRNA levels and serotonin transporter-specific ligand binding. *J. Biol. Chem.* **268** (1993) 21,626–21,631.

105. Ramamoorthy, S., Ramamoorthy, J. D., Prasad, P., Bhat, G. K., Mahesh, V. B., Leibach, F. H., and Ganapathy, V. Regulation of the human serotonin transporter by interleukin-1β. *Biochem. Biophys. Res. Comm.* **216** (1995) 560–567.

106. Riggs, D., Havill, A. M., Pitt, B. R., and Gillis, C. N. Pulmonary angiotensin-converting enzyme kinetics after acute lung injury in the rabbit. *J. Appl. Physiol.* **64** (1988) 2508–2516.

107. Rovescalli, A. C., Brunello, N., Riva, M., Galimberti, R., and Racagni, G. Effect of different photoperiod exposure on [^{3}H]imipramine binding and serotonin uptake in the rat brain. *J. Neurochem.* **52** (1989) 507–514.

108. Russo, A. F., Lanigan, T. M., and Sullivan, B. E. Neuronal properties of a thyroid C-cell line: Repression by dexamethasone and retinoic acid. *Mol. Endocrinol.* **6** (1992) 207–218.

109. Saito, N., Seno, K., Sakai, N., Murakami, N., and Honda, S. Modulation of serotonin transporter activity by interferon. *Soc. Neurosci. Abstr.* **21** (1995) 344.17.

110. Sakai, N., Morikawa, O., Ikegaki, N., Kobayashi, S., Fujimoto, M., and Saito, N. Cloning and characterization of the promoter region of the mouse serotonin transporter gene. *Soc. Neurosci. Abstr.* **21** (1995) 344.1.

111. Schroeter, S. and Blakely, R. D. Embryonic expression of biogenic amine transporters: studies on the cocaine and antidepressant-sensitive mouse serotonin transporter. *Cell. Mol. Mech. Drug Abuse: Cocaine, Ibogaines, Substituted Amphetamines* (1995) presented at the ISN Satellite meeting, Niigata, Japan, abstract 24.

112. Schroeter, S. and Blakely, R. D. Drug targets in the embryo: studies on the cocaine and antidepressant-sensitive serotonin transporter, *Ann. N. Y. Acad. Sci.* (1996), in press.

113. Shimada, S., Kitayama, S., Lin, C., Patel, A., Nanthakumar, E., Gregor, P., Kuhar, M., and Uhl, G. Cloning and expression of a cocaine-sensitive dopamine transporter complementary DNA. *Science* **254** (1991) 576–577.

114. Shuey, D. L., Sadler, T. W., and Lauder, J. M. Serotonin as a regulator of craniofacial morphogenesis: site specific malformations following exposure to serotonin uptake inhibitors. *Teratology* **46** (1992) 367–378.

115. Simpson, I. A. and Cushman, S. W. Hormonal regulation of mammalian glucose transport. *Ann. Rev. Biochem.* **55** (1986) 1059–1089.

116. Stoltz, J. F. Uptake and storage of serotonin by platelets. In Vanhoutte, P. M. (ed.), *Serotonin and the Cardiovascular System*, Raven, New York, 1985, pp. 37–42.

117. Tamir, H., Hsiung, S.-C., Liu, K.-P., Blakely, R. D., Russo, A. F., Nunez, E. A., and Gershon, M. D. Expression and development of a functional plasmalemmal 5-hydroxytryptamine transporter by thyroid follicular cells. *Endocrinology* (1996), in press.

118. Tecott, L., Shtrom, S., and Julius, D. Expression of a serotonin-gated ion channel in embryonic neural and nonneural tissues. *Mol. Cell. Neurosci.* **6** (1995) 43–55.

119. Usdin, T. B., Mezey, E., Chen, C., Brownstein, M. J., and Hoffman, B. J. Cloning of the cocaine-sensitive bovine dopamine transporter. *Proc. Natl. Acad. Sci. USA* **88** (1991) 11,168–11,171.

120. Van Hartesveldt, C., Moore, B., and Hartman, B. K. Transient midline raphe glial structure in the developing rat. *J. Comp. Neurol.* **253** (1986) 175–184.

121. Wade, P. R., Chen, J., Jaffe, B., Kassem, I. S., Blakely, R. D., and Gershon, M. D. Localization and function of a 5-HT transporter in crypt epithelia of the gastrointestinal tract. *J. Neurosci.* **16** (1996) 2352–2364.

122. Watanabe, K., Sakai, R. R., McEwen, B. S., and Mendelson, S. Stress and antidepressant effects on hippocampal and cortical 5HT1$_a$ and 5HT$_2$ receptors and transport sites for serotonin. *Brain Res.* **615** (1993) 87–94.

123. Whitaker-Azmitia, P. M., and Azmitia, E. C. Stimulation of astroglial serotonin receptors produces culture media which regulates growth of serotonergic neurons. *Brain Res.* **497** (1989) 80–85.

124. Whitaker-Azmitia, P. M., Murphy, R., and Azmitia, E. C. Stimulation of astroglial 5-HT$_{1A}$ receptors releases the serotonergic growth factor, protein S-100, and alters astroglial morphology. *Brain Res.* **528** (1990) 155–158.

125. White, L. A., Eaton, M. J., Castro, M. C., Klose, K. J., Globus, M. Y., Shaw, G., and Whittemore, S. R. Distinct regulatory pathways control neurofilament expression and neurotransmitter synthesis in immortalized serotonergic neurons. *J. Neurosci.* **14** (1994) 6744–6753.

126. Whitton, P. S., Sarna, G. S., O'Connell, M. T., and Curzon, G. The effect of the novel antidepressant tianeptine on the concentration of 5-hydroxytryptamine in rat hippocampal dialysates in vivo. *Neuropharmacology* **30** (1991) 1–4.

127. Wirz-Justice, A., Hackmann, E., and Lichtsteiner, M. The effect of oestradiol dipropionate and progesterone on monoamine uptake in rat brain. *J. Neurochem.* **22** (1974) 187–189.

128. Yavarone, M. S., Shuey, D. L., Sadler, T. W., and Lauder, J. M. Serotonin uptake in the ectoplacental cone and placenta of the mouse. *Placenta* **14** (1993) 149–161.

129. Yu, A., Yang, J., Pawlyk, A. C., and Tejani-Butt, S. Acute depletion of serotonin downregulates serotonin transporter mRNA in raphe neurons. *Brain Res.* **688** (1996) 209–212.

130. Zsilla, G., Barbaccia, M. L., Gandolf, O., Knoll, J., and Costa, E. (–)-Deprenyl, a selective MAO "B" inhibitor, increases [3H] imipramine binding and decreases beta-adrenergic receptor function. *Eur. J. Pharmacol.* **89** (1983) 111–117.

CHAPTER 3

Mechanisms of Biogenic Amine Neurotransmitter Transporters

Gary Rudnick

Introduction

The biogenic amine transporters, as described in Chapters 1, 4, 5, and 12 terminate the action of released biogenic amine neurotransmitters. These transporters utilize norepinephrine (NE), dopamine (DA), and serotonin (5-HT), and are referred to as NET, DAT, and SERT, respectively. Interruption of their function by agents, such as antidepressants and stimulants, causes profound changes in mood and behavior. In addition to their importance in regulating the extracellular concentration of neurotransmitters, these proteins are fascinating molecular machines that utilize the energy from transmembrane ion gradients to accumulate intracellular neurotransmitters. The pharmacology and molecular biology of these proteins is well covered in Chapters 1, 9, 11, and 12. This chapter focuses on the mechanism of neurotransmitter transport. Researchers are still far from completely understanding how these proteins work; however, recent advances give insight into the mechanism and encourage the hope that more understanding of the transport mechanism will issue from current and future research.

Na⁺, K⁺, and Cl⁻ ions Are Cofactors for Transport

Like many mammalian plasma membrane transport systems, the biogenic amine transporters require the presence of external Na^+ ions. This phenomenon was observed first for epithelial transporters, such as those for glucose and amino acids (10). The transport of NE into peripheral nerve endings was also found to be Na^+ dependent

Neurotransmitter Transporters: Structure, Function, and Regulation
Ed. M. E. A. Reith Humana Press Inc., Totowa, NJ

(24), as was 5-HT transport into platelets (68). When synaptosomes were established as an experimental system for studying presynaptic mechanisms, the Na^+ dependence of neurotransmitter uptake became firmly established, as each system in turn demonstrated its dependence on extracellular Na^+ (3,11,23,35,36,39). In all these cases, replacement of Na^+ with any other ion results in a loss of transport activity.

The importance of this Na^+ requirement became more apparent as the energetics of transport were studied. The Na^+ requirement provided a way to understand how the energy of adenosine triphosphate (ATP) hydrolysis drives transport. ATP is utilized by the Na^+ pump to move Na^+ ions out of, and K^+ into, the cell. By incorporating Na^+ into the transport reaction, the neurotransmitter transporters couple the energy released by ATP hydrolysis to the downhill Na^+ flux that accompanies transmitter accumulation (Fig. 1). Given that K^+ is pumped by the ATPase, it is not surprising that some neurotransmitter transporters also utilize internal K^+ in the transport process. The most notable are the 5-HT and glutamate transporters (29,60) and it is possible that other systems also take advantage of K^+ concentrated inside cells by the Na^+ pump. The requirement for internal K^+ can be fulfilled by H^+ in the case of the 5-HT transporter (30), but efforts to demonstrate this phenomenon with glutamate transporters resulted in the opposite conclusion, namely, that H^+ equivalents were moving with the flow of substrate rather than against it (46).

Another consequence of Na^+ pump action is related to the fact that three Na^+ ions are pumped out for each two K^+ ions pumped into the cell, leading to the generation of a transmembrane electrical potential. In itself, this potential can be used by neurotransmitter transporters, but more specifically, the potential leads to the loss of Cl^- ions from the cell. Many neurotransmitter transporters utilize this asymmetric Cl^- distribution. With the exception of glutamate transporters, all of the neurotransmitter transporters, and many related transporters, require Cl^- as well as Na^+ (37). It is a characteristic of the neurotransmitter transporter gene family that Cl^- is required for their activity; it is often referred to as the NaCl-coupled transporter family (26). The glutamate transporters represent a separate gene family.

Transport and Binding Requirements

One advantage to the study of biogenic amine transporters is that, unlike other members of the family, high-affinity ligands are available. Tricyclic antidepressants, such as imipramine and desipramine,

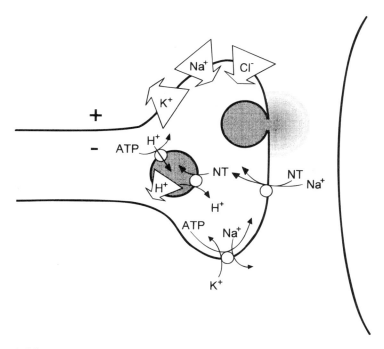

Fig. 1. Neurotransmitter recycling at the nerve terminal. Neurotransmitter (NT) is released from the nerve terminal by fusion of synaptic vesicles with the plasma membrane. After release, the transmitter is transported across the plasma membrane by a Na^+-dependent transporter in the plasma membrane. Transmitter delivered into the cytoplasm is further sequestered in synaptic vesicles by a vesicular transporter using the transmembrane H^+ gradient as a driving force. This driving force, shown by the arrow pointing in the direction of downhill H^+ movement, is generated by an ATP-dependent H^+ pump in the vesicle membrane. The Na^+ and K^+ gradients across the plasma membrane are generated by the Na^+/K^+-ATPase. This enzyme also creates a transmembrane electrical potential (negative inside) that causes Cl^- to redistribute. Neurotransmitter transport across the plasma membrane is coupled to the Na^+, Cl^-, and K^+ gradients generated by the ATPase. Reprinted with permission from Elsevier from ref. *58a*.

bind to SERT and NET and have been used to investigate the ion dependence of the binding process. SERT requires both Na^+ and Cl^- ions for maximal [³H]imipramine binding (*74*), although repeated attempts to demonstrate any effect of K^+ have been negative. Similar results have been obtained with [³H]desipramine and NET (*38*). Antidepressant binding differs from transport, however. The Na^+ dependence of [³H]imipramine binding to SERT and imipramine inhibition of transport were both sigmoidal, suggesting that two or more Na^+ ions participate in the reaction (73). In contrast, the Na^+ dependence of 5-HT transport and 5-HT inhibition of [³H]imipramine binding showed simple saturation behavior consistent with only one Na^+ ion being involved in 5-HT binding and transport (73). Similar results were obtained with NET. Transport is a simple saturable function of Na^+ (55), but [³H]desipramine binding shows a sigmoidal Na^+ dependence (38).

When binding of other ligands was examined, the difference between substrates and inhibitors became even more obvious. Paroxetine and the cocaine analogs 2β-carbomethoxy-3β-(4-fluorophenyl) tropane (CFT) and 2β-carbomethoxy-3β-(4-iodophenyl) tropane (β-CIT) bind to SERT and inhibit transport. This binding process was stimulated by Na^+ but not by Cl^- (8,22,61), despite the fact that Cl^- is required for transport. The DA transporter also binds cocaine and its analogs (57,77), and also demonstrated a different ion dependence for transport and β-CIT binding (77). For both SERT and DAT, β-CIT binding was stimulated by Na^+ but not by Cl^-, and β-CIT binding was inhibited at low pH for both transporters (77). In contrast, the binding of 5-HT or DA was stimulated by Cl^- and not affected by low pH (77). In at least one aspect, β-CIT binding paralleled substrate transport better than did imipramine binding. The Na^+ dependence of DA transport and β-CIT binding by DAT are both sigmoidal, suggesting the participation of two or more Na^+ ions, and β-CIT binding by SERT shares the same simple Na^+ dependence with 5-HT transport (77). From these and other studies, it is clear that inhibitor binding may be similar, in some aspects, to substrate binding. However, the two processes are distinct in their ionic dependence. Despite the differences, interactions between inhibitors and substrates at 5-HT, NE, and DA transporters is competitive, at least in equilibrium binding studies. Thus, a single binding site, or a set of overlapping binding sites, could account for substrate and inhibitor binding.

The sensitivity of β-CIT binding to displacement by substrate has allowed measurements of substrate binding under conditions in which direct substrate binding measurements are impossible. Using [¹²⁵I]β-CIT, 5-HT binding to SERT was measured in the absence of Na^+ and Cl^- and the individual effects of these ions were determined (22). Although Cl^- stimulated 5-HT binding by itself, Na^+ alone actually decreased 5-HT binding affinity. Maximal 5-HT affinity was observed only in the presence of both Na^+ and Cl^-, suggesting that 5-HT binds to the transporter together with these two ions (22).

Ion Gradients Drive Biogenic Amines Across the Membrane

Influence of Ion Gradients on 5-HT Transport

Studies with synaptosomes and platelets indicated that the biogenic amine transport systems possessed an impressive ability to concentrate DA, NE, and 5-HT. These preparations, however, contained intracellular amine storage organelles (synaptic vesicles or dense granules) that sequester most of the intracellular amine. The ability of the plasma membrane amine transporters to concentrate their substrates was not appreciated until platelet membrane vesicles were introduced. These vesicles accumulated internal 5-HT to concentrations hundreds of times higher than the external medium, when appropriate transmembrane ion gradients were imposed (58). The vesicle experiments demonstrated conclusively that the plasma membrane transporters generated gradients of their substrate amines using the energy of transmembrane Na^+, Cl^-, and K^+ ion gradients.

Na⁺

When a Na^+ concentration gradient (out > in) was imposed across the platelet plasma vesicle membrane in the absence of other driving forces, this gradient was sufficient to drive 5-HT accumulation (58). Coupling between Na^+ and 5-HT transport follows from the fact that Na^+ could drive transport only if its own gradient is dissipated. Thus, Na^+ influx must accompany 5-HT influx. Na^+-coupled 5-HT transport into membrane vesicles is insensitive to inhibitors of other Na^+ transport processes, such as ouabain and furosemide, supporting the hypothesis that Na^+ and 5-HT fluxes are coupled directly by the transporter (47,58). Many of these results have been reproduced in membrane vesicle systems from cultured rat basophilic leukemia cells (28), mouse brain synaptosomes (50), and human placenta (2).

Cl⁻

The argument that Cl^- is cotransported with 5-HT is somewhat less direct, since it has been difficult to demonstrate 5-HT accumulation with only the Cl^- gradient as a driving force. However, the transmembrane Cl^- gradient influences 5-HT accumulation when a Na^+ gradient provides the driving force. Thus, raising internal Cl^- decreases the Cl^- gradient, and inhibits 5-HT uptake. External Cl^- is required for 5-HT uptake, although Cl^- can be replaced by Br^-, to a lesser extent by SCN^-, NO_3^-, and NO_2^-, and not at all by SO_4^{2-}, PO_4^{3-}

and isethionate (*49*). In contrast, 5-HT efflux requires internal but not external Cl⁻ (*49*). The possibility that Cl⁻ stimulated transport by electrically compensating for electrogenic (charge-moving) 5-HT transport was ruled out by the observation that a valinomycin-mediated K^+ diffusion potential (interior negative) was unable to eliminate the external Cl⁻ requirement for 5-HT influx (*49*).

K^+

The ability of internal K^+ to stimulate 5-HT transport was not immediately obvious, for two reasons. First, there was no absolute requirement for K^+ in transport and, second, no Na^+ cotransport system had ever been shown to be coupled also to K^+. Initially, it was proposed that a membrane potential generated by K^+ diffusion was responsible for driving electrogenic 5-HT transport (*58*). Subsequent studies, however, showed that K^+ stimulated transport even if the membrane potential was close to zero (*48,60*). In the absence of a K^+ gradient, the addition of 30 mM K^+ simultaneously to both the internal and external medium increased the transport rate 2.5-fold (*48*). Moreover, hyperpolarization of the membrane by valinomycin in the presence of a K^+ gradient had little or no effect on transport. There were two conclusions from these results. First, the transport process was probably electrically silent. Second, since the K^+ gradient did not seem to act indirectly through the membrane potential, it was likely to act directly by exchanging with 5-HT.

The reason 5-HT transport still occurred in the absence of K^+ became apparent in a study of the pH dependence of 5-HT transport. In the absence of K^+, internal H^+ ions apparently fulfill the requirement for a countertransported cation (*30*). Even when no other driving forces were present (NaCl in = out, no K^+ present), a transmembrane pH difference (ΔpH, interior acid) could serve as the sole driving force for transport. ΔpH-driven 5-HT accumulation required Na^+ and was blocked by imipramine or by high K^+ (in = out), indicating that it was mediated by the 5-HT transporter, and was not a result of nonionic diffusion (*30*). From all of these data, it was concluded that inwardly directed Na^+ and Cl⁻ gradients, and outwardly directed K^+ or H^+ gradients, served as driving forces for 5-HT transport (Fig. 2).

Electrical Consequences

Although studies using platelet plasma membrane vesicles provided direct evidence that 5-HT transport was electrically silent (*48,60*), evidence relating the membrane potential to 5-HT transport has been

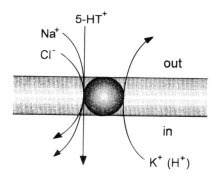

Fig. 2. Driving forces for 5-HT transport. Na^+ and Cl^- on the outside of the cell are transported inward with the cationic form of 5-HT. In the same catalytic cycle, K^+ is transported out from the cytoplasm. In the absence of internal K^+, H^+ ions take the place of K^+. The energy released by downhill movement of Na^+, Cl^-, and K^+ provides the driving force for 5-HT accumulation against its concentration gradient.

mixed in other systems. Kanner and Bendahan (*28*) found that 5-HT transport into plasma membrane vesicles from rat basophilic leukemia cells was stimulated by a K^+ diffusion potential. However, other workers studying plasma membrane vesicles from mouse brain and human placenta concluded that 5-HT transport in these tissues was not driven by a transmembrane electrical potential ($\Delta\psi$, interior negative) (*9,56*).

One might expect that electrogenicity could be easily tested if cells expressing the 5-HT transporter could be directly impaled with microelectrodes. This has been done by Mager et al. (*42*), using *Xenopus* oocytes injected with 5-HT transporter mRNA, with somewhat surprising results. A simple prediction is that current should not flow across the membrane during 5-HT transport if the transporter is electroneutral. In fact, a 5-HT-dependent current has been measured, but closer inspection of its properties suggests that it does not represent electrogenic 5-HT transport, but, rather, a conductance that is stimulated by transport. The key finding is that the transport-associated current is voltage dependent. Thus, the inward current increases as the inside of the cell is made more negative. In the same cells, however, [^{3}H]5-HT transport is independent of membrane potential. It is, therefore, very unlikely that the voltage-dependent current represents the 5-HT transport process. Instead, as will be discussed, the current results from a newly discovered ion channel property of neurotransmitter transporters.

5-HT and NE Transporters Use the Protonated Form of the Substrate

Since 5-HT, DA, and NE exist primarily in the protonated form at physiological pH, many workers have assumed that these substrates are transported as cations. However, a small fraction of these amines exist in the neutral or zwitterionic form at neutral pH, and it is important to assess the possibility that these forms are the true substrates for transport. In the case of the vesicular monoamine transporter (VMAT), the ionic form of the substrate is a matter of some controversy. Different investigators have reached opposite conclusions (33,34,66). If the neutral form is transported, one consequence might be that the K_m for transport will be pH dependent. As the pH increases, the mole fraction of biogenic amine in the neutral or zwitterionic form will increase sharply, but below pH 8–9, the majority of the substrate will be in the cationic form and the mole fraction of that form will not change significantly. The K_m for total substrate (cationic and neutral) will, therefore, appear to decrease if the neutral form is the substrate, but will be pH independent if the cationic form is transported. Results with the 5-HT and NE transporters (17,59) show no change in K_m with pH and suggest that the cationic form is the true substrate.

There is another consequence if the neutral or zwitterionic form is transported. The substrate would need to dissociate a H^+ ion before transport, and then would bind H^+ after transport. By imposing a ΔpH, the equilibrium amine distribution across the membrane could be influenced. In seeming agreement with this prediction, 5-HT accumulation by platelet plasma membrane vesicles is increased (in the absence of K^+) when the vesicle interior is acidified (30). However, this phenomenon represents the ability of H^+ to replace K^+ in 5-HT countertransport, and not an influence on 5-HT protonation. In the presence of K^+, ΔpH does not stimulate 5-HT uptake, although it should stimulate if the neutral form of 5-HT is the true substrate (30).

Overall 5-HT Stoichiometry

The number of Na^+, Cl^-, and K^+ ions transported with 5-HT transporter has been estimated by imposing known Na^+, Cl^-, and K^+ concentration gradients across the plasma membrane as a driving force, and measuring the 5-HT concentration gradient accumulated in response to that driving force at equilibrium. This is essentially a thermodynamic measurement balancing a known driving force against a measured gradient of substrate. Technically, such measurements require that the imposed ion gradients are relatively stable, so that the available driving force is known at a given time after imposition of the ion gradient.

Transport Kinetics Can Suggest, but Not Determine, Stoichiometry

Kinetic techniques also have been used to assess the Na^+, Cl^-, and K^+ stoichiometry for 5-HT, NE, and DA transport. One technique, which is technically simple, is to measure the dependence of transport rate (or its kinetic determinants K_m or V_{max}) on Na^+, Cl^-, or K^+ concentration, and to calculate a Hill coefficient for that ion. Using this analysis for the 5-HT and NE transporters yields $n = 1$ for both Na^+ and Cl^- in membrane vesicles *(14,21,54)*, where initial rates of transport showed a simple hyperbolic dependence on Na^+ or Cl^-; this is consistent with a Na^+:Cl^-:substrate stoichiometry of 1:1:1.

However, steady-state kinetics do not necessarily provide accurate information on cotransport stoichiometry. It is possible that more than one Na^+ ion is required for substrate binding or even translocation (as reflected in the Hill coefficient calculated from rate measurements), but that only one of those Na^+ ions is actually cotransported. It is also possible that a substrate is cotransported with two Na^+ ions, but that the affinities or rates of association of the two Na^+ ions are so disparate that the initial rate of transport is dependent on only the weaker binding or slower associating of the two, leading to an apparent Hill coefficient of 1. These difficulties are inherent in any kinetic method, whether transport is measured directly, by tracer flux, or indirectly, by measurements of electrical currents that may accompany transport. Similarly, the dependence of transport rate on the concentration of a given ion may suggest a transport stoichiometry, but cannot provide proof for it.

A still more direct method is to measure the flux of driving ions, as well as the flux of substrate. Usually, the basal levels of ion fluxes are too fast relative to the rates of substrate transport, but Kanner and coworkers *(31,32,53)* were able to measure Na^+ and Cl^- flux, along with GABA flux by the GABA transporter, in a purified, reconstituted system. In this case, when both thermodynamic and direct kinetic data exist, both methods indicate a Na^+:Cl^-:GABA stoichiometry of 2:1:1.

Thermodynamic Approach

Because kinetic approaches may be experimentally difficult or misleading, it is essential to confirm the stoichiometry by a thermodynamic measurement. In the thermodynamic method, known Na^+, Cl^-, or K^+ concentration gradients are imposed across the plasma membrane as a driving force, and the substrate concentration gradient in equilibrium with that driving force is measured. By varying the concentration gradient of the driving ion, and measuring the effect on substrate accumulation, the stoichiometry can be calculated. For a simple system where two solutes, A and B, are cotransported, a plot of $\ln(A_{in}/A_{out})$ vs $\ln(B_{out}/B_{in})$ gives the B:A stoichiometry as its slope. As a special case, if the stoichiometry is 1:1, then a plot of A_{in}/A_{out} vs B_{in}/B_{out} will be a straight line. Using this method, a 1:1 coupling was determined for 5-HT transport with both Na^+ (*73*) and K^+ (*58*). The Cl^- stoichiometry was deduced from the fact that 5-HT transport was not affected by imposition of a $\Delta\psi$ (interior negative), and was, therefore, likely to be electroneutral. Given that 5-HT is transported in its cationic form (*30,59*), only a $5\text{-}HT^+:Na^+:Cl^-:K^+$ stoichiometry of 1:1:1:1 is consistent with all the known facts. Obviously, this analysis requires an experimental system, like membrane vesicles, where the composition of both internal and external media can be controlled. In addition, this method relies on the ability to measure, or at least to estimate, an equilibrium substrate gradient under conditions when the ion gradients are known.

Each Transporter Has a Characteristic Coupling of Ion Flux to Substrate Flux

NET

Although no membrane vesicle systems containing DAT have been described, two plasma membrane vesicle systems have emerged for studying NET: the placental brush-border membrane (*54*) and cultured PC-12 cells (*19*). Harder and Bonisch (*19*) concluded that NE transport into PC12 vesicles was coupled to Na^+ and Cl^-, and was electrogenic, but they failed to arrive at a definitive coupling stoichiometry because of uncertainties about the role of K^+. According to their analysis, stimulation of NE influx by internal K^+ resulted either from direct K^+ countertransport, as occurs with SERT (*48*), or from a K^+ diffusion potential that drives electrogenic NE influx, as occurs with GAT-1 (*27*). Ramamoorthy and coworkers (*54*) studied NET-mediated transport of both NE and DA into placental membrane vesicles (DA is utilized by NET as a substrate [*18*]). They reached similar conclusions regarding ion coupling, but also were left with some ambiguity regarding K^+. In fact, the effects of ions on NET-mediated DA accumulation were similar to those observed with SERT-mediated 5-HT transport in the same membranes and the two activities were distinguished only by their inhibitor sensitivities (55). Part of the difficulty in interpreting and comparing these data stems from the fact that they were obtained in various cell types, with unknown, and potentially very different, conductances to K^+.

Two further problems made it difficult to interpret previous data on NET ion coupling. Both previous studies assumed that the cationic form of the catecholamine substrate was transported (19,54) and did not consider the possibility that the neutral or zwitterionic form was the true substrate. Moreover, previous studies estimated NET stoichiometry using kinetic, rather than thermodynamic, measurements. The number of Na^+ ions cotransported with each catecholamine substrate was estimated from the dependence of transport rate on Na^+ concentration (19,54).

The author and coworkers recently established LLC-PK$_1$ cell lines stably expressing the biogenic amine transporters SERT, NET, and DAT, as well as the GABA transporter GAT-1. Using these cell lines, we have characterized and compared the transporters under the same conditions and in the same cellular environment (18). One attractive advantage of LLC-PK$_1$ cells is that it has been possible to prepare plasma membrane vesicles that are suitable for transport studies (5). We took advantage of this property to prepare membrane vesicles containing transporters for GABA, 5-HT, and NE, all in the same LLC-PK$_1$ background. These vesicles should have identical composition, except for the heterologously expressed transporter. Moreover, these vesicles are suitable for estimating equilibrium substrate accumulation in response to imposed ion gradients. This property helped to define the ion coupling stoichiometry for NET using the known stoichiometries for GAT-1- and SERT-mediated transport as internal controls.

The results for SERT and GAT-1 are consistent with previously reported determinations of ion-coupling stoichiometry. For NET, accumulation of [^{3}H]DA (DA) was stimulated by imposition of Na^+ and Cl^- gradients (out > in) and by a K^+ gradient (in > out). To determine the role that each of these ions and gradients play in NET-mediated transport, the influence of each ion on transport was measured when that ion was absent, present at the same concentration internally and externally, or present asymmetrically across the membrane. The presence of Na^+ or Cl^-, even in the absence of a gradient, stimulated DA accumulation by NET, but K^+ had little or no effect in the absence of a K^+ gradient. Stimulation by a K^+ gradient was markedly enhanced by increasing the K^+ permeability with valinomycin, suggesting that net positive charge is transported together with DA. The cationic form of DA is likely to be the substrate for NET, since varying pH did not affect the K_m of DA for transport. The Na^+:DA stoichiometry was estimated by measuring the effect of internal Na^+ on peak accumulation of DA. Taken together, the results suggest that NET catalyzes cotransport of one cationic substrate molecule with one Na^+ ion, and one Cl^- ion, and that K^+ does not participate directly in the transport process (17).

DAT

DAT has a ion dependence different from that of SERT or NET. Although initial rates of DA transport were found to be dependent on a single Cl^-, two Na^+ ions were apparently involved in the transport process (18,45). Thus, the initial rate of DA transport into suspensions of rat striatum was a simple hyperbolic function of $[Cl^-]$, but depended on $[Na^+]$ in a sigmoidal fashion. These data are consistent with a Na^+:Cl^-:DA stoichiometry of 2:1:1. These differences in Na^+ stoichiometry have been reproduced with the cloned transporter cDNAs stably expressed in LLC-PK$_1$ cell lines, indicating that they are intrinsic properties of the transporters and not artifacts a result of the different cell types used (17). Although the precautions discussed earlier in this chapter prevent any firm conclusions about the ion coupling stoichiometry of DAT, the ion dependence differs from that of both SERT and NET, suggesting that each of these three biogenic amine transporters has a unique stoichiometry of coupling.

Amphetamines Are Substrates for Biogenic Amine Transporters

Amphetamine Action

Amphetamines represent a class of stimulants that increase extracellular levels of biogenic amines. Their mechanism differs from simple inhibitors like cocaine, although it also involves biogenic amine transporters. Amphetamine derivatives are apparently substrates for biogenic amine transporters, and lead to transmitter release by a process of transporter-mediated release from intracellular stores (13,62,72). Both catecholamine and 5-HT transporters are affected by amphetamines. In particular, compounds, such as p-chloroamphetamine (PCA) and 3,4-methylenedioxymethamphetamine (MDMA, also known as ecstasy), preferentially release 5-HT (52,69), and also cause degeneration of serotonergic nerve endings (44). Other amphetamine derivatives, such as methamphetamine, preferentially release catecholamines.

Actions at the Plasma Membrane Transporter

The process of exchange stimulated by amphetamines results from two properties of amphetamine and its derivatives. These compounds are substrates for biogenic amine transporters (62–64,67) and they also are highly permeant across lipid membranes (64,67,72). As substrates, they are taken up into cells expressing the transporters, and as permeant solutes, they rapidly diffuse out of the cell without requiring participation of the transporter. The result is that an amphetamine derivative will cycle between the cytoplasm and the cell exterior in a process that allows Na^+ and Cl^- to enter the cell, and in some cases K^+ to leave, each time the protonated amphetamine enters. Additionally, a H^+ ion will remain inside the cell if the amphetamine leaves as the more permeant neutral form (Fig. 3). This dissipation of ion gradients and internal acidification may possibly be related to the toxicity of amphetamines in vivo. The one-way utilization of the transporter (only for influx) leads to an increase in the availability of inward-facing transporter binding sites for efflux of cytoplasmic 5-HT, and, together with reduced ion gradients, results in net 5-HT efflux.

Actions at the Vesicular Membrane

In addition, the ability of amphetamine derivatives to act as weak base ionophores at the dense granule membrane leads to leakage of vesicular biogenic amines into the cytoplasm (64,72). Weakly basic amines are able to raise the internal pH of acidic organelles by dissociating into the neutral, permeant form, entering the organelle, and binding an internal H^+ ion. Weakly basic amines, such as ammonia and methylamine, have been used to raise the internal pH of chromaffin granules, for example (25). Although amphetamine derivatives are certainly capable of dissipating transmembrane ΔpH by this mechanism, they are much more potent than simple amines when tested in model systems. For example, PCA and MDMA are 5–10 times more potent than NH_4Cl in dissipating ΔpH in chromaffin granule membrane vesicles (62,64). This result suggests that not only are these compounds crossing the membrane in their neutral form, but also as protonated species. By cycling into the vesicle as an uncharged molecule and back out in the protonated form, an amphet-

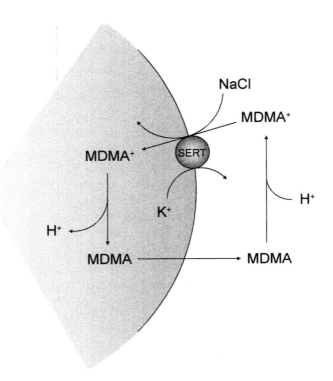

Fig. 3. Interaction of MDMA with the 5-HT transporter. MDMA is a substrate for SERT and, like 5-HT, is transported into cells together with Na^+ and Cl^-, and in exchange for K^+. Since it is membrane permeant in its neutral form, MDMA deprotonates intracellularly and leaves the cell, at which time it can reprotonate and serve again as a substrate for SERT. This futile transport cycle may lead to dissipation of cellular Na^+, Cl^-, and K^+ gradients and acidification of the cell interior.

amine derivative could act as a classical uncoupler to increase the membrane permeability to H^+ ions.

In addition to this uncoupling activity, amphetamine derivatives have affinity to the vesicular monoamine transporter, VMAT. Binding of various amphetamine derivatives to VMAT has been observed with both native and heterologously expressed VMAT (*51*). Despite the affinity of many amphetamines to VMAT, at least one compound, PCA, has no demonstrable binding to VMAT (*67*), despite its robust ability to release stored biogenic amines (*64*). Thus, the ability of amphetamines to dissipate vesicular pH differences is sufficient to explain their effects on vesicular release.

Sulzer et al. (*71*) extended this hypothesis by measuring the effects of intracellularly injected amphetamine and DA. Using the *Planorbis corneus* giant DA neuron, they demonstrated that amphetamine could act intracellularly to release DA from the cell. Moreover, injections of DA directly into the cytoplasm led to DA efflux that was sensitive to nomifensine, suggesting that it was mediated by the plasma membrane transporter. According to the hypothesis put forward by Sulzer et al. (*71*), amphetamine action at the vesicular membrane is sufficient to account for amphetamine-induced amine release. These results would also appear to explain the observation that blockade of plasma membrane transporters prevents the action of amphetamines (*1,13*).

The Amphetamine Permeability Paradox

If amphetamine derivatives act only by uncoupling at the level of biogenic amine storage vesicles, then classical uncouplers, such as 2,4-dinitrophenol, should act as psychostimulants like amphetamine. However, no such action has been reported for uncouplers or other weakly basic amines. Moreover, all of the amphetamine derivatives that were tested bind to plasma membrane amine transporters (*62–65,67,76*). What role could the plasma membrane transporters play in amphetamine action? One possibility is that they serve merely to let amphetamine derivatives into the cell. This would account for the specificity of various amphetamine derivatives. For example, the preferential ability of methamphetamine to release DA, while MDMA and fenfluramine release 5-HT, could result from their relative ability to be transported by SERT or DAT. However, it seems unlikely that amphetamines, which are so permeant that they act as uncouplers at the vesicle membrane, are unable to cross the plasma membrane without the aid of a transporter. If this is truly the role of the plasma membrane transporters in amphetamine action, it would seem that the vesicular and plasma membranes have vastly different permeabilities to amphetamines.

An alternative possibility, however, is that the ability of amphetamines to serve as substrates for plasma membrane transporters is important in their action, even if the membrane does not constitute a barrier to amphetamine diffusion. In this view, futile cycling of the plasma membrane transporter is induced by transporter-mediated influx followed by diffusion back out of the cell. As described, this process will lead to dissipation of Na^+, Cl^-, and, in some cases, K^+, gradients, and possibly also acidify the cell interior. As a result of the lower gradients and the appearance of cytoplasmic binding sites following amphetamine dissociation on the cell interior, biogenic amine efflux via the transporter will be stimulated. Clearly, the issues of amphetamine permeation across the plasma membrane and the specificity of amphetamine action need to be explored further.

The Mechanism of Translocation Involves Conformational Changes

Mechanisms for Ion Coupling

It is interesting to consider how the biogenic amine transporters, with predicted molecular weights of 60–80 kDa, are able to couple the fluxes of substrate, Na^+, Cl^-, and, in some cases, K^+, in a stoichiometric manner. The problem faced by a coupled transporter is more complicated than that faced by an ion channel, since a channel can function merely by allowing its substrate ions to flow across the lipid bilayer. Such uncoupled flux will dissipate the ion gradients and will not utilize them to concentrate another substrate. However, the structural similarities between transporters and ion channels may give a clue to the mechanism of transport (Fig. 4). Just as ion channels are thought to have a central aqueous cavity surrounded by amphipathic membrane-spanning helices, neurotransmitter transporters may have a central binding site that accommodates Na^+, Cl^-, and substrate. The difference in mechanism between a transporter and a channel may be that, though a channel assumes open (conducting) and closed (nonconducting) states, a transporter can also assume two states that differ only in the accessibility of the central binding site. In each of these states, the site is exposed to only one face of the membrane, and the act of substrate translocation represents a conformational change to the state in which the binding site is exposed on the opposite face (Fig. 4). Thus, the transporter may behave like a channel with a gate at each face of the membrane, but only one gate is usually open at any point in time.

For this mechanism to lead to cotransport of ions with substrate molecules, the transporter must obey a set of rules governing the conformational transition between its two states (Fig. 5). For cotransport of Na^+, Cl^-, and 5-HT, the rule would allow a conformational change when the binding site was occupied with Na^+, Cl^-, and substrate. To account for K^+ countertransport with 5-HT, the reverse conformational change to external-facing form would occur only when the binding site contained K^+. This simple model of a binding site exposed alternately to one side of the membrane or the other can

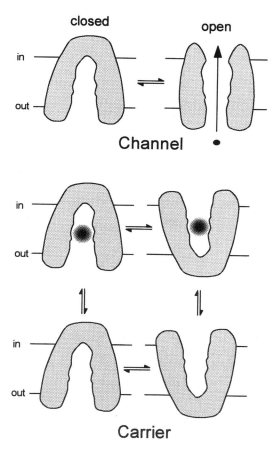

Fig. 4. Channels and carriers may have similar structures. A single structural model can account for transport by carriers and channels. In a channel (above), one or more gates, or permeability barriers, open to allow free passage for ions from one side of the membrane to the other. A carrier can be thought of as a channel with two gates. Normally only one is open at a time. By closing one gate and opening another, the carrier allows a solute molecule, bound between the two gates, to cross the membrane. Reprinted with permission from Elsevier from ref. *58a.*

explain most carrier-mediated transport. However, the model makes specific predictions about the behavior of the transport system.

In particular, this model requires that the substrate is transported in the same step as Na^+ and Cl^-, but in a different step than a countertransported ion, such as K^+. As described earlier in this chapter, there is ample evidence from studies measuring binding of 5-HT and

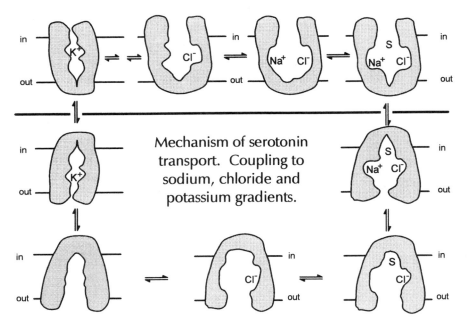

Fig. 5. Mechanism of 5-HT transport. Starting at the lower left and continuing counterclockwise, the transporter binds Cl⁻, 5-HT (S), and Na⁺. These binding events permit the carrier to undergo a conformational change to the form in the upper right hand corner. This internal-facing form dissociates Na⁺, Cl⁻, and 5-HT to the cytoplasm. On binding internal K⁺, another conformational change allows the carrier to dissociate K⁺ on the cell exterior, generating the original form of the transporter, which can initiate another round of transport by binding external Na⁺, Cl⁻, and 5-HT. Reprinted with permission from Elsevier from ref. *58a*.

inhibitors that Na⁺ and Cl⁻ bind to the transporter together with 5-HT (*22*). There is also evidence that 5-HT and K⁺ are transported in different steps. The exchange of internal and external 5-HT does not require the K⁺-dependent step that is rate-limiting for net 5-HT flux. The steps required for 5-HT binding, translocation, and dissociation, therefore, do not include the steps (where K⁺ is translocated) that become rate-limiting in the absence of K⁺ (*48*).

Structural Correlates of Conformational Changes

As detailed in Chapters 1 and 2, the biogenic amine transporters are composed of alternating hydrophobic and hydrophilic stretches of amino acid residues. The schematic mechanism of transport outlined in Fig. 5 ultimately needs to be reconciled with a structure that may contain 12 helical transmembrane segments connected by alternating extracellular and cytoplasmic loops. The conformational changes that are believed to convert substrate accessibility from extracellular to cytoplasmic and back again are triggered by binding events that presumably occur within the transmembrane segments of a transport protein. However, the conformational changes themselves may involve more than transmembrane domains. Recent experiments using a chimeric 5-HT transporter, in which a portion of the second putative extracellular loop was replaced with the corresponding sequence from the NE transporter, suggest that this loop may be involved in the conformational transitions required for 5-HT transport (*70*). Although this chimera is expressed on the surface of transfected cells at levels similar to wild-type SERT, the rate at which it transports 5-HT is 10% that of the wild type. The transport deficit is not because of defective binding of 5-HT, since the ability of 5-HT to displace β-CIT and the Na^+ dependence of binding are unchanged in the chimeric mutant. It is likely, therefore, that the chimeric transporter binds 5-HT, Na^+, and Cl^- normally, but cannot easily undergo the reorientation that exposes these bound solutes to the cytoplasmic surface of the plasma membrane. Experiments like these highlight the possibility that external loops may be more than simply passive links between helices, but, rather, may be active participants in the transport process.

Biogenic Amine Transporters Are Related to Pumps, Receptors, and Channels

What Is the Difference Between a Channel and a Carrier?

The proteins responsible for accumulating biogenic amines are commonly called transporters, but they are more precisely referred to as carriers. Carriers and pumps are proteins that move solutes across membranes by a mechanism that requires a conformational change for every molecule or ion transported. Although carriers can couple the transmembrane movement of more than one solute, they are distinguished from pumps by their lack of coupling to metabolic energy. Pumps are quite similar to carriers in mechanism, but in addition to moving solutes, pumps also mediate a chemical reaction, such as ATP hydrolysis, decarboxylation, or a redox or photochemical reaction that is coupled to the conformational changes in a way that utilizes the energy source to drive solute transport. Both carriers and pumps have the ability to use an energy source for solute accumulation, and this property sets them apart from channels, which only allow their substrate ion to flow down its electrochemical gradient.

The characteristic that most clearly distinguishes channels from carriers is the phenomenon of counterflow. In carrier-mediated transport, it is common for the influx of a substrate into a cell or vesicle to be insensitive to, or even stimulated by, substrate efflux from the same cell. The movement of substrate in one direction does not interfere with movement in the opposite direction. This happens because the step that translocates substrate into the cell is distinct from the step that translocates substrate out. In a channel, where the two processes of influx and efflux both require the same aqueous pathway through the open channel, it is inevitable that influx will inhibit efflux and vice versa. An analogous situation in everyday macroscopic life is the difference between a stairway and an elevator in a multi-story building. If many people are rushing down the stairs, it is more difficult to climb upward against the crowd. However, if the same crowd is using the elevator to descend, it is even more likely to find an elevator waiting on the ground floor than when nobody is going down.

In this simplistic discussion, the author has assumed that a given protein can be either a carrier or a channel, but recent evidence suggests that some proteins act like both. The 5-HT, NE, and GABA transporters all seem to mediate uncoupled ion fluxes in addition to their ability to catalyze substrate accumulation (6,15,16,42,43). These transporters may not be unique in possessing more than one activity. There are reports that cystic fibrosis membrane conductance regulator (CFTR) and P-glycoprotein of multidrug resistance (MDR) can operate as both channels and pumps (20). It is important to distinguish the two activities, however. The ability of a biogenic amine carrier to conduct ions as a channel represents a distinct activity of the protein. Though there may be conditions under which carrier and channel activity influence each other, uphill substrate accumulation cannot result from channel activity and rapid ion conductance is unlikely to be caused by carrier activity.

How Is a Carrier Like a Receptor?

The triggering of conformational changes by substrate binding is one of the key events postulated to result in coupling of solute fluxes. For example, SERT does not transport 5-HT in the absence of Na^+ or Cl^-, presumably because all three solutes must be bound together on the transporter to trigger the conformational change that exposes them to the other side of the membrane. This process is not unlike the one in which a surface receptor undergoes a conformational change in response to agonist binding. In a receptor, that conformational change could open an ion channel or stimulate nucleotide exchange or tyrosine kinase activity in an associated intracellular protein. In a carrier, the conformational change acts on the agonist (substrate) itself to change its accessibility from the internal and external faces of the membrane. From the perspective of evolution, carriers were much more important for primitive unicellular organisms (to ingest foodstuffs and excrete wastes) than were channels and receptors. It is tempting to speculate that the structure and function of carriers were adapted to carry out the activities of channels and receptors, as organisms developed the need for cell–cell communication.

Transporters Mediate Uncoupled Ionic Currents in Addition to Transport Currents

What Is the Relationship Between Uncoupled and Transport Current?

It has become apparent recently that in addition to the coupled flux of Na^+, Cl^-, and, in some cases, K^+, the 5-HT, GABA, and NE transporters also catalyze uncoupled ion flux (6,16,42). Recent evidence for each of these three transporters demonstrates the appearance of ion channel activity either by direct observation of single channels or by analysis of current noise (7,15,41). The uncoupled flux is likely, therefore, to represent events in which the transporter transiently operates like an ion channel instead of operating like a carrier. From the amount of current that flows with each channel event, and the frequency of channel events, it was possible to estimate that, for the 5-HT transporter, channels open very rarely relative to the number of times that a given transporter molecule goes through its catalytic cycle. These channel events are not an integral part of the transport process, but rather are analogous to a side reaction that occurs infrequently in an enzymatic reation. The uncoupled current, however, has important implications for the use of current recording techniques in transporter studies.

Studies that attempt to measure solute transport by recording the electrical current associated with transport can be confounded by the uncoupled ion flux. For example, even though 5-HT transport is electroneutral, addition of 5-HT to oocytes expressing SERT leads to an inward current (42). Measurements of substrate accumulation, as opposed to current, depend on imposed ion gradients and, in some cases, electrical potentials, but they are not likely to be influenced by uncoupled currents carried by the transporter. The total current will be the sum of any current associated with ion-coupled substrate transport plus the uncoupled current that flows through any channels that open during the time of the measurement. Since the uncoupled current is frequently stimulated by substrate binding or transport (7,15,41), it is difficult to estimate the proportion of the total current that is coupled or uncoupled. The danger of assuming that all transporter-mediated current represents substrate flux is illustrated by the case of the glutamate transporter. This transporter has an associated uncoupled anion channel that is stimulated by glutamate (12,75). Previous studies of glutamate-stimulated current unknowingly assumed that the anion current actually represented glutamate influx, and prematurely concluded that anion efflux was coupled stoichiometrically to glutamate influx (4).

What Do Electrogenic and Electroneutral Really Mean?

The recent demonstration that neurotransmitter transporters also mediate uncoupled ion flux (6,12,16,42), has cast a measure of confusion on the terms used to describe these proteins and their properties. If, as seems likely, these transporters transiently form conductive channels through the membrane, a distinction must be made between the types of electrical currents caused by channel activity and substrate transport. The term *electrogenic* has traditionally been used to describe a coupled transport process in which net charge crosses the membrane. In the absence of ion gradients, an electrogenic transporter should generate an electrical potential in response to an imposed transmembrane substrate gradient. In contrast, the channel activity of such a transporter can only mediate energetically downhill ion flux. Thus, though SERT and GAT-1 both conduct ions by virtue of their intermittant channel activity, GAT-1 is an electrogenic transporter because it transports net charge with GABA (27), and SERT is electroneutral because the 5-HT transport cycle itself does not move net charge across the membrane (60).

What Do Uncoupled Currents Tell Us?

Transporter-mediated currents fall into three categories. The first and simplest are transport currents themselves, which result from electrogenic movement of ions during the transport reaction. Second, the individual steps in the transport cycle also may be associated with charge movement that appears as a transient current when the transporter redistributes between two states. These transient currents have been very useful in demonstrating and characterizing electrogenic binding of Na^+ to the GABA transporter (40,42). The third category is the uncoupled currents that seem, at least in some cases, to be caused by a channel activity of a transporter that normally functions only as a carrier. If, as recent results suggest, these channel openings occur very rarely in relation to the normal transport cycle, one might question whether they can tell us anything at all about the transporters. Perhaps they are just an epiphenomenon that has nothing to do with normal transport or physiological function. It is too early to tell for sure, but there are reasons to believe that these uncoupled fluxes may allow insight into the transporters that would be difficult to obtain in any other way.

The most interesting issue is the relationship between the aqueous pore through which ions permeate during channel activity and the pathway that substrates take as they are transported across the membrane. The binding site for substrates is thought of as a potential channel through the core of the transporter, which is normally separated from one surface of the membrane or the other by permeability barriers (or gates). It is possible that if the barriers are both open, an aqueous channel through the membrane will be formed. If the ion channel does represent the substrate transport pathway, it will provide support for the concept that transport substrates bind in a channel closed at one end or the other by gates. To learn if the transport pathway and the ion channel are identical, it would be helpful to know if substrates are bound during the time that the transporter is acting like a channel. Substrate stimulates channel activity by 5-HT, NE, and glutamate transporters (12,15,40). On the surface, this result might suggest that the channel opens when substrate is bound, and that the transport pathway, occupied by bound substrate, could not function as the channel. An alternative explanation, however, is that the transport of substrate and its release to the cytoplasm leaves the transporter in a conformation with a higher probability of opening as a channel.

To distinguish between these possibilities, it must be known if the requirements for substrates to stimulate channel activity are at all different from those for transport. If conditions are found in which a substrate cannot be transported but does stimulate channel activity, it will suggest that substrate binding opens a separate channel as in a ligand-gated ion channel. Alternatively, if substrate binds within the ion channel, but dissociates from that site to leave the transporter in a state with a higher probability of opening for uncoupled ion flux, then substrate stimulation of channel activity would be observed only when substrate transport occurs.

Aside from the issue of the ion channel being the substrate site, there are other ways that channel activity may provide useful information about transporters. The properties of the channel, either its conductance, or opening or closing kinetics, might differ between states of the transporter. For example, the conductance of substrate-stimulated channels in a mutant 5-HT transporter is different from that of the channels observed in the absence of substrate (40). It may be possible to identify intermediates in the transport cycle with specific ion channel properties. These properties could then be used to analyze the presence of those intermediates under specific conditions or in mutant transporters. The true impact of channel activity by transporters will be likely to modify our understanding of transport mechanism as more of its details are explored.

References

1. Azzaro, A. J., Ziance, R. J., and Rutledge, C. O. The importance of neuronal uptake of amines for amphetamine-induced release of ^{3}H-norepinephrine from isolated brain tissue. *J. Pharmacol. Exp. Ther.* **189** (1974) 110–118.
2. Balkovetz, D. F., Tirruppathi, C., Leibach, F. H., Mahesh, V. B., and Ganapathy, V. Evidence for an imipramine-sensitive serotonin transporter in human placental brush-border membranes. *J. Biol. Chem.* **264** (1989) 2195–2198.
3. Bennett, J. P., Jr., Logan, W. J., and Snyder, S. H. Amino acid neurotransmitter candidates: sodium-dependent high-affinity uptake by unique synaptosomal fractions. *Science* **178** (1972) 997–999.
4. Bouvier, M., Szatkowski, M., Amato, A., and Attwell, D. The glial cell glutamate uptake carrier countertransports pH-changing anions. *Nature* **360** (1992) 471–474.
5. Brown, C. D., Bodmer, M., Biber, J., and Murer, H. Sodium-dependent phosphate transport by apical membrane vesicles from a cultured renal epithelial cell line (LLC-PK1). *Biochim. Biophys. Acta* **769** (1984) 471–478.
6. Cammack, J. N., Rakhilin, S. V., and Schwartz, E. A. A GABA transporter operates asymmetrically and with variable stoichiometry. *Neuron* **13** (1994) 949–960.
7. Cammack, J. N. and Schwartz, E. A. Channel behavior in a GABA transporter. *Proc. Natl. Acad. Sci. USA* **93** (1996) 723–727.
8. Cool, D. A., Leibach, F. H., and Ganapathy, V. High-affinity paroxetine binding to the human placental serotonin transporter. *Am. J. Physiol.* **259** (1990) C196–C204.
9. Cool, D. R., Leibach, F. H., and Ganapathy, V. Modulation of serotonin uptake kinetics by ions and ion gradients in human placental brush-border membrane vesicles. *Biochemistry* **29** (1990) 1818–1822.

10. Crane, R. K., Forstner, G., and Eichholz, A. Studies on the mechanism of the intestinal absorption of sugars. *Biochim. Biophys. Acta* **109** (1965) 467–477.

11. Curtis, D. and Johnston, G. Amino acid transmitters in the mammalian central nervous system. *Rev. Physiol. Biochem. Exp. Pharm.* **69** (1974) 97–188.

12. Fairman, W. A., Vandenberg, R. J., Arriza, J. L., Kavanaugh, M. P., and Amara, S. G. An excitatory amino-acid transporter with properties of a ligand-gated chloride channel. *Nature* **375** (1995) 599–603.

13. Fischer, J. F. and Cho, A. K. Chemical release of dopamine from striatal homogenates: evidence for an exchange diffusion model. *J. Pharm. Exp. Therap.* **208** (1979) 203–209.

14. Friedrich, U. and Bonisch, H. The neuronal noradrenaline transport system of PC-12 cells: kinetic analysis of the interaction between noradrenaline, Na^+ and Cl^- in transport. *Naunyn-Schmiedegergs Arch. Pharmacol.* **333** (1986) 246–252.

15. Galli, A., Blakely, R. D., and DeFelice, L. J. Norepinephrine transporters have channel modes of conduction. *Proc. Natl. Acad. Sci. USA* (1996) in press.

16. Galli, A., DeFelice, L. J., Duke, B. J., Moore, K. R., and Blakely, R. D. Sodium-dependent norepinephrine-induced currents in norepinephrine-transporter-transfected Hek-293 cells blocked By cocaine and antidepressants. *J. Exp. Biol.* **198** (1995) 2197–2212.

17. Gu, H. H., Wall, S. C., and Rudnick, G. Ion coupling stoichiometry for the norepinephrine transporter in membrane vesicles from stably transfected cells. *J. Biol. Chem.* **271** (1996), 6911–6916.

18. Gu, H. H., Wall, S. C., and Rudnick, G. Stable expression of biogenic amine transporters reveals differences in ion dependence and inhibitor sensitivity. *J. Biol. Chem.* **269** (1994) 7124–7130.

19. Harder, R. and Bonisch, H. Effects of monovalent ions on the transport of noradrenaline across the plasma membrane of neuronal cells (PC-12 cells), *J. Neurochem.* **45** (1985) 1154–1162.

20. Higgins, C. Volume-activated chloride currents associated with the multidrug resistance P-glycoprotein. *J. Physiol. (Lond.)* **482** (1995) 31S–36S.

21. Humphreys, C. J., Beidler, D., and Rudnick, G. Substrate and inhibitor binding and translocation by the platelet plasma membrane serotonin transporter. *Biochem. Soc. Trans.* **19** (1991) 95–98.

22. Humphreys, C. J., Wall, S. C., and Rudnick, G. Ligand binding to the serotonin transporter: equilibria, kinetics and ion dependence. *Biochemistry* **33** (1994) 9118–9125.

23. Iversen, L. L. Neuronal uptake processes for amines and amino acids. *Adv. Biochem. Psychopharmacol.* **2** (1970) 109–132.

24. Iversen, L. L. *The Uptake and Storage of Noradrenaline in Sympathetic Nerves.* Cambridge University Press, Cambridge, UK, 1967.

25. Johnson, R. G. and Scarpa, A. Protonmotive force and catecholamine transport in isolated chromaffin granules. *J. Biol. Chem.* **254** (1979) 3750–3760.

26. Jones, E. M. C. Na^+- and Cl^--dependent neurotransmitter transporters in bovine retina—identification and localization by *in situ* hybridization histochemistry. *Vis. Neurosci.* **12** (1995) 1135–1142.

27. Kanner, B. I. Active transport of γ-aminobutyric acid by membrane vesicles isolated from rat brain. *Biochemistry* **17** (1978) 1207–1211.

28. Kanner, B. I. and Bendahan, A. Transport of 5-hydroxytryptamine in membrane vesicles from rat basophillic leukemia cells. *Biochim. Biophys. Acta* **816** (1985) 403–410.

29. Kanner, B. I. and Sharon, I. Active transport of L-glutamate by membrane vesicles isolated from rat brain. *Biochemistry* **17** (1978) 3949–3953.

30. Keyes, S. R. and Rudnick, G. Coupling of transmembrane proton gradients to platelet serotonin transport. *J. Biol. Chem.* **257** (1982) 1172–1176.

31. Keynan, S. and Kanner, B. I. γ-aminobutyric acid transport in reconstituted preparations from rat brain: coupled sodium and chloride fluxes. *Biochemistry* **27** (1988) 12–17.

32. Keynan, S., Suh, Y. J., Kanner, B. I., and Rudnick, G. Expression of a cloned γ-aminobutyric acid transporter in mammalian cells. *Biochemistry* **31** (1992) 1974–1979.

33. Knoth, J., Isaacs, J., and Njus, D. Amine transport in chromaffin granule ghosts. pH dependence implies cationic form is translocated. *J. Biol. Chem.* **256** (1981) 6541–6543.

34. Kobold, G., Langer, R., and Burger, A. Does the carrier of chromaffin granules transport the protonated or the uncharged species of catecholamines? *Nauyn-Schmiedegergs Arch. Pharmacol.* **331** (1985) 209–219.

35. Krnjevic, K. Chemical nature of synaptic transmission in vertebrates. *Physiol. Rev.* **54** (1974) 418–540.

36. Kuhar, M. J. Neurotransmitter uptake: a tool in identifying neurotransmitter-specific pathways. *Life Sci.* **13** (1973) 1623–1634.

37. Kuhar, M. J. and Zarbin, M. A. Synaptosomal transport: a chloride dependence for choline, GABA, glycine and several other compounds. *J. Neurochem.* **31** (1978) 251–256.

38. Lee, C. M., Javitch, J. A., and Snyder, S. H. Characterization of [³H]desipramine binding associated with neuronal norepinephrine uptake sites in rat brain membranes. *J. Neurosci.* **2** (1982) 1515–1525.

39. Levi, G. and Raiteri, M. Synaptosomal transport processes. *Int. Rev. Neurobiol.* **19** (1976) 51–74.

40. Lin, F., Lester, H. A., and Mager, S. Single channel currents at the serotonin transporter reveal an amino acid in the permeation pathway. Submitted for publication (1996).

41. Lin, F., Lester, H. A., and Mager, S. Single channel studies of the serotonin transporter: (A) Different conducting states and (B) An amino acid in the permeation pathway. *Soc. Neurosci. Abstract* **21** (1995) 781.

42. Mager, S., Min, C., Henry, D. J., Chavkin, C., Hoffman, B. J., Davidson, N., and Lester, H. A. Conducting states of a mammalian serotonin transporter. *Neuron* **12** (1994) 845–859.

43. Mager, S., Naeve, J., Quick, M., Labarca, C., Davidson, N., and Lester, H. A. Steady states, charge movements, and rates for a cloned GABA transporter expressed in *Xenopus* oocytes. *Neuron* **10** (1993) 177–188.

44. Mamounas, L. A., Mullen, C., Ohearn, E., and Molliver, M. E. Dual serotoninergic projections to forebrain in the rat—morphologically distinct 5-HT axon terminals exhibit differential vulnerability to nerutotoxic amphetamine derivatives. *J. Comp. Neurol.* **314** (1991) 558–586.

45. McElvain, J. S. and Schenk, J. O. A multisubstrate mechanism of striatal dopamine uptake and its inhibition by cocaine. *Biochem. Pharmacol.* **43** (1992) 2189–2199.

46. Nelson, P. J., Dean, G. E., Aronson, P. S., and Rudnick, G. Hydrogen ion cotransport by the renal brush border glutamate transporter. *Biochemistry* **22** (1983) 5459–5463.

47. Nelson, P. J. and Rudnick, G. Anion-dependent sodium ion conductance of platelet plasma membranes. *Biochemistry* **20** (1981) 4246–4249.

48. Nelson, P. J. and Rudnick, G. Coupling between platelet 5-hydroxytryptamine and potassium transport. *J. Biol. Chem.* **254** (1979) 10,084–10,089.

49. Nelson, P. J. and Rudnick, G. The role of chloride ion in platelet serotonin transport. *J. Biol. Chem.* **257** (1982) 6151–6155.

50. O'Reilly, C. A. and Reith, M. E. A. Uptake of [^{3}H]serotonin into plasma membrane vesicles from mouse cortex. *J. Biol. Chem.* **263** (1988) 6115–6121.

51. Peter, D., Jimenez, J., Liu, Y. J., Kim, J., and Edwards, R. H. The chromaffin granule and synaptic vesicle amine transporters differ in substrate recognition and sensitivity to inhibitors. *J. Biol. Chem.* **269** (1994) 7231–7237.

52. Peyer, M. and Pletscher, A. Liberation of catecholamines and 5-hydroxytryptamine from human blood-platelets. *Naunyn Schmiedebergs Arch. Pharmacol.* **316** (1981) 81–86.

53. Radian, R. and Kanner, B. I. Stoichiometry of Na$^+$ and Cl$^-$ coupled GABA transport by synaptic plasma membrane vesicles isolated from rat brain. *Biochemistry* **22** (1983) 1236–1241.

54. Ramamoorthy, S., Leibach, F. H., Mahesh, V. B., and Ganapathy, V. Active transport of dopamine in human placental brush-border membrane vesicles. *Am. J. Physiol.* **262** (1992) C1189–C1196.

55. Ramamoorthy, S., Prasad, P., Kulanthaivel, P., Leibach, F. H., Blakely, R. D., and Ganapathy, V. Expression of a cocaine-sensitive norepinephrine transporter in the human placental syncytiotrophoblast. *Biochemistry* **32** (1993) 1346–1353.

56. Reith, M. E. A., Zimanyi, I., and O'Reilly, C. A. Role of ions and membrane potential in uptake of serotonin into plasma membrane vesicles from mouse brain. *Biochem. Pharmacol.* **38** (1989) 2091–2097.

57. Ritz, M. C., Lamb, R. J., Goldberg, S. R., and Kuhar, M. J. Cocaine receptors on dopamine transporters are related to self-administration of cocaine. *Science* **237** (1987) 1219–1223.

58. Rudnick, G. Active transport of 5-hydroxytryptamine by plasma membrane vesicles isolated from human blood platelets, *J. Biol. Chem.* **252** (1977) 2170–2174.

58a. Rudnick, G. and Clark, J. From synapse to vesicle: the reuptake and storage of biogenic amine neurotransmitters. *Biochim. Biophys. Acta* **1144** (1993) 249–263.

59. Rudnick, G., Kirk, K. L., Fishkes, H., and Schuldiner, S. Zwitterionic and anionic forms of a serotonin analog as transport substrates. *J. Biol. Chem.* **264** (1989) 14,865–14,868.

60. Rudnick, G. and Nelson, P. J. Platelet 5-hydroxytryptamine transport an electroneutral mechanism coupled to potassium. *Biochemistry* **17** (1978) 4739–4742.

61. Rudnick, G. and Wall, S. C. Binding of the cocaine analog 2-beta-[H-3] carbomethoxy-3-beta-[4-fluorophenyl]tropane to the serotonin transporter. *Mol. Pharm.* **40** (1991) 421–426.

62. Rudnick, G. and Wall, S. C. The molecular mechanism of ecstasy [3,4-methyl-enedioxymethamphetamine (MDMA)]—serotonin transporters are targets for MDMA-induced serotonin release. *Proc. Natl. Acad. Sci. USA* **89** (1992) 1817–1821.

63. Rudnick, G. and Wall, S. C. Non-neurotoxic amphetamine derivatives release serotonin through serotonin transporters. *Molecular Pharmacology* **43** (1993) 271–276.

64. Rudnick, G. and Wall, S. C. *p*-Chloroamphetamine induces serotonin release through serotonin transporters. *Biochemistry* **31** (1992) 6710–6718.

65. Rudnick, G. and Wall, S. C. The platelet plasma membrane serotonin transporter catalyzes exchange between neurotoxic amphetamines and serotonin. *Ann. NY Acad. Sci* **648** (1992) 345–347.

66. Scherman, D. and Henry, J.-P. pH Dependence of the ATP-dependent uptake of noradrenaline by bovine chromaffin granule ghosts. *Eur. J. Biochem.* **116** (1981) 535–539.

67. Schuldiner, S., Steiner-Mordoch, S., Yelin, R., Wall, S. C., and Rudnick, G. Amphetamine derivatives interact with both plasma membrane and secretory vesicle biogenic amine transporters. *Mol. Pharmacol.* **44** (1993) 1227–1231.

68. Sneddon, J. M. Sodium-dependent accumulation of 5-hydroxytryptamine by rat blood platelets. *Br. J. Pharmacol.* **37** (1969) 680–688.

69. Steele, T., Nichols, D., and Yim, G. Stereochemical effects of 3,4-methylene-dioxymethamphetamine (MDMA) and related amphetamine derivatives on inhibition of uptake of [^{3}H]monoamines into synaptosomes from different regions of rat brain. *Biochem. Pharmacol.* **36** (1987) 2297–2303.

70. Stephan, M. M., Chen, M. A., and Rudnick, G. An extracellular loop region of the serotonin transporter may be involved in the translocation mechanism. Submitted for publication (1996).

71. Sulzer, D., Chen, T. K., Lau, Y. Y., Kristensen, H., Rayport, S., and Ewing, A. Amphetamine redistributes dopamine from synaptic vesicles to the cytosol and promotes reverse transport. *J. Neurosci.* **15** (1995) 4102–4108.

72. Sulzer, D. and Rayport, S. Amphetamine and other psychostimulants reduce pH gradient in midbrain dopaminergic neurons and chromaffin granules: a mechanism of action. *Neuron* **5** (1990) 797–808.

73. Talvenheimo, J., Fishkes, H., Nelson, P. J., and Rudnick, G. The serotonin transporter-imipramine "receptor": different sodium requirements for imipramine binding and serotonin translocation. *J. Biol. Chem.* **258** (1983) 6115–6119.

74. Talvenheimo, J., Nelson, P. J., and Rudnick, G. Mechanism of imipramine inhibition of platelet 5-hydroxytryptamine transport. *J. Biol. Chem.* **254** (1979) 4631–4635.

75. Wadiche, J. I., Amara, S. G., and Kavanaugh, M. P. Ion fluxes associated with excitatory amino acid transport. *Neuron* **15** (1995) 721–728.

76. Wall, S. C., Gu, H. H., and Rudnick, G. Biogenic amine flux mediated by cloned transporters stably expressed in cultured cell lines: amphetamine specificity for inhibition and efflux. *Mol. Pharmacol.* **47** (1995) 544–550.

77. Wall, S. C., Innis, R. B., and Rudnick, G. Binding of the cocaine analog [^{125}]-2β-carbomethoxy-3β-(4-iodophenyl) tropane (β-CIT) to serotonin and dopamine transporters: different ionic requirements for substrate and β-CIT binding. *Mol. Pharmacol.* **43** (1993) 264–270.

CHAPTER 4

Cloned Sodium- (and Chloride-) Dependent High-Affinity Transporters for GABA, Glycine, Proline, Betaine, Taurine, and Creatine

Joshua W. Miller, Daniel T. Kleven,
Barbara A. Domin, and Robert T. Fremeau, Jr.

Introduction

For many decades it has been recognized that a variety of endogenous molecules are taken up by central nervous tissue through structurally specific, high-affinity, sodium-dependent, plasma membrane transport processes. Only recently, however, through the development of modern molecular cloning techniques, has it been realized that despite significant variability in the chemical and biochemical natures of these substances, there is remarkable similarity between the proteins and mechanisms responsible for their transport. High-affinity transport proteins have been cloned from brain and spinal cord tissue, not only for the biogenic amine neurotransmitters as described in Chapter 1, but also for the inhibitory neurotransmitters γ-aminobutyric acid (GABA) and glycine. In addition, transport proteins have been cloned for several other small mol-wt compounds, including proline, betaine, taurine, and creatine. Each of these transporters share strikingly common putative structural features consisting of approx 12 transmembrane α-helical domains, cytoplasmic amino and carboxyl termini, and a large glycosylated extracellular loop separating putative transmembrane domains 3 and 4 (Fig. 1). Moreover, these transporters share ≥40% primary sequence identity (Fig. 2), which establishes them as a distinct gene family.

Neurotransmitter Transporters: Structure, Function, and Regulation
Ed. M. E. A. Reith Humana Press Inc., Totowa, NJ

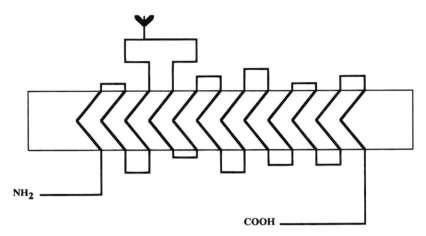

Fig. 1. Schematic model of the putative transmembrane topology of the Na$^+$-(and Cl$^-$-) dependent transporter(s). Common structural components include 12 transmembrane α-helical domains, cytoplasmic amino and carboxyl termini, and a glycosylated extracellular loop separating TMDs 3 and 4.

In this chapter, we discuss recent advances in our understanding of the molecular and pharmacological properties, localization, structure–function relationships, and physiological and clinical relevance of the cloned, nonbiogenic amine members of this transporter family. The primary goal of this review is to provide specific, up-to-date information about each transporter, with an emphasis on their known and/or potential roles in central nervous system (CNS) function. It will become clear, however, that the similarities and differences among these transporters provide a broader view of how nature has utilized an effective mechanism, Na$^+$- (and Cl$^-$-) dependent translocation, and adapted it for varied, yet specific functions with both common and wide-ranging pharmacological and physiological characteristics. These functions include, but are not limited to, the termination of neural signals. Consequently, these transporters are recognized as potential targets for therapeutic and pathological alterations of both neurological and non-neurological physiological functions.

GABA Transporters

The accumulation of exogenously administered GABA into mammalian brain tissue was first described over 30 yr ago (*32,147*). A decade later, Iversen and colleagues (*55,56,92*) provided detailed char-

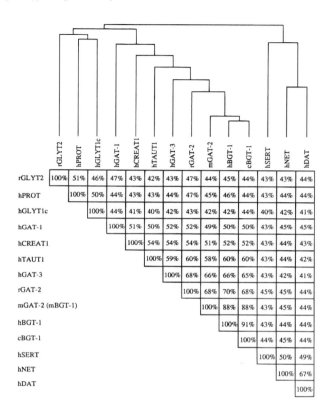

Fig. 2. Amino acid sequence relationships between various members of the Na$^+$- (and Cl$^-$-) dependent transporter gene family. The percent amino acid sequence identity between pairs of transporters is presented. The human homologs for each transporter are shown except in cases where no human sequence has been published. Canine BGT-1 and mouse GAT-2 are included for comparison to human BGT-1. As shown in the dendogram, three distinct subfamilies can be resolved based on amino acid sequence identities: the subfamily of amino acid (glycine and proline) transporters; the subfamily of GABA, betaine, taurine, and creatine transporters; and the subfamily of biogenic amine (serotonin, norepinephrine, and dopamine) transporters. rGLYT2, rat brain glycine transporter 2 (71); hPROT, human brain proline transporter (123); hGLYT1c, human brain glycine transporter 1c (62), hGAT-1, human brain GABA transporter 1 (94); hCREAT1, human brain creatine transporter 1 (129); hTAUT1, human brain taurine transporter 1 (57); hGAT-3, human brain GABA transporter 3 (9); rGAT-2, rat brain GABA transporter 2 (12); mGAT-2, mouse brain GABA transporter 2 (80); hBGT-1, human brain betaine/GABA transporter 1 (11); cBGT-1, canine kidney betaine/GABA transporter 1 (155); hSERT, human brain serotonin transporter (111); hNET, human brain norepinephrine transporter (102); hDAT, human brain dopamine transporter (42).

acteristics of this process: GABA uptake in rat cortical slices was found to be structurally specific, Na^+- and temperature-dependent, and saturable, with an experimentally determined K_m (22 μM) indicative of high-affinity transport. These studies provided convincing evidence that a plasma membrane transport protein existed in mammalian brain that was specific for GABA. Moreover, subsequent experiments indicated that there appeared to be two GABA transporter subtypes that were distinguished by their differential sensitivities to the GABA uptake inhibitors cis-1,3-aminocyclohexane carboxylic acid (ACHC) (14) and β-alanine (55). It was further suggested that these inhibitor sensitivities indicated localization of these transport proteins to specific cell types within the brain (i.e., the ACHC-sensitive subtype was thought to be expressed in neuronal cells, whereas the β-alanine-sensitive subtype was thought to be expressed in glial cells). Today, with the application of modern molecular characterization and localization techniques, we now know that this pharmacological classification of GABA transporter subtypes as "neuronal" and "glial" is insufficient. We also now recognize that there are at least four distinct high-affinity GABA transporter subtypes that exhibit distinct pharmacologies and unique temporal and spatial patterns of expression. They also are not exclusively expressed in the CNS.

Molecular and Pharmacological Characterization and Localization

The molecular and pharmacological characterization of GABA transport proteins began with the pioneering work of Kanner and colleagues (50,108) who first purified and cloned a high affinity GABA transporter from rat brain (GAT-1). On expression in *Xenopus* oocytes, GAT-1 was found to be highly selective for GABA with a K_m of 7 μM. An absolute dependence on extracellular Na^+ ions for transport was demonstrated, consistent with the findings in rat cortical slices. A dependence on extracellular Cl^- ions was also shown. In addition, GAT-1 was found to be strongly inhibited by the GABA uptake inhibitors ACHC, nipecotic acid, and 2,4-diaminobutyric acid (DABA), but only weakly inhibited by β-alanine and 4,5,6,7-tetrahydroisoxazolo[4,5-c]pyridin-3-ol (THPO). The authors then went on to show that the protein encoded by GAT- 1 crossreacted with an antiserum against the purified native rat brain GABA transporter and that immunoprecipitation produced a major product with a molecular weight similar to that of the GABA transporter core protein. Moreover, Northern blot analysis revealed that GAT-1 was localized throughout the brain, including the cerebrum, cerebellum, and brain stem, but was not found in liver. With these findings, GAT-1 became the first member of the Na^+- (and Cl^--) dependent transporter family to be cloned and characterized.

Shortly after this landmark effort, high-affinity GAT-1 transporters were cloned from human (94), mouse (74), and *Torpedo californica* (136) brains which exhibited 97, 99, and 84% sequence identity with rat GAT-1, respectively. Mouse GAT-1 (74) and *Torpedo* GAT-1 (136) were pharmacologically characterized and found to have substrate affinities, rates of transport, and inhibitor sensitivity profiles consistent with those observed for rat GAT-1, supporting their designations as GAT-1 transporters. Transporters with GAT-1 properties were also cloned from and/or localized to mouse (119) and rat (18) retinas, rat spinal motor neurons (128), and the *T. californica* electric lobe (136). These findings dispelled the notion that the GAT-1 transporter was exclusive to the brain. Furthermore, reports have indicated that GAT-1 transporters are localized to both pre- and postsynaptic neurons (128,135), as well as to glial cells (18,86,109,136). This latter finding dismissed the traditional distinction of the GAT-1 transporter as "neuronal" as was initially suggested by uptake inhibitor sensitivities and by immunolocalization (82).

In 1992, López-Corcuera et al. (80) isolated a novel high-affinity GABA transporter, GAT-2, that exhibited 49% identity with the GAT-1 GABA transporter. When expressed in *Xenopus* oocytes, mouse GAT-2 exhibited distinct pharmacological properties. It had an approx 10-fold lower affinity for GABA ($K_m = 79\ \mu M$) compared to GAT-1 ($K_m = 7\ \mu M$), and it exhibited different sensitivities to the GABA uptake inhibitors nipecotic acid and β-alanine; IC_{50} values for nipecotic acid were <100 μM and >1 mM for mouse GAT-1 and -2, respectively, whereas IC_{50} values for β-alanine were >2 mM and ~2 mM, respectively. Moreover, mouse GAT-2 was shown to be significantly inhibited by the osmolyte and methyl donor betaine. This finding was meaningful in that mouse GAT-2 was found to have 88% sequence identity with a transporter (BGT-1) that had recently been cloned from canine kidney cells and had been shown to transport both GABA and betaine with relatively high affinity (155). Human versions of BGT-1 also have been cloned from brain (11) and kidney (115), which exhibit 87 and 91% sequence identity with mouse GAT-2 and canine BGT-1, respectively. This has led to some discussion of the true identity and function of mouse GAT-2. Is it a product of the same gene as BGT-1? Is its biological function to transport GABA, or betaine, or both? These issues have not been definitively resolved and are discussed in more detail in the section on betaine transporters.

Around the same time, reports were made of two additional high-affinity GABA transporters that were themselves distinct from GAT-1 and mouse GAT-2, and that caused some confusion as to nomenclature. First, Clark et al. (*22*) described the cloning and expression of "GAT-B" from rat midbrain. GAT-B was found to have 50% sequence identity with rat GAT-1 and 63% identity with canine BGT-1. On transient expression into HeLa cells, GAT-B transported GABA with a K_m of 2.3 µM. The transport was strongly inhibited by β-alanine ($IC_{50} \sim 6.7$ µM) and nipecotic acid ($IC_{50} \sim 53$ µM), and mildly to weakly inhibited by DABA, THPO, taurine, and ACHC (IC_{50} values ranged from 100–800 µM). Northern analyses and *in situ* hybridization demonstrated that GAT-B was localized almost exclusively to nervous tissue and predominately to neurons. Thus, GAT-B could not be classified as "glial" as might be suggested by its sensitivity to β-alanine. Shortly thereafter, Borden et al. (*12*) isolated two cDNA high-affinity GABA transporter clones from rat brain. These were designated "GAT-2" and "GAT-3," and exhibited 52.5 and 52% sequence identity with rat GAT-1, and 68 and 65% identity with canine BGT-1, respectively. It was with these designations that the nomenclature became confused. The molecular and pharmacological profile for the rat GAT-2 isolated by Borden et al. (*12*) was significantly different from the mouse GAT-2 isolated by López-Corcuera et al. (*80*). After transient expression in COS cells, rat GAT-2 was found to have a significantly lower K_m for GABA (8 µM) than mouse GAT-2 (79 µM), and it was found to be sensitive to inhibition by β-alanine, but not betaine. Through Northern blot analysis and polymerase chain reaction (PCR) techniques, mRNAs for rat GAT-2 were localized to brain, retina, liver, and kidney. As for rat GAT-3, comparison of its amino acid sequence, pharmacological properties, inhibitor sensitivities, and tissue localization indicated that this transporter was the same as the GAT-B transporter isolated by Clark et al. (*22*).

In the meantime, Liu et al. (*72*) cloned two high-affinity GABA transporters from mouse brain that were designated "GAT-3" and "GAT-4," thus confounding the nomenclature further. However, a careful comparison of the amino acid sequences, pharmacological properties, inhibitor sensitivities, and tissue localization of these two mouse proteins reveals that mouse GAT-3 and rat GAT-2 are probable species homologs, as are mouse GAT-4 and rat GAT-3 (GAT-B). And more recently, Borden et al. (9) cloned a human GABA transporter with characteristics indicating that it is a species homolog of mouse GAT-4 and rat GAT-3 (GAT-B). For clarity, the mammalian GABA transporter clones described are summarized in Table 1. We have also included in this table a gentle suggestion for modification of the nomenclature. A comparison of the primary sequences of the GABA transporters, along with the sequences for the betaine, taurine, and creatine transporters described later in this chapter, is shown in Fig. 3.

Lastly, Mbungu et al. (85) reported the cloning of a high-affinity GABA transporter from *Manduca sexta* (moth) embryos (MasGAT). MasGAT has 50–58% sequence identity with the known mammalian GABA transporters, and pharmacologically most resembles the mammalian GAT-1 transporter, as determined after expression of MasGAT in *Xenopus* oocytes. However, MasGAT is apparently insensitive to ACHC, which distinguishes it from mammalian GAT-1. Therefore, MasGAT potentially represents a fifth GAT subtype.

Structure–Function Relationships

With the significant advances in molecular and pharmacological characterization and localization, researchers are now turning their attention toward identifying the structural components of high-affinity GABA transporters which are essential for function. Of interest are which amino acid residues are important for substrate specificity and affinity; substrate and ion translocation; transport inhibition; and protein synthesis, targeting, and conformation. The search for these functionally important structural components not only will provide significant insight into the mechanisms of GABA transport, but in many cases will provide information generalizable to the entire Na^+- (and Cl^--) dependent transporter family.

The substrates translocated by the GAT transporters—GABA, sodium, and chloride—are charged species. Consequently, charged and polar amino acids residing in GAT membrane-spanning domains were singled out as potentially important components involved in the recognition and/or translocation of these substrates (103). Precedent for this assumption came from work with cloned adrenergic receptors (131,150) and the cloned dopamine transporter (63) in which charged amino acids lying in hydrophobic domains were implicated in catecholamine binding and dopamine transport, respectively. With this insight, Pantanowitz et al. (103) identified five charged residues within the 12 membrane-spanning domains of the GAT-1 transporter and, using site-directed mutagenesis, determined

Table 1
Cloned Mammalian GABA Transporters

Original clone	Suggested name	Substrates, K_m	Inhibitors, (IC_{50})[a]	Refs.
Mouse GAT-1	mGAT-1	GABA (5.9 µM)	NIP (<100 µM) GUV (<100 µM) DABA (~500 µM)	74,80 72
Rat GAT-1	rGAT-1	GABA (7.3 µM)	NIP (~10 µM) GUV (~ 10 µM) ACHC (~100 µM) DABA (~100 µM)	12,50
Human GAT-1	hGAT-1	GABA (5 µM)	NIP (8 µM) GUV (14 µM)	9,94
Mouse GAT-2	mBGT-1	GABA (79 µM) Betaine[b]	Betaine (~200 µM)	72,80
Canine BGT-1	cBGT-1	GABA (93, 120 µM)[c] Betaine (398, 480 µM)[c]	nd	155
Human BGT-1	hBGT-1	GABA (18–36 µM) Betaine[b]	DABA (354 µM)	11,115
Mouse GAT-3	mGAT-2	GABA (18 µM) β-ALA (28 µM) Taurine (540 µM)	β-ALA (~10 –100) µM	72
Rat GAT-2	rGAT-2	GABA (5–8 µM)	β-ALA (19 µM) NIP (39 µM) GUV (58 µM) DABA (~100 µM)	9,12

Mouse GAT-4	GABA (0.65 μM) β-ALA (99 μM) Taurine (1.4 mM)	GUV (<100 μM) β-ALA (~10 –100 μM) NIP (~100 μM)	72
Rat GAT-B	GABA (2.3 μM)	β-ALA (~6.7 μM) GUV (~22 μM) NIP (~53 μM) DABA (~109 μM) Taurine (~459 μM)	22
Rat GAT-3	GABA (12 μM)	β-ALA (<100 μM)	12
Human GAT-3	GABA (7 μM)	β-ALA (58 μM) NIP (106 μM) GUV (119 μM)	9

[a]Includes selected inhibitors with experimentally determined IC$_{50}$ values ≤ 500 μM.
[b]Betaine transport is assumed, but never actually determined with radioactive substrate.
[c]K_m values for cBGT expressed in both *Xenopus* oocytes and MDCK cells, respectively.
Abbreviations: ACHC, cis-1,3-aminocyclohexane carboxylic acid; β-ALA, β-alanine; DABA, 2,4-diaminobutyric acid; nd, not determined; GUV, guvacine; NIP, nipecotic acid.

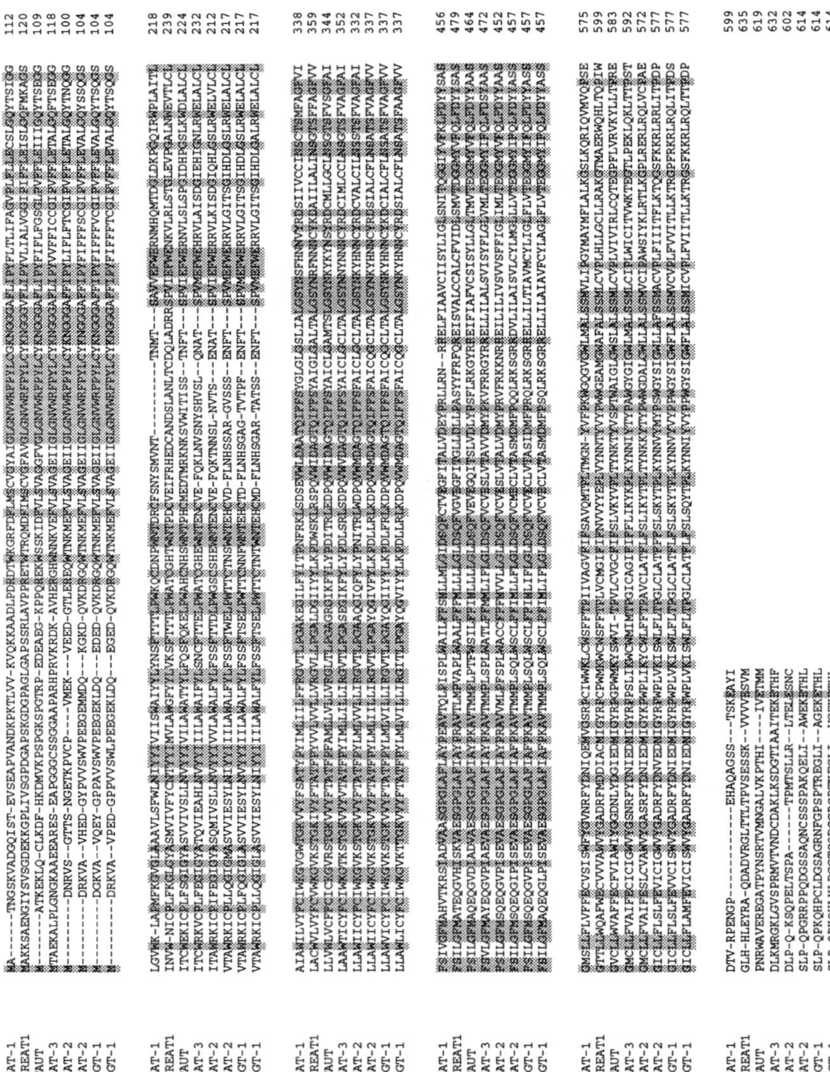

Fig. 3. Alignment of predicted amino acid sequences encoding the subfamily of GABA, betaine, taurine, and creatine Na⁺- (and Cl⁻) dependent transporter(s). Shaded residues represent those amino acids absolutely conserved for all members of the subfamily. For abbreviations, *see* Fig. 2.

that only one, an arginine located at position 69 in transmembrane domain 1 (TMD-1), was essential for transport. Interestingly, this arginine residue is completely conserved, not only within the GABA transporter subtypes, but also throughout the entire Na^+- (and Cl^--) dependent transporter family, including those transporters for the biogenic amines (dopamine, norepinephrine, serotonin). Because the biogenic amines do not contain a negatively charged carboxyl group such as that found in GABA, it is unlikely that this arginine residue plays a specific role in GABA transport, such as substrate recognition. More likely, it may participate in the binding of ions such as Cl^-, or some other function shared by all members of this transporter family.

Along the same lines, it was recognized that amino acids capable of electrostatic interactions with positive charges, such as aromatic tryptophan residues, could be candidates for the binding of Na^+ ions or of the amino group of GABA (64). Kleinberger-Doron and Kanner (64) identified 10 tryptophan residues located in the TMDs of GAT-1 and determined their roles in transport, again by site-directed mutagenesis. Three tryptophans, located at positions 68 (TMD-1), 222 (TMD-4), and 230 (TMD-4), were found to be essential for transport. Tryptophan 68, like arginine 69, is completely conserved throughout the Na^+- (and Cl^--) dependent transporter family, and therefore further emphasizes the importance of TMD-1 in the function of these proteins. Tryptophan 222 also is conserved throughout the transporter family, except in the biogenic amine transporters. This suggests that this residue is involved in the recognition of a motif (i.e., positively charged amino groups shared by GABA, amino acids and their analogs, but not by the biogenic amines). Contrasted with tryptophans 68 and 222, the effect of tryptophan 230 on transport was somewhat different; mutations at this position eliminated uptake by affecting the targeting of the transporter to the plasma membrane. Interestingly, this residue is conserved throughout the transporter family, except in the glycine and proline transporters described elsewhere in this chapter. Whether or not this residue affects the targeting of the rest of the transporter family remains to be determined.

As indicated by tryptophan 230, the subcellular expression of the GABA transporters (or any member of the Na^+- [and Cl^--] dependent transporter family), particularly within neurons, is of significant functional interest. To participate in the rapid termination of synaptic signaling, a transporter presumably must be localized at or near a nerve terminal with a relatively high local density. Little is known, however, about the mechanisms by which transporters are sorted to functionally relevant subcellular locales (i.e., neuronal and glial plasma membranes). The cloning of the Na^+- (and Cl^--) dependent transporters provides the opportunity to determine structural motifs within the proteins that are important for subcellular targeting, such as tryptophan 230.

Though not neuronal in origin, a good model for this purpose may be the Madin-Darby canine kidney (MDCK) cell line. It was from these cells that the BGT-1 transporter was initially cloned (*155*) (*see* section on betaine transporters). Under appropriate cell culture conditions, MDCK cells form a polarized bilayer consisting of basolateral and apical membranes. Pietrini et al. (*107*) observed that BGT-1 expressed in MDCK cells accumulated primarily at the basolateral membrane, supporting earlier work by Yamauchi et al. (*154*). Pietrini et al. (*107*) then found that on stable transfection in MDCK cells, GAT-1 accumulated primarily in the apical membrane. Thus, BGT-1 and GAT-1 were targeted to different subcellular locations within this cell type. Earlier studies were cited (*30,31*) suggesting that similar mechanisms were employed within epithelial cells and neurons for the sorting of proteins. Therefore, MDCK cells were concluded to be a potential model for the neuronal targeting of the GABA transporters.

This hypothesis was the basis of a more recent study by Ahn et al. (*3*) that looked at the expression of GAT transporters in MDCK cells and cultured hippocampal neurons. In MDCK cells, the GAT-2 transporter was found to localize to the basolateral membrane, like BGT-1, whereas GAT-3 was found to localize to the apical membrane, like GAT-1. Similar sorting phenomena were observed in hippocampal neurons microinjected with GABA transporter DNA; BGT-1 was found only in somatodendritic membranes, whereas GAT-3 was found in axons as well as cell bodies and dendrites. The subcellular distributions of GAT-1 and -2 within hippocampal neurons were not determined, but based on the MDCK data it was predicted that their expressions would follow those observed for BGT-1 and GAT-3, respectively. Since the GABA transporters share ≥50% sequence identity, it is probable that the differences in primary structure between these transporter subtypes determine the observed differential targeting.

Continued investigation into the roles of charged amino acid residues in GAT-1-mediated transport led to identification of a glutamate at position 101, located on the carboxyl terminal side of putative TMD-2. Keshet et al. (*60*) found that the conversion of glutamate 101 to an aspartate produced a transporter with only 1% of the activity of the wild type, whereas conversion of the residue to a glycine, alanine, or glutamine produced a transporter with no detectable activity at all. Glutamate 101 is conserved throughout the transporter family, and thus it was suggested that this residue was involved in the binding of Na$^+$ ions. However, more detailed analysis showed that increasing the extracellular concentrations of Na$^+$ and Cl$^-$ ions did not increase the percent transport observed for the aspartate 101 mutant. Keshet et al. (60) therefore speculated that glutamate 101 was somehow involved in the presumed conformational changes that occur during, and are essential for, a complete translocation cycle. A second, related possibility is that the mutations caused a significant change in the tertiary structure of the transporter. Either of these possibilities might result if the mutations resulted in the disruption of a structurally important salt bridge between the negatively charged glutamate 101 and a positively charged residue, such as a lysine, arginine, or histidine.

Using a different strategy, Tamura et al. (141) recognized that all the GABA transporter subtypes were sensitive to inhibition by β-alanine except GAT-1. It was suggested that this differential sensitivity to inhibition was caused by structural differences between GAT-1 and the other GAT subtypes in the substrate binding domain. Tamura et al. looked for amino acid sequences within the putative six external loops (1 – 6) of these transporters that were identical in each subtype except GAT-1. Then, by site-directed mutagenesis, they created GAT-1 mutants in which the identified amino acids were changed to the corresponding residues found in the other subtypes. Mutations in external loops 4 and 6 were found to affect substrate binding affinity, whereas changes in external loop 5 affected the sensitivity to β-alanine inhibition. It was concluded that the three external loops (4, 5, and 6) of GABA transporters formed a "pocket" that constituted the substrate binding domain for these proteins.

In experiments that addressed the importance of other domains of the GAT-1 transporter, Kanner and colleagues (6,83) focused on the cytoplasmic amino and carboxyl termini. Bendahan and Kanner (6) created deletion mutants of GAT-1 in which the amino and carboxyl termini had been removed. Despite these truncations, it was found on transient expression into HeLa cells that these mutants still retained GABA transport capability. Therefore, it was concluded that these regions of the transporter were unessential for transport.

A different aspect of Na$^+$- (and Cl$^-$-) dependent transporter structure–function relationships that has received some attention is the potential for dynamic regulation of uptake activity. The short-term up- or downregulation of transporter efficiency could be a significant mechanism for altering synaptic physiology in response to rapidly changing neural requirements. The process of protein phosphorylation may function in this capacity. Analysis of GAT protein primary sequences indicates that there are three putative cytoplasmic protein kinase C (PKC) phosphorylation sites. Several research groups have attempted to define the role of phosphorylation and second messenger systems in GABA transport by assessing the effects of phosphorylation activators and phosphatase inhibitors. Corey et al. (24) showed that activation of PKC by phorbol esters, and inhibition of phosphatase, increased GABA uptake by GAT-1 expressed in *Xenopus* oocytes. Interestingly, removal of the putative PKC sites in GAT-1 by site-directed mutagenesis had no effect on the regulation of transport by the phosphorylation modulators, suggesting that the their effects were occurring at a nonconsensus phosphorylation site or were not related to phosphorylation, at all. Corey et al. also showed that the phosphorylation modulators apparently affected transport by causing a redistribution of the GABA transporter from a cytoplasmic location to the plasma membrane. This was supported by kinetic analysis that showed that the primary effect was on the V_{max} of transport, rather than substrate affinity, consistent with an increase in the number of cell surface transporters. In addition, it was suggested that the modulation of transport may involve the conversion of the transporter between active and inactive conformations. Consistent with these findings is the study of Cupello et al. (27) that showed that the V_{max} of GABA uptake into rat brain synaptosomes is increased 58–74% by the PKC activators phorbol 12-myristate 13-acetate (PMA) and oleyl-acetyl glycerol (OAG).

Other studies, however, have obtained conflicting results. Activation of PKC by phorbol esters and diacylglycerol analogs was found to decrease GABA uptake into rat synaptosomes (*101*), GAT-1 transfected *Xenopus* oocytes (*101*), and rat cortex primary glial cultures (*43*). Kinetic analysis revealed the effect of the PKC activators in these systems was to increase the K_m value for GABA. Moreover, the phosphatase inhibitor okadaic acid was found to significantly decrease GABA uptake into rat synaptosomes (*143*). In this study, it was also shown that activation of cyclic adenosine monophosphate (AMP)-dependent protein kinase (PKA) inhibited synaptosomal GABA uptake. Finally, one study (*43*) showed that PKC activation had no effect on the uptake of GABA into rat embryo primary neuronal cultures. Taken together, these studies suggest that the regulation of high-affinity GABA transport by phosphorylation is a complex phenomenon that may be dependent on assay conditions, the choice of phosphorylation modulator, and both specific and nonspecific effects. In addition, the observed differences between these studies may represent differential regulation expressed by the four GAT subtypes. Further studies are needed to resolve these issues.

Two other aspects of GABA transporter structure–function relationships that have received attention are N-glycosylation and ion-dependence. Common to all the GAT protein subtypes are potential N-linked asparagine glycosylation sites in the putative extracellular loop that spans between TMD-3 and TMD-4. All of the subtypes and species homologs have three N-glycosylation sites within this extracellular region (9,12,22,50,72,94), except mouse GAT-2 (80), canine/human BGT-1 (11,115,155), and MasGAT (85), which have only two sites. MasGAT also has one potential N-glycosylation site located in the extracellular loop that spans between TMD-5 and TMD-6. The functional role of N-glycosylation has been preliminarily examined in GAT-1 by Keynan et al. (61). Incubation of GAT-1 expressing L- and Hela cells with tunicamycin, a specific inhibitor of N-glycosylation, caused a decrease in GABA transport that was dependent on the time of exposure to the inhibitor. How the inhibition of N-glycosylation affected transport was not determined, however. It was postulated that N-linked oligosaccharides could be involved in the processing, targeting, stability, and/or function of the transporter, but nonspecific effects of tunicamycin, such as inhibition of protein synthesis, could not be discounted. Evaluation of the role(s) of N-glycosylation for the other GAT subtypes has not been carried out.

All the GAT subtypes, like the rest of the Na^+- (and Cl^--) dependent neurotransmitter transporter family, have an absolute requirement for extracellular Na^+. Replacement of Na^+ in GABA transport assays with lithium, choline, potassium, or Tris leads to a >90% reduction in GABA uptake (12,22,25,46,50,80,85,108,115,119,136,155). The requirement for extracellular Cl^- is less specific, however, with significant uptake activity retained when Cl^- is replaced by certain anions. Interestingly, the capacity of these anions to substitute for Cl^- seems to be related to their ionic radii (46). Close to 100% GABA uptake is retained when Cl^- is replaced with bromide which has a relatively small ionic radius (46,80). Reduced, but detectable uptake is observed when Cl^- is replaced with nitrate, succinate, gluconate, glucuronate, fluoride, or iodide which have intermediate radii (12,22,25,46,50,80,85,115,136,155). No uptake is seen if Cl⁻ is replaced with sulfate which has a relatively large radius (*46*). This pattern is generally consistent among the GAT subtypes. However, an interesting difference between the subtypes has been found in regards to the anion acetate. Essentially no uptake of GABA has been observed in GAT-1 assays in which acetate has been substituted for Cl⁻ (*25,46,50,119*), whereas reduced, but significant activity has been observed for assays of rat GAT-2 and -3 (*12*). Moreover, 100% activity is retained by MasGAT (*85*). These observations suggest that differences in the amino acid sequences between these subtypes will account for these contrasting data and that these differences might be exploited to identify the putative Cl⁻ binding site in these proteins.

Much work remains to be done to tease out the structural components of GABA transporters that are essential for function. Ultimately, the three-dimensional orientation within the plasma membrane is the major goal. However, purification of these proteins to the extent required for X-ray crystallographic analysis of the three-dimensional structure is difficult and may not be accomplished soon. In the meantime, the continuing use of carefully focused site-directed mutagenesis should continue to provide important clues about structure–function relationships. So far, these efforts have mostly centered on the GAT-1 transporter. Expanding efforts to include the other GAT subtypes and species homologs should help determine the structural components responsible for their differences in substrate affinities and inhibitor sensitivities. This could prove to be clinically important in the design of drugs that are targeted to specific members of the GAT transporter subfamily, as discussed in the following section.

Clinical and Behavioral Correlates

GABA is the major inhibitory neurotransmitter in the mammalian CNS and decreased GABAergic neurotransmission has been implicated in the pathophysiology of several CNS disorders, in particular epilepsy (*65*). As a consequence, much research has centered on novel pharmacological approaches to increase GABAergic function. One potentially effective strategy has been the development of orally active inhibitors of GABA transport. Theoretically, such inhibitors would cross the blood–brain barrier and enhance GABAergic neurotransmission by increasing the time GABA remains in the synapse. Inhibitors such as nipecotic acid are not particularly lipid soluble, do not cross the blood–brain barrier, and consequently have very little effect in vivo. However, the addition of lipophilic side chains to the nitrogen atom of some of the known GABA transport inhibitors has resulted in the identification of several compounds that are active in vivo. These include: SK&F 89976-A (*10,70,138,149,156*), CI-966 (*10,110,146*), NNC-711 (*10,133*), and the most widely tested compound tiagabine (*4,10,16,37,47,96,106,134*), among others. Some or all of these drugs have been shown to act as anticonvulsants in laboratory animals (*4,16,106,133,134,138,156*), to increase extracellular levels of GABA in brain (*37,134,142,149*), and perhaps most interestingly to be highly specific for the GAT-1 transporter subtype (*10*). Tiagabine is currently in phase II/III clinical trials for the treatment of epilepsy in Europe and the United States (*47,134*) and has been found to be significantly effective in decreasing seizure frequency in a dose-dependent manner (*26,47,117,118,134*).

Recently, a novel GAT inhibitor, (S)-SNAP-5114, has been identified which apparently is highly specific for human GAT-3 (*9,21,29*). (S)-SNAP-5114 is a lipophilic compound which inhibits human GAT-3 with an IC_{50} of 5 μM. In contrast, IC_{50} values for rat GAT-2, human GAT-1, and human BGT-1 were 21 μM, >200 μM, and >100 μM, respectively. Presumably, though it apparently has not been determined, (S)-SNAP-5114 will inhibit the species homologs of human GAT-3 (mouse GAT-4 and rat GAT-3 [GAT-B]) with the same specificity as for human GAT-3. If so, this compound should be useful in determining the physiological roles of these homologous subtypes. Lipophilic inhibitors that are specific for the remaining two GAT subtypes (mouse GAT-3/rat GAT-2 and mouse GAT-2/canine, human BGT-1) remain to be synthesized and/or identified.

In addition to epilepsy, there is evidence for a role of GABA transporters in several clinically important conditions. First, there is data indicating that some anesthetics can inhibit the rate of uptake of GABA into striatal synaptosomes and that this effect may play a role in the mechanism of anesthesia for these agents (*84*). Second, postmortem analysis of schizophrenic brains has revealed a decreased number of GABA uptake sites in subcortical regions, suggesting that GABAergic mechanisms are abnormal in schizophrenia (*124*). Third, advanced liver disease can impair high-affinity GABA uptake into liver, thus increasing circulating GABA levels (*87*). This has been postulated as being responsible for hepatic encephalopathy and hypotension during advanced liver disease. Also, high circulating levels of GABA caused by GABA-synthesizing bacterial pathogens have been implicated in the decreased levels of consciousness observed during bacterial sepsis (*87*). Fourth, the rabies virus has been shown to increase GABA release and decrease GABA uptake in primary cortical neuronal cultures, thus suggesting an involvement of GABA in the neuropathological sequelae of rabies virus infection (*69*). Fifth, tiagabine has been shown to have analgesic (*122,134*) and anxiolytic effects (*94,134*) in rodents. This latter relationship may be indicative of the observed effects of a variety of stressors on GABA uptake in rodent brains (*1,34–36*). Rats exposed to novel environments and novel social interactions exhibit increased GABA uptake into hippocampal and/or cortical slices (*35,36*), whereas rats exposed to more negative stressors, such as cat odor (*35*), chronic noise and vibrations (*34*), or chronic cold stress (*1*), exhibit decreased GABA uptake into these and other brain regions. Last, the nonsteroidal anti-inflammatory drug indomethacin has been shown to be a noncompetitive inhibitor of mouse cortical synaptosomal GABA uptake (*152*). This has been postulated to be responsible for some CNS side effects of indomethacin, including the impairment of psychomotor functions.

Clearly, further study is required to elucidate the physiological relationships between GABA uptake and pathological conditions. Perhaps the most intriguing possibility is that the four GABA transporter subtypes may be differentially related to these conditions. This implies that pharmacological agents might be developed that target specific subtypes and consequently have highly specific primary effects and little or no side effects. The availability of cDNA clones for the GABA transporters should advance this research significantly.

Glycine Transporters

Prior to the molecular cloning of the first Na^+- (and Cl^--) dependent transporter, high-affinity, sodium-dependent uptake of glycine into mammalian central nervous tissue had been extensively studied by several research groups over three decades (*8,33,59,67,76,93,125,158*). Interestingly, the elucidation of the properties of glycine transport closely mirrored that of the GABA transporters. First, experimental evidence indicated the existence of more than one glycine transporter subtype with distinctive pharmacological properties (*59,76*). Second, a potent inhibitor of glycine uptake, sarcosine (*N*-methylglycine), was identified (*158*) which later proved to differentially affect the glycine transporter subtypes. Then, the isolation of molecular clones revealed that there were in fact four glycine transporter subtypes with distinct pharmacologies and unique temporal and spatial patterns of expression, as had been seen for the GABA transporters. In addition, glycine transporter subtypes were found to be expressed in both the CNS and peripheral tissues.

Molecular and Pharmacological Characterization and Localization

In 1992, Smith et al. (*126*) reported the first molecular cloning and characterization of a high-affinity glycine transporter. Low stringency screening of a rat brain cDNA library with probes derived from the rat GAT-1 transporter led to the isolation of complementary DNA which exhibited 45% sequence identity with rat GAT-1. Pharmacological analysis of this clone after transient expression in COS cells revealed that it specifically transported glycine with a K_m of 123 µM. Glycine transport in this system was dependent on both extracellular Na^+ and Cl^-. No other neurotransmitters or amino acids, including closely related alanine, were found to be transported. The screening of potential uptake blockers revealed that only glycine derivatives were potent inhibitors, with sarcosine being the most significant ($IC_{50} \sim 50$ µM). Sarcosine was not tested as a substrate.

A short time later, similar probing efforts led to the independent cloning and characterization of Na^+- and Cl^--dependent glycine transporters from mouse and rat brains by Liu et al. (*75*) and Guastella et al. (*49*), respectively. These transporters were expressed in *Xenopus* oocytes and found to have somewhat different kinetics than the transporter isolated by Smith et al. (*126*). Specifically, mean K_m values for these transporters were four- to fivefold lower than that described by Smith et al. (*126*) (20 and 33 µM for mouse and rat, respectively). The three transporters did, however, share similar sensitivities to sarcosine. Subsequent comparison of the primary sequences of these isoforms showed that they differed only in the amino terminus; the protein encoded by the Smith et al. transporter had an initial 15-residue sequence that was distinct from the initial 10-residue sequence found in the Liu et al. (*75*) and Guastella et al. (*49*) transporters (*49,62,75,126*) (Fig. 4A). Appropriately, the nomenclature for these transporters was later defined with those of Liu et al. (*75*) and Guastella et al. (*49*) assigned the name GLYT1a, and that of Smith et al. (*126*) assigned GLYT1b (*62*).

In 1994, Kim et al. (*62*) reported the cloning of a human version of GLYT1b, as well as a third subtype termed GLYT1c. These isoforms were found, after transient expression in COS cells, to transport glycine with K_m values of 72 and 90 µM, respectively. Sarcosine was found to inhibit GLYT1b, as had been shown for the rat version (*126*), but its effect on GLYT1c was not determined. Comparison of the primary sequences of the three isoforms again showed differences exclusive to the amino termini; GLYT1c had an initial 15-residue sequence that was equivalent to that of GLYT1b, but that was followed by a unique 54-residue sequence that was not found in the other two isoforms (Fig. 4). Beside these amino terminal differences, the three isoforms shared a high degree of sequence identity which suggested they were all products of the same genetic loci. This was supported by the efforts of Liu et al. (*71*) and Adams et al. (*2*) who determined that the gene encoding the GLYT1 transporters was subjected to alternate splicing and/or separate promoters which gave rise to the distinct isoforms. Kim et al. (*62*) localized the GLYT1 gene to human chromosome 1p31.3–p32 and mouse chromosome 4.

As the isoforms of GLYT1 were being cloned and characterized, a fourth Na^+- and Cl^--dependent high-affinity glycine transporter was isolated from rat brain (GLYT2) by Liu et al. (*71*). This subtype exhibited only 48% identity with mouse GLYT1a. On expression in *Xenopus* oocytes, GLYT2 was found to transport glycine with a K_m of 17 µM. Unlike the GLYT1 isoforms, GLYT2 was not sensitive to inhibition by sarcosine. Therefore, GLYT2 was considered to be pharmacologically discrete and to be a product of a distinct genetic loci. A comparison of the primary sequences of the glycine transporters, along with the sequence for the closely related proline transporter described in the next section, is shown in Fig. 4.

The four cloned GLYT subtypes not only feature differences in primary structure and pharmacological characteristics, but also exhibit differential expression patterns in various brain regions and peripheral tissues. This has been extensively studied using both Northern analyses and *in situ* hybridization. GLYT1a mRNA from the rat has been localized to various brain regions, as well as to pancreas, uterus, stomach, spleen, liver, and lung (*13*). However, rat GLYT1b and human GLYT1c have been found only in the brain and CNS (*13,62*). Interestingly, the use of probes designed to detect mRNA for all three GLYT1 subtypes has detected expression in mouse and/or human brain, kidney, pancreas, lung, placenta, liver, heart, and muscle (*2,62*). This is in contrast to the data from the rat where the heart and kidney show no mRNA for GLYT1a, -b, or -c (*13,62,126*). Whether this is the result of failure to detect signal in the rat, indication of yet another isoform, or differences between the species, is not known (*2*). GLYT2 has been found only in the brain and spinal cord of the rat (*71*). No other species have been examined for GLYT2 expression.

```
rGLYT2   MDCSAPKEMNKPPTNILEATVPGHRDSPRAPRTSPEQDLPAAAPAAAVQPPRVPRSASTGAQTFQSADARACEAQRPGVGFCKLSSPQAQATSAALRDLS   100
hPROT    M----------------KKLQG---A---------HL----R-----------------------------------------KPVT-----------    14
hGLYT1c  M----------------AAAHG----PVAPSSPEQVTLLPVQRSFFLPP------------FSGA-----------------TPSTSLAESVLKVWH    48

rGLYT2   EGHSAQANPPSGAAGAGNALHCKIPALRGPEEDENVSVAKGTLEHNNTPPVGWVNMSQSTVVLGTDGIASVLPGSVATTTIPEDEQGDENKARGNWSSKL   200
hPROT    -----------------------PDL--------------------------L----MTPSDQ-------GDVDLDV---DFAAH----RGNWTGKL    44
hGLYT1c  GAY------------NSGL---LPQL--------------------------MAQHSLAMAQN-------GAVPSEATKRDQNLK----RGNWGNQI    93

rGLYT2   DFILSMVGYAVGLGNVWRFPYLAFQNGGGAFLIPYLMMLALAGLPIFFLEVSLGQFASQGPVSVWKAIPALQGCGIAMLIISVLIAIYYNVIICYTLFYL   300
hPROT    DFLLSCIGYCVGLGNVWRFPYRAYTNGGGAFLVPYFLMLAICGIPLFFLELSLGQFSSLGPLAVWKISPLFKGAGAAMLLIVGLVAIYYNMIIAYVLFYL   144
hGLYT1c  EFVLTSVGYAVGLGNVWRFPYLCYRNGGGAFMFPYFIMLIFCGIPLFFMELSFGQFASQGCLGVWRISPMFKGVGYGMMVVSTYIGIYYNVVICIAFYYF   193

rGLYT2   FASFVSVLPWGSCNNPWNTPECKDKTKLLLDSCVIGDHPKIQIKNSTFCMTAYPNLTMVNFTSQANKTFVSGSEEYFKYFVLKI--SAGIEYPGEIRWPL   398
hPROT    FASLTSDLPWEHCGNWWNTERC-------LEHRVSKDGN--GA------LP----LN---LTCTV-----SPSEEYWSRYVLHIQGSQGIGRPGEIRWNL   217
hGLYT1c  FSSMTHVLPWAYCNNPWNTHDCAG----VLDASNLTNGSRPAA------LP--SNLSHL-LNHSLQRT--SPSEEYWRLYVLKL--SDDIGNFGEVRLPL   276

rGLYT2   PFCLFLAWVIVYASLAKGIKTSGKVVYFTATFPYVVLVILLIRGVTLPGAGAGIWYFITPKWEKLTDATVWKDAATQIFFSLSAAWGGLITLSSYNKFHN   498
hPROT    CLCLLLAWVIVFLCILKGVKSSGKVVYFTATFPYLILLMLLVRGVTLPGAWKGIQFYLTPQFHHLLSSKVWIEAALQIFYSLGVGFGGLLTFASYNTFHQ   317
hGLYT1c  LGCLGVSWLVVFLCLIRGVKSSGKVVYFTATFPYVVLTILFVRGVTLEGAFDGIMYYLTPQWDKILEAKVWGDAASQIFYSLACAWGGLITMASYNKFHN   376

rGLYT2   NCYRDTLIVTCTNSATSIFAGFVIFSVIGFMANERKVNIENVADQGPGIAFVVYPEALTRLPLSPFWAIIFFLMLLTLGLDTMFATIETIVTSISDEFPK   598
hPROT    NIYRDTFIVTLGNAITSILAGFAIFSVLGYMSQELGVPVDQVAKAGPGLAFVVYPQAMTMLPLSPFWSFLFFFMLLTLGLDSQFAFLETIVTAVTDEFPY   417
hGLYT1c  NCYRDSVIISITNCATSVYAGFVIFSILGFMANHLGVDVSRVADHGPGLAFVAYPEALTLLPISPLWSLLFFFMLILLGLGTQFCLLETLVTAIVDEVGN   476

rGLYT2   YLRTHKPVF-TLGCCICFFIMGFPMITQGGIYMFQLVDTYAASYALVIIAIFELVGISYVYGLQRFCEDIEMMIGFQPNIFWKVCWAFVTPTILTFILCF   697
hPROT    YLRPKKAVFSGL-ICVAMYLMGLILTTDGGMYWLVLLDDYSASFGLMVVVITTCLAVTRVYGIQRFCRDIHMMLGFKPGLYFRACWLFLSPATLLALLVY   516
hGLYT1c  EWILQKKTYVTLGVAVAGFLLGIPLTSQAGIYWLLLMDNYAASFSLVVISCIMCVAIMYIYGHRNYFQDIQMMLGFPPPLFFQICWRFVSPAIIFFILVF   576

rGLYT2   SFYQWEPMTYGSYRYPNWSMVLGWLMLACSVIWIPIMFVIKMYLAPG-RFIERLKLVCSPQPDWGPFLAQHRGERYKNMIDPL-GTSSLGL---------   786
hPROT    SIVKYQPSEYGSYRFPPWAELLGILMGLLSCLMIPAGMLVAVLREEG-SLWERLQQASRPAMDWGPSLEENRTGMYVATLAGSQSPKPLMVHMRKYGGIT   615
hGLYT1c  TVIQYQPITYNHYQYPGWAVAIGFLMALSSVLCIPLYAMFRLCRTDGDTLLQRLKNATKPSRDWGPALLEHRTGRYAPTIAPS-PEDGFEVQ-SLHPDKA   674

rGLYT2   ---KLPV---KDL--ELGTQC   799
hPROT    SFENTAIEVDREIAEEEESMM   636
hGLYT1c  ---QIPIVGSNGSSRLQDSRI   692
```

Fig. 4. Alignments of predicted amino acid sequences encoding the amino termini of the three isoforms of the GLYT1 transporter, and the subfamily of glycine and proline Na^+- (and Cl^--) dependent transporter. Shaded residues represent those amino acids absolutely conserved for all members of the subfamily. For abbreviations, *see* Fig. 2.

Within the CNS, transcripts arising from the GLYT1 gene have been shown to be expressed throughout the brain and in the spinal cord. The expression of GLYT1 mRNA and protein are highest in the caudal regions of the cerebellum, brain stem, and spinal cord, whereas more rostral areas show more variable expression (*13,157,159*). As for cellular localization, it has been suggested that GLYT1 is only expressed in glial cells (*2*), even though Borowsky et al. (*13*) described neuronal GLYT1 labeling using *in situ* hybridization. More recent data, however, lend more support for some neuronal expression. In particular, Zafra et al. (*157*) localized GLYT1 to amacrine neurons within the retina by immunocytochemistry using an antibody that would recognize all three GLYT1 subtypes. Nonetheless, taking into consideration all the available data, it can be concluded that GLYT1 expression is predominately glial. The expression of GLYT2 is more restricted. GLYT2 is found only in the pons medulla, cerebellum, and the spinal cord (*81,157,159*). Unlike GLYT1, GLYT2 appears to be expressed solely in neurons with the noted exception being Golgi cells of the granular cell layer in the cerebellum (*157*).

More detailed localization of the GLYT subtypes within the brain has suggested specific functional roles. The expression pattern of GLYT2 within the hindbrain and spinal cord has been found to overlap [^{3}H]strychnine binding sites, colocalizing GLYT2 with strychnine-sensitive glycine receptors (*81*). Furthermore, high levels of GLYT2 protein have been detected in putative glycinergic nerve terminals (*157*). This strongly suggests that GLYT2 functions to terminate glycinergic neurotransmission. In contrast, it has been suggested that GLYT1 is involved in both glycinergic and N-methyl-D-aspartate (NMDA) receptor-mediated glutamatergic pathways. Glycine has been shown to be a coagonist at NMDA receptors (*58*) and GLYT1 expression has been observed within areas not associated with glycinergic pathways (*13,71,75,81,126,157,159*). However, a precise overlap with glutamatergic pathways does not exist (*13,71,75,81,126,157,159*). Moreover, high levels of GLYT1 have been detected in glial cells surrounding putative glycinergic synapses (*157*). It may be that a specific isoform of GLYT1 is associated with NMDA receptor-expressing pathways whereas other variants are associated with glycinergic pathways.

The developmental expression patterns of GLYT1 and GLYT2 are also distinct. Both variant types have been shown to be expressed in prenatal embryos. GLYT1 mRNA in the mouse has been seen early in development with a peak at embryonic stages E13 to E15 (*2*). In the rat, maximal GLYT1 mRNA levels have not been observed until postnatal d 14–21, with protein levels lagging slightly behind (*159*). GLYT2 expression patterns are significantly different, but have only been examined in the rat (*159*). Peak GLYT2 mRNA expression has been observed early in postnatal life, but then decreases after 21 d. The protein levels peak similarly, but do not show a substantial decrease after postnatal d 21.

Structure–Function Relationships

A limited number of structure–function studies have been reported for the glycine transporters. The studies have centered around the physical properties of the purified transporter, regulation of transport by PKC, and analysis of the role of *N*-glycosylation.

Like for GAT-1, the importance of the amino and carboxyl termini of GLYT1b in glycine transport has been assessed through site-directed mutagenesis. Olivares et al. (*99*) transiently expressed amino and carboxyl terminal rat GLYT1b deletion mutants in COS cells. They found that most of the amino terminus and a significant portion of the carboxyl terminus are not required for transport. However, more extensive deletions in the carboxyl terminus yielded inactive transport owing to improper protein targeting to the plasma membrane, indicating the importance of this domain in GLYT1b function. It may be postulated that this finding is generalizable to the other two GLYT1 isoforms based on their high degree of primary sequence identity. This remains to be determined.

Two studies on the effect of PKC modulators, one by Sato et al. (*120*) and the other by Gomeza et al. (*44*), showed that activation of PKC inhibits transport of glycine by GLYT1. Sato et al. used PMA to activate PKC in HEK 293 cells expressing mouse GLYT1b. The cells treated with PMA exhibited a 60% reduction in [^{3}H]-glycine uptake. The effect of PMA was on the rate of translocation and not affinity, as reflected by a significant decrease in V_{max}, but no change in K_m. In addition, PKC inhibitors were found to block the effect of PMA on uptake. Sato et al. also identified four consensus intracellular PKC phosphorylation sites and mutated them individually and together through site-directed mutagenesis. It was assumed that this would abolish direct phosphorylation of the transporter by PKC. PMA treatment of HEK 293 cells expressing these mutants continued to show reduced uptake indicating that PKC activation was actually occurring at a cryptic nonconsensus phosphorylation site or was unrelated to phosphorylation entirely. (PMA might have affected protein synthesis, processing, targeting, or stability.) Consistent with these findings is the work of Gomeza et al. (44) using glioblastoma cells. Glycine uptake in these cells is inhibited by sarcosine, indicating that they naturally express the GLYT1 transporter, but not the GLYT2 subtype (158). Activation of PKC by the phorbol ester 12-O-tetrade-canoylphorbol 13-acetate (TPA) caused a reduction in glycine uptake similar to that seen in the studies by Sato et al. (120).

GLYT1 cDNA encodes for seven potential N-linked glycosylation sites, with four of these sites presumed to be extracellular. These four sites are present in the large extracellular domain between TMDs 3 and 4. To establish the functional role of these N-glycosylation sites, Aragón and colleagues (79,98,100) determined the effects of deglyco-sylation on transporter function using glycosidase treatments and site-directed mutagenesis. Deglycosylation assays on a purified glycine transporter confirmed the presence of N-linked carbohydrates while not revealing any O-linked carbohydrate modifications (98). Reconsti-tution of the purified protein in liposomes followed by treatment with deglycosylating enzymes led to reduced uptake with only 25% the activity of the fully glycosylated transporter (98). Treatment of GLYT1 expressed in COS cells with the N-glycosylation inhibitor tunicamycin produced a protein of 46-kDa (100). Site-directed mutagenesis of the four putative extracellular asparagine glycosylation sites also reduced the GLYT1 protein to a 46-kDa mobility (100). Successively higher mobilities were observed for mutations of 3, 2, 1, and 0 asparagines, respectively, indicating the presence of as many as four N-linked sug-ars in the native protein (100). Immunofluorescence studies of the GLYT1 mutant lacking all four glycosylation sites showed abnormal targeting to the plasma membrane, thus establishing the importance of N-linked sugars to the proper subcellular sorting of this transporter (80). Because all Na^+- (and Cl^--) dependent transporters contain poten-tial glycosylation sites in the same extracellular region, the importance of N-glycosylation on protein targeting and sorting may apply to the entire transporter family.

Remarkably little work has been done utilizing site-directed muta-genesis to identify specific amino acid residues and domains within the glycine transporters that are essential for substrate affinity and translocation, and for sarcosine inhibition. Because it is such a simple, nonpolar amino acid, narrowing the field of residues that potentially can interact with glycine during substrate binding and/or transloca-tion may be proving to be difficult. One initial strategy that is sure to be exploited is the construction of chimeric mutants. Such chimeras between the GLYT1 and GLYT2 subtypes may lead to the residues involved in the inhibition of GLYT1 by sarcosine. In addition, the high-affinity proline transporter (PROT) is closely related to GLYT1 (*see* Proline Transporter section). GLYT1 does not transport proline and PROT does not transport glycine, but both transporters are significantly inhibited by sarcosine. Chimeras made from these transporters may therefore lead to the identification of the residues involved in substrate binding and/or translocation, and sarcosine inhibition for both GLYT1 and PROT.

Potential Physiological and Pathophysiological Roles

In the CNS, glycine has a variety of functions. First, like GABA, glycine is a major inhibitory neurotransmitter, particularly in the brain stem and spinal cord. Second, as stated, glycine also serves as a co-agonist for NMDA receptors indicating an additional role in glutamatergic neurotransmission. Third, glycine is an important intermediate in one-carbon metabolism by virtue of its biochemical interconversion with serine. Finally, glycine serves as an amino acid component of proteins. Taken together, these functions imply that it is important to regulate extracellular glycine concentrations for effective neural signaling and biochemical synthesis. This is the putative function of the glycine transporters. However, how the regulation of extracellular glycine levels by the GLYT subtypes affects physiological and pathophysiological conditions remains to be determined.

Glycinergic and NMDA-mediated glutamatergic neural pathways are known to be involved in the control and regulation of motor functions, arousal states, and cognitive processes such as memory storage. Presumably, disruption of glycine transport would affect one or more of these processes. Support for this supposition may come from the genetic mouse neurological disorder *clasper*. This abnormality has been mapped to mouse chromosome 4 (*62,137*), very near the loci of the GLYT1 gene (*62*). Moreover, the phenotype of the *clasper* mouse is very similar to that of a second mouse strain that has the genetic neurological disorder *spastic* (*62,151*). Although the molecular basis of the *clasper* mouse has apparently not been elucidated, the *spastic* mouse has been shown to exhibit significantly reduced numbers of strychnine-positive glycine receptors (*62,151*), thus implicating an abnormality in glycinergic neurotransmission. It remains to be determined if the *clasper* and/or *spastic* mice have abnormalities in high-affinity glycine transport.

The development of in vivo-acting GLYT-specific inhibitors, perhaps related to sarcosine, may help delineate the importance of high-affinity glycine transport. Such inhibitors may also prove to be significant as anticonvulsants and antispastics. High-affinity glycine transport may be important in certain human genetic disorders, such as nonketotic hyperglycinemia and sarcosinemia, both of which present with CNS pathology. Peripheral localization suggests a non-neural function for some GLYT subtypes.

L-Proline Transporter

It has been known for more than 20 yr that mammalian brain synaptosomes express high-affinity, Na^+-dependent L-proline uptake which exhibits properties similar to the synaptosomal uptake activities identified for the amino acid neurotransmitters GABA, glycine, and L-glutamate (7,105). This has suggested that L-proline may serve a synaptic function in the mammalian CNS (reviewed in ref. 38). However, identification of a role for L-proline in neurotransmission has been hampered by the inability to associate this imino acid with specific nerve pathways, its complex excitatory and/or inhibitory actions on neurons in different brain regions (reviewed in ref. 54), and the lack of specific inhibitors that block its biosynthesis or high-affinity transport in nervous tissue. With the cloning of the mammalian high-affinity L-proline transporter, an important tool for addressing these issues has been isolated. Initial efforts have led to several observations that have brought us significantly closer to identifying the putative function of proline in neurotransmission. These include the exclusive localization of the proline transporter to a subset of glutamate neurons and the identification of the enkephalins and their des-tyrosyl derivatives as competitive inhibitors of high-affinity proline uptake.

Molecular and Pharmacological Characterization and Localization

We isolated human (123) and rat (38) brain cDNA clones that code for a novel high-affinity, Na^+- (and Cl^--) dependent L-proline transporter (PROT). Mammalian brain PROT was found to exhibit significant amino acid sequence identity (42–50%) with the rest of the gene family of Na^+- (and Cl^--) dependent plasma membrane transport proteins (Fig. 2), and was found to be most closely related to the glycine transporters (~50% amino acid sequence identity with the three isoforms of human GLYT1 and rat GLYT2) (Fig. 4). The substrate specificity, pharmacological properties, kinetics, and inorganic ion requirements of L-proline uptake in PROT-transfected HeLa cells clearly distinguished PROT from the other mammalian Na^+-dependent plasma membrane carriers that transport L-proline including the intestinal brush border "imino" carrier (130) and the system "A" and system "ASC" neutral amino acid carriers (20). In transiently transfected HeLa cells, PROT transported L-proline with a K_m of ~5–10 µM (38,123), which is within the range of values observed for L-proline uptake by rat hippocampal synaptosomes (40,89). In contrast, the system "A," system "ASC," and intestinal imino carriers transport L-proline with low apparent affinity (K_m values exceeding 230 µM) (20,130). Interestingly, mammalian brain PROT exhibited a narrow range of substrate specificity with striking selectivity for L-proline (38,123). In contrast, the system "A," and system "ASC" neutral amino acid carriers transport a wide range of neutral (dipolar) amino acids in addition to L-proline (reviewed in ref. 20). Furthermore, sarcosine (N-methylglycine) was found to compete with high apparent affinity for PROT-induced L-proline uptake (K_i ~24 µM) (38,123) but was found to only weakly inhibit L-proline transport by the rabbit jejunum brush border imino carrier (K_m ~8700 µM) (130).

Multiple tissue Northern blot analysis revealed brain-specific expression of PROT mRNA in human (123) and rat (148) tissues (Fig. 5). A ~4.0 kb hPROT mRNA transcript was heterogeneously distributed in different regions of human brain, but was not detected in human heart, placenta, lung, liver, kidney, skeletal muscle, or pancreas. Similarly, a 68-kDa hPROT immunoreactive protein was detected in crude synaptosomal membranes from various regions of human brain, but not in membranes prepared from human liver, kidney, or heart (123). This apparent brain-specific expression of PROT is interesting because other members of the Na$^+$- (and Cl$^-$-) dependent transporter family do not show this degree of brain specificity. For example, multiple mRNAs for the human serotonin transporter have been detected in human placenta and lung in addition to serotonergic neurons in human brain (5,111). Similarly, as described in this chapter, mRNAs for GABA, glycine, betaine, taurine, and creatine transporters are all variously expressed in mammalian peripheral tissues, in addition to brain. The brain-specific expression and transport properties of PROT indicate that this novel transporter may serve an important and unique physiological role in the mammalian brain.

Although little is known about the putative physiological roles of high-affinity L-proline uptake in nervous tissue, several lines of evidence support the hypothesis that such uptake modulates excitatory synaptic transmission in specific glutamatergic nerve terminals. First, *in situ* hybridization of rat brain sections and cultured neurons

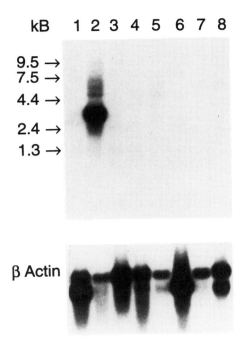

Fig. 5. Brain-specific localization of mRNA for the mammalian high-affinity L-proline transporter (PROT) *(123)*. Data represent an autoradiograph (4 d) of hybridization of a rat PROT cDNA probe to a rat multiple tissue Northern blot (Clontech, Palo Alto, CA). The blot contained poly(A)⁺ RNA (2 µg/lane) from the following rat tissues: heart (lane 1), brain (lane 2), spleen (lane 3), lung (lane 4), liver (lane 5), skeletal muscle (lane 6), kidney (lane 7), and testis (lane 8). Reproduced with permission from ref. *148*.

revealed that PROT mRNA is localized to specific subpopulations of glutamatergic neurons (Fig. 6), *(38,148)*. Second, functional autoradiography studies localized high-affinity L-proline uptake to a subset of hippocampal glutamate pathways *(90)*. Specifically, terminal fields of the Schaffer collateral, commissural, and ipsilateral associational fibers in areas CA1, CA3, and the lateral perforant path, and associational-commissural projections in the dentate molecular layer exhibit prominent high-affinity L-proline uptake. In contrast, the medial perforant path and mossy fiber pathway, which also use L-glutamate as their excitatory transmitter, exhibit little, or no high affinity L-proline uptake. Third, we have recently obtained direct ultrastructural evidence that the PROT protein is localized to certain glutamatergic nerve terminals in mammalian brain *(39)*. We used an affinity-purified antibody directed against a unique peptide sequence in the carboxy-terminus of PROT (*148*) for the light and electron microscopic immunolocalization of the PROT protein in rat brain. Intense immunoperoxidase staining was localized in punctate, varicose processes in the neuropil of brain regions that receive dense glutamatergic innervation including the olfactory bulb, piriform cortex, hippocampal formation, amygdala, and caudate-putamen (*39*). In the hippocampal formation, a laminar immunolabeling pattern was observed that corresponded quite well with the expected distribution based on the *in situ* hybridization and functional autoradiography studies. Electron microscopic ultrastructural studies revealed that the punctate labeling observed at the light level corresponded to the specific labeling of a subset of presynaptic axon terminals forming asymmetric "excitatory-type" synapses with postsynaptic dendritic spines in the stratum oriens of the CA1 region of the hippocampus, caudate nucleus, and somatosensory cortex. The differential expression of PROT in specific subpopulations of glutamatergic nerve terminals provides molecular and anatomic evidence supporting the functional heterogeneity of the presynaptic component of individual glutamatergic synapses. Fourth, L-proline appears to enhance excitatory synaptic transmission at one synapse where PROT is localized to the corresponding presynaptic excitatory nerve terminals: the Schaffer collateral-commissural synapse in hippocampal area CA1 (*39*). Proline-induced potentiation (PIP) of excitatory transmission at this synapse is long-lasting, requires the activation of NMDA receptors, and is separable from electrically evoked long-term potentiation (LTP). Future studies will examine whether high affinity L-proline uptake modulates PIP at these synapses.

Definitive studies of the physiological role(s) of high-affinity L-proline uptake in nervous tissue have been precluded by the lack of specific uptake inhibitors. We recently identified a potent and selective peptide inhibitor of mammalian brain PROT (*40*) by extending the earlier work of Rhoads et al. (*116*). Leu- and met-enkephalin, and their des-tyrosyl derivatives, potently and selectively inhibited high-affinity L-proline uptake in HeLa cells transfected with the recombinant PROT cDNA. High concentrations (100 μM) of the opiate receptor antagonists, naloxone and naltrexone, could not reverse this inhibitory action of the enkephalins. Furthermore, the opiate receptor-inactive peptide fragment, des-tyrosyl-leu-enkephalin (GGFL), was the most potent inhibitor of the recombinant transporter (IC$_{50}$ ~0.26 μM). Therefore, opioid receptors do not mediate this inhibitory action of the enkephalins.

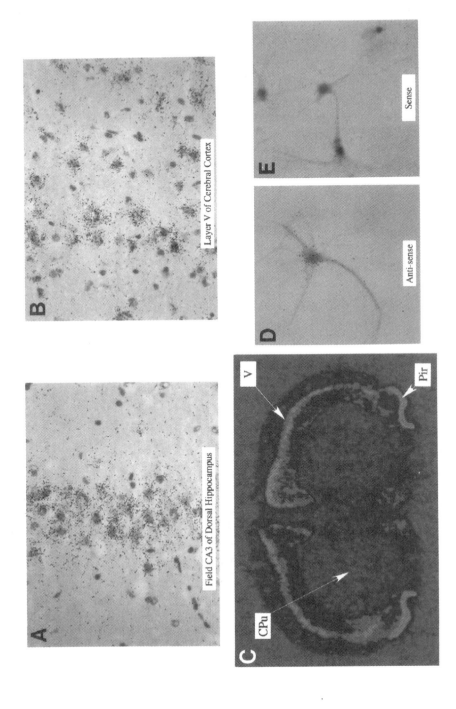

B Layer V of Cerebral Cortex

A Field CA3 of Dorsal Hippocampus

C CPu V Pir

D Anti-sense

E Sense

GGFL elevated the apparent K_m of L-proline transport in PROT-transfected HeLa cells without altering the V_{max}. In contrast, GGFL did not inhibit the transport activities of several structurally related transporters expressed in HeLa cells, ruling out nonspecific inhibitory actions of the enkephalins. Finally, GGFL selectively inhibited the high-affinity component of L-proline uptake in rat hippocampal synaptosomes (IC$_{50}$ ~0.34 mM). These results indicate that enkephalins competitively inhibit mammalian brain PROT through a direct interaction with the transporter protein at, or near, the L-proline binding site. The high potency and specificity of GGFL makes this compound a useful tool for elucidating the structure–function properties and physiological role(s) of PROT.

We recently made a surprising discovery: The mammalian brain PROT protein is predominantly localized to synaptic vesicles in specific glutamatergic nerve terminals (*39*). Two lines of evidence support this conclusion. First, electron microscopic ultrastructural studies demonstrated that immunogold-silver particles were predominantly localized over synaptic vesicles in labeled excitatory nerve terminals in both the caudate nucleus and in the stratum oriens of the CA1 region of the hippocampus. In most cases, at least one or two gold particles were also found near the plasma membrane, adjacent to the synapse. Second, subcellular fractionation studies revealed that PROT is substantially enriched in a highly purified synaptic vesicle fraction compared to markers for the plasma membrane, such as the NMDA glutamate receptor subtype. We estimate that ~80–90% of the immunoreactive PROT protein is vesicular, whereas the remaining 10–20% is on the presynaptic plasma membrane. These results raise the intriguing possibility that the major function of PROT may be vesicular. Future stud-

---

Fig. 6. (*previous page*) Regional and neuronal localization of mRNA for the mammalian high-affinity L-proline transporter in rat brain by *in situ* hybridization (*148*). A and B, coronal rat brain sections hybridized with ^{35}S-labeled anti-sense RNA derived from rat PROT cDNA. Specific labeling of the CA3 pyramidal neurons in the hippocampus and layer V pyramidal neurons in the cerebral cortex is apparent. No specific labeling was observed when the adjacent sections were hybridized with a sense-strand control probe. C, X-ray film autoradiograph of a coronal rat brain section hybridized with the same ^{35}S-labeled anti-sense RNA probe. There is a distinct lack of labeling over the caudate putamen. D and E, rat hippocampal neurons cultured for 14 d and then hybridized with either the ^{35}S-labeled antisense rat PROT cDNA probe (D) or an ^{35}S-labeled sense-control probe (E). CPu, caudate putamen (striatum); V, layer V of the cerebral cortex; Pir, piriform cortex. Reproduced with permission from ref. *148*.

ies will attempt to discover a functional role for vesicular PROT. It should be possible to immunoisolate the PROT-containing vesicles and examine the neurotransmitter phenotype and biochemical properties of this unique subpopulation of synaptic vesicles. Are the PROT-containing vesicles "prolinergic" or "glutamatergic," or do they have another function in specific glutamatergic nerve terminals? Does PROT function as a high affinity L-proline transporter in these vesicles? If so, does L-proline move into or out of the vesicles? Do the PROT-containing vesicles represent intermediates in the exo- and endocytotic recycling of synaptic vesicles? Do they represent a cryptic pool of intracellular transporters that can be recruited to the nerve terminal membrane in response to neuronal activity and/or alterations in second messengers? There is no precedent for the existence of any high-affinity, Na^+-dependent transporter in synaptic vesicles.

We have recently observed that in stably transfected MDCK cells, PROT also is localized predominantly in intracellular vesicles. We were surprised by this result because earlier studies had demonstrated that the structurally related GABA transporter subtype, GAT-1, is targeted specifically to the apical plasma membrane domain in MDCK cells (107). No vesicular labeling was reported. These results indicate that the primary amino acid sequence of the PROT protein contains information necessary for targeting this transporter to intracellular vesicles, even in non-neural cells. Little is known about how proteins are targeted to synaptic vesicles. Our studies indicate PROT may be a valuable model system with which to elucidate sorting signals which target proteins to intracellular vesicles.

Potential Physiological and Pathophysiological Roles

It is generally accepted that L-glutamate is the excitatory transmitter used by the vast majority of excitatory pathways in the mammalian brain. Since the mammalian brain-specific PROT protein has been localized to specific excitatory nerve terminals, where it is enriched in synaptic vesicles, high-affinity L-proline uptake may modulate some aspect of excitatory synaptic transmission in specific glutamatergic nerve terminals. Glutamatergic synapses have been implicated in diverse physiologic process including synapse formation, synaptic plasticity, memory and learning, and neuroendocrine regulation (19). Furthermore, abnormalities of glutamatergic transmission have been implicated in the pathophysiology of neurologic disorders in which excitotoxic processes are thought to play a role including cerebral strokes, epilepsy, and head trauma (19). Therefore, an understanding of the functional role of PROT in specific gluta-matergic nerve terminals may provide new insights into presynaptic regulatory mechanisms involved in synaptic plasticity and excito-toxic nerve cell damage. Certain glutamatergic nerve terminals appear to coexpress high affinity L-proline and L-glutamate trans-porters. The pharmacological selectivity of mammalian brain PROT (*38,123*) may provide a new therapeutic strategy for the selective modulation of one component of a neurons excitatory innervation. Compounds that target high-affinity L-proline uptake, such as GGFL, may have therapeutic utility in excitotoxic neurological disorders.

Betaine, Taurine, and Creatine Transporters

As is the case for proline, direct roles for betaine, taurine, and cre-atine in neurotransmission have not been identified. Nonetheless, high-affinity, Na^+- (and Cl^--) dependent transporters specific for these substrates have been isolated from mammalian brains. This suggests that these transporters have roles in the brain independent of the termination of neurotransmission. It remains to be determined whether one or more of these substrates may function in neural sig-naling in some unrecognized capacity.

Betaine Transporter

The first high-affinity, Na^+- (and Cl^--) dependent betaine trans-porter (BGT-1) was isolated by Yamauchi et al. (*155*) from MDCK cells by expression cloning. On expression in *Xenopus* oocytes, BGT-1 was found to transport betaine with a K_m of 398 µM. This substrate affinity was similar to that calculated for betaine uptake into native MDCK cells (480 µM). Betaine, however, was not the only high-affin-ity substrate for BGT-1, because Yamauchi et al. found that it also transported GABA. In fact, the K_m for GABA transport in *Xenopus* oocytes (98 µM) and native MDCK cells (120 µM) was significantly lower than for betaine. Despite this marked difference in substrate affinity, it was concluded that BGT-1 was primarily a betaine trans-porter based on two observations: First, tissue localization through Northern analysis detected BGT-1 mRNA in canine kidney, but not brain. Second, significant levels of betaine, but not GABA, were found to accumulate in the kidney because of a large difference in plasma concentrations (~180 µM and <1 µM for betaine and GABA, respectively) (*155*). Yamauchi et al. also found that BGT-1 was rela-tively insensitive to the GABA uptake inhibitors nipecotic acid, β-alanine, and DABA (IC_{50} values > 1 mM). These observations, along with a higher K_m for GABA, pharmacologically distinguished BGT-1 from the previously cloned rat brain GAT-1 transporter (*50*). Nonetheless, when primary structures were compared, BGT-1 surprisingly shared significant sequence identity with GAT-1 (53%). BGT-1 also shared significant identity with the previously cloned human brain norepinephrine transporter, NET (46%) (*102*). These observations established BGT-1 as a novel member of the Na^+-(and Cl^--) dependent transporter family.

Subsequently, López-Corcuera et al. (*80*) isolated mouse brain GAT-2 that exhibited 88% sequence identity with canine BGT-1 and had similar pharmacological properties. As described in the GABA transporters section, GABA transport by mouse GAT-2 had a K_m (79 μM) that was similar to BGT-1 (98 μM). In addition, GABA uptake by mouse GAT-2 was inhibited by betaine, a finding that was assumed to mean that betaine was a substrate for this transporter. (Demonstration of this assumption with radioactively labeled betaine was not carried out.) These observations, along with the localization by Northern analysis of mouse GAT-2 to kidney (in addition to brain), suggested that the two transporters were products of the same gene. However, López-Corcuera et al. questioned this conclusion citing several observations: First, the 88% identity between mouse GAT-2 and canine BGT-1 was high, but not as high as the ≥97% identity shared by the human, mouse, and rat GAT-1 transporters. Second, Northern analysis yielded a single mRNA transcript of 5 kb that hybridized with mouse GAT-2, whereas a doublet of 3 and 2.4 kb had been previously reported for canine BGT-1 (*155*). Third, no homology was observed in the 3'-nontranslated cDNA sequences between the transporters. Based on these findings, López-Corcuera et al. (*80*) concluded that mouse GAT-2 and canine BGT-1 were distinct gene products.

Subsequently, BGT-1 transporters were cloned from human brain (*11*) and kidney (*115*) which exhibited ≥87% sequence identity with mouse GAT-2 and canine BGT-1, and shared similar pharmacological properties. Based on these findings it appears likely that the human and canine BGT-1 proteins and the mouse GAT-2 protein are products of the same gene (*11,115*). This was bolstered by the finding that transcripts arising from the canine BGT-1 gene are expressed in brain (*139*), contrary to the first report of Yamauchi et al. (*155*). However, as for mouse GAT-2, direct demonstration of betaine as a substrate for human BGT-1 was not carried out using a radioactive label, though betaine was shown to weakly inhibit [^{3}H]GABA uptake. Therefore, the conclusion that human BGT-1 and mouse GAT-2 are betaine transporters remains only a strong assumption.

Because of the localization of the putative betaine transporter to both brain and peripheral tissues (human BGT-1 has also been shown to be expressed in liver, heart, skeletal muscle, and placenta [115]), speculation has centered on its true physiological function. In the renal medulla, betaine serves as one of the major osmolytes used for volume regulation and the betaine transporter is thought to be a central component of this function. Indeed, BGT-1 mRNA is induced by hypertonicity (139,140,146). Recently, a small 5'-flanking region has been identified upstream of the BGT-1 promotor that harbors a hypertonicity responsive enhancer element (TonE) (140). Thus, it appears that BGT-1 plays a significant role in volume homeostasis. Volume regulation may be the function of the betaine transporter in other organs, as well. However, in the brain, the betaine transporter might also function as a GABA transporter and consequently play a role in modulation of GABAergic transmission (11,115). It must be noted, though, that the distribution of human BGT-1 in the brain does not match the localization pattern of GABAergic pathways (11). It may be the case that this transporter sequesters GABA that has diffused away from synaptic regions (11). Alternatively, it may not function to transport GABA at all. Last, the brain localization may be indicative of an unrecognized role for betaine in neurotransmission.

Taurine Transporter

In 1992, several species homologs of a high affinity, Na$^+$- (and Cl$^-$-) dependent taurine transporter (TAUT) were cloned and characterized, with the first isolated by Smith et al. (127) from rat brain. On transient expression in COS cells, TAUT was found to transport taurine with a K_m of 43 µM. Transport was strongly inhibited by hypotaurine and β-alanine (IC$_{50}$ values between 10 and 100 µM), and weakly inhibited by GABA (IC$_{50}$ ~1 mM). Northern analysis indicated that TAUT was expressed in a variety of tissues, including brain, retina, liver, kidney, heart, spleen, and pancreas. Shortly thereafter, TAUT cDNA's were cloned from MDCK cells (144,145) and mouse brain (73), followed by human placenta (114), thyroid (56), and retinal epithelial pigment cells (112). These clones shared >90% sequence identity with rat TAUT, slightly higher affinities for taurine (K_m values ranging from 4.5–12 µM), and similar sensitivities to inhibition by hypotaurine and β-alanine. β-Alanine was also shown to be a substrate (*73*). Additional tissues in which TAUT was found to be expressed were ileal mucosa, epididymis (*144*), lung (*127*), skeletal muscle (*114*), breast, colon, and ovary (*57*).

Several human cell lines have also been shown to express high affinity, Na^+- (and Cl^--) dependent taurine transport (*41*). These have been exploited to identify other factors that regulate taurine uptake, in particular PKC and calmodulin. In both placental-derived (*68*) and intestinal-derived (*17*) cell lines, treatment with the PKC activator PMA resulted in the specific inhibition of TAUT. This effect of PMA was blocked by staurosporin, a potent inhibitor of PKC. Detailed analysis in one of the intestinal cell lines (*17*) indicated that the effect of PMA was not on protein synthesis or its targeting to the plasma membrane. It was therefore concluded that phosphorylation of TAUT through the activity of PKC causes the inhibition of transport. Consistent with this interpretation is the presence of six potential PKC recognition sites within the primary sequence of the transporter (*114*). Similar studies have found that taurine transport is decreased by calmodulin inhibitors (*41,97,112,113*). Although many of these calmodulin inhibitors may have differential effects on PKC, at least one, CGS 9343 B, is highly selective for calmodulin (*97,112*). Therefore, this implicates calmodulin as an activator of TAUT. Its effect was shown not to involve transcriptional processes (*97*), but whether it affects protein synthesis, protein targeting, substrate affinity, and/or substrate translocation has not been determined.

The physiological functions of high-affinity TAUT are not well understood. Like BGT-1, the expression of TAUT in MDCK cells is regulated by hypertonicity supporting a role for taurine and its transporter in osmoregulation. However, taurine is involved in a number of other important physiological processes, including bile acid conjugation in hepatocytes, detoxification, membrane stabilization, and modulation of calcium flux and neural excitability (*132*). This latter function, along with the localization of TAUT in the CNS, strongly suggests some role for TAUT in neurotransmission, particularly since free taurine is found in millimolar concentrations in excitable tissues (*153*). Also indicative of potential functions for TAUT are the observed effects of taurine deficiency, which include retinal blindness, and abnormalities in immune, cardiac, and reproductive functions (*132*). In addition, the TAUT gene has been mapped to human chromosome 3p24–p25 (*104,114*), a region associated with mental retardation and other neurological defects. The availability of TAUT cDNA clones and the potential for the development of specific TAUT inhibitors will be invaluable for understanding the disease states associated with taurine deficiency, as well as a possible neurotransmitter role for this substrate.

Creatine Transporter

In 1993, Guimbal et al. (*51*) isolated and characterized a high affinity, Na^+- (and Cl^--) dependent creatine transporter from rabbit brain and muscle. In separate experiments, this clone was found to have a K_m for creatine ranging from 27–43 μM when transiently expressed in COS cells. This range was in agreement with previous creatine uptake affinities determined in a variety of tissues and cell types (*28,66,77,78,88*). Various creatine-related compounds were assessed for their inhibitory capacity, with 3-guanidinopropionate and 4-guanidinobutyrate being the most potent (IC_{50} values < 5 mM). Northern analysis found mRNA for the transporter expressed in kidney, heart, skeletal muscle, brain, lung, epididymis, and testis. Later, creatine transporter cDNAs were isolated from rat brain (*15,45,53,121*), and human kidney (*91*) brain stem/spinal cord (*129*), and striatum (*129*). In this latter study, the brain stem/spinal cord and striatum clones were found to differ by two amino acids, suggesting possible allelic variation. The two residue differences did not have an effect on the pharmacological profiles of the two variants, and therefore their significance is unclear.

The primary sequence identity between the creatine transporter species homologs is very high (98–99%), whereas identity with BGT-1 and TAUT is ~50%. Because BGT-1 and TAUT do not transport creatine, comparisons of the primary sequences should suggest which amino acid domains are involved in substrate binding. In this regard, Nash et al. (*91*) proposed that TMDs 9, 10, and 11 are likely to be responsible for the observed differences in substrate affinities. Moreover, a creatine transporter has been cloned by Guimbal and Kilimann (*52*) from *T. marmorata* which has 64% identity with the mammalian creatine transporter proteins. Inclusion of this species homolog in the comparison of primary structures suggested that only a few residues are candidates for involvement in creatine substrate specificity (*52*). It is anticipated that site-directed mutagenesis will be employed to answer these predictions.

The creatine transporter is widely expressed in a variety of mammalian tissues, including adrenal gland, intestine, colon, prostate, thymus, ovary, spleen, pancreas, placenta, umbilical cord, thyroid, tongue, pharynx, vertebral discs, jaw, and nasal epithelium (*15,45,51,53,91,121,129*). Creatine transporter expression has also been observed in a variety of brain regions, including cerebellum, hippocampus, pontine nuclei, the trapezoid body, white matter fiber tracts, brain stem nuclei, and others (*15,45,53,121*). This diverse tissue expression is consistent with a general metabolic role for creatine as a substrate for the creatine kinase-catalyzed biosynthesis of phospho-creatine, a reaction which is critical for maintaining adenosine triphosphate homeostasis. This interpretation is supported by the dif-fuse localization of the transporter in the brain which corresponds well with the CNS distribution of creatine kinase (*53*). There is no indication that creatine participates in neurotransmission. A poten-tial role for the creatine transporter in genetic disease is suggested by its mapping to human chromosome Xq28 (*48,91*). This genetic loci has been linked to several skeletoneuromuscular disorders. The avail-ability of cDNA for this transporter provides the opportunity to more fully investigate its roles in normal physiological function and genetic disease.

Future Directions

The molecular identification of the high-affinity, Na^+-(and Cl^--) dependent transporters has unveiled an exciting area of biological research with significant physiological and clinical relevance. Of pri-mary interest has been the putative role of the transporters in the ter-mination of neural signals through the uptake of neurotransmitters from the synaptic cleft. It is apparent, however, that these proteins subserve a diversity of function beyond the regulation of neural events, as exemplified by their expression in both the CNS and peripheral tissues, and by their affinities for substrates with no known neurotransmitter roles. The goal of future research will be to elucidate these varied physiological functions.

In regard to the putative roles of these transporters in neurotrans-mission, the present chapter has illustrated several significant and intriguing findings which should influence and focus future study. First, the multiple GABA and glycine transporter subtypes, with their varied pharmacologies and expression patterns, suggest a remarkable synaptic heterogeneity. These subtypes may provide a basis for differential neural signaling using the same neurotransmit-ter. Moreover, this heterogeneity may be exploitable for the targeting of therapeutic agents with reduced side-effect profiles in the treatment of neuropsychiatric disorders. Second, at least two mechanisms are utilized for generating the molecular diversity displayed by these subtypes—transcription of separate genes and alternative post-transcriptional splicing of single genes. Third, the presumed function of these transporters is substrate translocation across plasma membranes, but at least one member of the family (the proline transporter PROT) is unusually expressed in synaptic vesicles in certain glutamatergic nerve terminals. This has prompted a fundamental question: What is the function of vesicular PROT? Does PROT function in these vesicles in some "prolinergic" or "glutamatergic" capacity? Does PROT actually transport proline in or out of these vesicles, or do the vesicles represent a cryptic PROT pool that can be recruited to the nerve terminal membrane in response to neuronal activity and/or alterations in second messengers? This unprecedented finding provides an exciting impetus for future investigation into presynaptic regulatory mechanisms in excitatory neurotransmission. Fourth, differences in primary amino acid sequence between the transporters and their subtypes not only determine substrate specificity and affinity, but also apparently determine subcellular expression patterns. In addition to the vesicular localization of PROT, a good example of this is the differential expression of the GABA transporter subtypes in neurons (somatodendritic vs axonal). These observations are important clues into the nature of neuronal subcellular protein targeting mechanisms. Finally, the intrinsic activities of these transporters may be dynamically regulated by transient post-translational modifications, such as protein kinase-mediated phosphorylation.

Taken together, these findings indicate that this transporter family subserves a diversity of physiological functions within the CNS. This, in turn, leads to the recognition of these transporters as important targets for therapeutic and pathological alterations of neurotransmission. For example, as discussed elsewhere in this book, cocaine, amphetamines, and tricyclic antidepressants block biogenic amine transport and produce dramatic behavioral changes. In addition, the ability of the biogenic amine transporters to accumulate certain neurotransmitter-like toxins, including N-methyl-4-phenylpyridine (MPP$^+$), 6-hydroxydopamine, and 5,6-dihydroxytryptamine, suggests a role for these transporters in the selective vulnerability of specific classes of neurons to exogenous agents. Undoubtedly, similar functional relationships exist for the non-biogenic amine members of this transporter family. Indeed, specific GABA uptake inhibitors are being developed as potential antiepileptic agents, as discussed in this chapter. Beyond these examples, however, very little is known about the functional relationships between this family of transporters and neurotransmission. Future research will undoubtedly focus on the elucidation of the varied physiological functions of these proteins. Moreover, the availability of cDNA clones for these transporters provides the opportunity to investigate whether hereditary genetic variations contribute to neuropsychiatric disorders.

References

1. Acosta, G. B., Losada, M. E. O., and Rubio, M. C. Area-dependent changes in GABAergic function after acute and chronic cold stress. *Neurosci. Lett.* **154** (1993) 175–178.
2. Adams, R. H., Sato, K., Shimada, S., Tohyama, M., Püschel, A. W., and Betz, H. Gene structure and glial expression of the glycine transporter GLYT1 in embryonic and adult rodents. *J. Neurosci.* **15** (1995) 2524–2532.
3. Ahn, J., Mundigl, O., Muth, T. R., Rudnick, G., and Caplan, M. J. Polarized expression of GABA transporters in Madin-Darby canine kidney cells and cultured hippocampal neurons. *J. Biol. Chem.* **271** (1996) 6917–6924.
4. Andersen, K. E., Braestrup, C., Grønwald, F. C., Jørgensen, A. S., Nielsen, E. B., Sonnewald, U., Sørensen, P. O., Suzdak, P. D., and Knutsen, L. J. S. The synthesis of novel GABA uptake inhibitors: 1. elucidation of the structure–activity studies leading to the choice of (R)-l-[4,4-Bis(3-methyl-2-thienyl)-3-butenyl]-3-piperidinecarboxylic acid (tiagabine) as an anticonvulsant drug candidate. *J. Med. Chem.* **36** (1993) 1716–1725.
5. Austin, M. C., Bradley, C. C., Mann, J. J., and Blakely, R. D. Expression of serotonin transporter messenger RNA in the human brain. *J. Neurochem.* **62** (1994) 2362–2367.
6. Bendahan, A. and Kanner, B. I. Identification of domains of a cloned rat brain GABA transporter which are not required for its functional expression. *FEBS Lett.* **318** (1993) 41–44.
7. Bennett, J. P., Jr., Logan, W. J., and Snyder, S. H. Amino acid neurotransmitter candidates: sodium-dependent high-affinity uptake by unique synaptosomal fractions. *Science* **178** (1972) 997–999.
8. Blasberg, R. G. Specificity of cerebral amino acid transport: a kinetic analysis. *Prog. Brain Res.* **29** (1968) 245–258.
9. Borden, L. A., Dhar, T. G. M., Smith, K. E., Branchek, T. A., Gluchowski, C., and Weinshank, R. L. Cloning of the human homologue of the GABA transporter GAT-3 and identification of a novel inhibitor with selectivity for this site. *Recept. Channels* **2** (1994) 207–213.
10. Borden, L. A., Dhar, T. G. M., Smith, K. E., Weinshank, R. L., Branchek, T. A., and Gluchowski, C. Tiagabine, SK&F 89976-A, CI-966, and NNC-711 are selective for the cloned GABA transporter GAT-1. *Eur. J. Pharmacol.–Mol. Pharmacol. Sec.* **269** (1994) 219–224.

11. Borden, L. A., Smith, K. E., Gustafson, E. L., Branchek, T. A., and Weinshank, R. L. Cloning and expression of a betaine/GABA transporter from human brain. *J. Neurochem.* **64** (1995) 977–984.

12. Borden, L. A., Smith, K. E., Hartig, P. R., Branchek, T. A., and Weinshank, R. L. Molecular heterogeneity of the γ-aminobutyric acid (GABA) transport system: cloning of two novel high affinity GABA transporters from rat brain. *J. Biol. Chem.* **267** (1992) 21,098–21,104.

13. Borowsky, B., Mezey, É., and Hoffman, B. J. Two glycine transporter variants with distinct localization in the CNS and peripheral tissues are encoded by a common gene. *Neuron* **10** (1993) 851–836.

14. Bowery, N. G., Jones, G. P., and Neal, M. J. Selective inhibition of neuronal GABA uptake by *cis*-1,3-aminocyclohexane carboxylic acid. *Nature* **264** (1976) 281–284.

15. Bradley, C. C., Moore, K. R., Fremeau, R. T., Ramamoorthy, S., Ganapathy, V., Han, H., Yang-Feng, T., and Blakely, R. D. Molecular cloning, expression, and chromosomal localization of a rat brain creatine transporter. *Soc. Neurosci. Abstr.* **19** (1993) 220 (abstract).

16. Braestrup, C., Nielsen, E. B., Sonnewald, U., Knutsen, L. J. S., Andersen, K. E., Jansen, J. A., Frederiksen, K., Andersen, P. H., Mortensen, A., and Suzdak, P. D. (R)-N-[4,4-Bis(3-methyl-2-thienyl)but-3-en-1-yl]nipecotic acid binds with high affinity to the brain γ-aminobutyric acid uptake carrier. *J. Neurochem.* **54** (1990) 639–647.

17. Brandsch, M., Miyamota, Y., Ganapathy V., and Leibach, F. H. Regulation of taurine transport in human colon carcinoma cell lines (HT-29 and Caco-2) by protein kinase C. *Am. J. Physiol.* **264** (1993) G939–G946.

18. Brecha, N. S. and Weigmann, C. Expression of GAT-1, a high affinity gamma-aminobutyric acid plasmamembrane transporter in the rat retina. *J. Compar. Neurol.* **345** (1994) 602–611.

19. Choi, D. W. Bench to bedside: the glutamate connection. *Science* **258** (1992) 241–243.

20. Christensen, H. N. Role of amino acid transport and countertransport in nutrition and metabolism. *Physiol. Rev.* **70** (1990) 43–77.

21. Clark, J. A. and Amara, S. G. Stable expression of a neuronal γ-aminobutyric acid transporter, GAT-3, in mammalian cells demonstrates unique pharmacological properties and ion dependence. *Mol. Pharmacol.* **46** (1994) 550–557.

22. Clark, J. A., Deutch, A. Y., Gallipoli, P. Z., and Amara, S. G. Functional expression and CNS distributiion of a β-alanine-sensitive neuronal GABA transporter. *Neuron* **9** (1992) 337–348.

23. Cohen, S. M. and Nadler, J. V. Proline-induced potentiation of synaptic transmission is long-lasting and NMDA receptor-dependent. *Soc. Neurosci. Abstr.* **21** (1995) 1108 (abstract).

24. Corey, J. L., Davidson, N., Lester, H. A. Brecha, N., and Quick, M. W. Protein kinase C modulates the activity of a cloned γ-aminobutyric acid transporter expressed in *Xenopus* oocytes via regulated subcellular redistribution of the transporter. *J. Biol. Chem.* **269** (1994) 14,759–14,767.

25. Corey, J. L., Guastella, J., Davidson, N., and Lester, H. A. GABA uptake and release by a mammalian cell line stably expressing a cloned rat brain GABA transporter. *Mol. Membr. Biol.* **11** (1994) 23–30.

26. Crawford, P. M., Engelsman, M., Brown, S. W., et al. Tiagabine: phase II study of efficacy and safety in adjunctive treatment of partial seizures. *Epilepsia* **34(Suppl. 2)** (1993) 182 (abstract).

27. Cupello, A., Gasparetto, B., Mainardi, P., and Vignolo, L. Effect of protein kinase C activators on the uptake of GABA by rat brain synaptosomes. *Int. J. Neurosci.* **69** (1993) 131–136.

28. Daly, M. M. and Seifter, S. Uptake of creatine by cultured cells. *Arch. Biochem. Biophys.* **203** (1980) 317–324.

29. Dhar, T. G. M., Borden, L. A., Tyagarajan, S., Smith, K. E., Branchek, T. A., Weinshank, R. L., and Gluchowski, C. Design, synthesis and evaluation of substituted triarylnipecotic acid derivatives as GABA uptake inhibitors: identification of a ligand with moderate affinity and selectivity for the cloned human GABA transporter GAT-3. *J. Med. Chem.* **37** (1994) 2334–2342.

30. Dotti, C. G., Parton, R. G., and Simons, K. Polarized sorting of glypiated proteins in hippocampal neurons. *Nature* **349** (1991) 158–161.

31. Dotti, C. G. and Simons, K. Polarized sorting of viral glycoproteins to the axon and dendrites of hippocampal neurons in culture. *Cell* **62** (1990) 63–72.

32. Elliot, K. A. C. and van Gelder, N. M. Occlusion and metabolism of γ-aminobutyric acid by brain tissue. *J. Neurochem.* **3** (1958) 28–40.

33. Fedele, E. and Foster, A. C. [^{3}H]Glycine uptake in rat hippocampus: kinetic analysis and autoradiographic localization. *Brain Res.* **572** (1992) 154–163.

34. Fernandes, C. and File, S. E. Beware the builders: construction noise changes [^{14}C]GABA release and uptake from amygdaloid and hippocampal slices in the rat. *Neuropharmacology* **32** (1993) 1333–1336.

35. File, S. E., Zangrossi, H., and Andrews, N. Novel environment and cat odor change GABA and 5-HT release and uptake in the rat. *Pharmacol. Biochem. Behav.* **45** (1993) 931–934.

36. File, S. E., Zangrossi, H., and Andrews, N. Social interaction and elevated plus-maze tests: changes in release and uptake of 5-HT and GABA. *Neuropharmacology* **32** (1993) 217–221.

37. Fink-Jensen, A., Suzdak, P. D., Swedberg, M. D. B., Judge, M. E., Hansen, L., and Nielsen, P. G. The γ-aminobutyric acid (GABA) uptake inhibitor, tiagabine, increases extracellular brain levels of GABA in awake rats. *Eur. J. Pharmacol.* **220** (1992) 197–201.

38. Fremeau, R. T., Jr., Caron, M. G., and Blakely, R. D. Molecular cloning and expression of a high affinity L-proline transporter expressed in putative glutamatergic pathways of rat brain. *Neuron* **8** (1992) 915–926.

39. Fremeau, R. T., Jr., Chan, J., Pohorille, A., Nadler, J. V., Milner, T. A., and Pickel, V. Mammalian brain-specific L-proline transporter: preferential localization of transporter protein to glutamatergic nerve terminals. *Soc. Neurosci. Abst.* **21** (1995) 2062 (abstract).

40. Fremeau, R. T., Jr., Velaz-Faircloth, M., Miller, J. W., Henzi, V. A., Cohen, S. M., Nadler, J. V., Shafqat, S., Blakely, R. D., and Domin, B. A novel non-opioid action of enkephalins: competitive inhibition of the mammalian brain high affinity L-proline transporter. *Mol. Pharmacol.* (1996) in press.

41. Ganapathy, V. and Leibach, F. H. Expression and regulation of the taurine transporter in cultured cell lines of human origin, in *Taurine in Health and Disease* (Huxtable, R., and Michalk, D. V., eds.), Plenum, New York, 1994, pp. 51–57.

42. Giros, B., el Mestikawy, S., Godinot, N., Zheng, K., Han, H., Yang-Feng, T., Caron, M. G. Cloning, pharmacological characterization, and chromosome

assignment of the human dopamine transporter. *Mol. Pharmacol.* **42** (1992) 383–390.

43. Gomeza, J., Casado, M., Giménez, C., and Aragon, C. Inhibition of high-affinity γ-aminobutyric acid uptake in primary astrocyte cultures by phorbol esters and phospholipase C. *Biochem. J.* **275** (1991) 435–439.

44. Gomeza, J., Zafra, F., Olivares, L., Giménez, C., and Aragón C. Regulation by phorbol esters of the glycine transporter (GLYT1) in glioblastoma cells. *Biochim Biophys Acta* **1233** (1995) 41–46.

45. Gonzalez, A. M. and Uhl, G. R. "Choline/orphan V8-2-1/creatine transporter" mRNA is expressed in nervous, renal, and gastrointestinal systems. *Mol. Brain Res.* **23** (1994) 266–270.

46. Goncalves, P. P. and Carvalho, A. P. Effect of anions on the uptake and release of γ-aminobutyric acid by isolated synaptic plasma membranes. *Neurochem. Int.* **25** (1994) 483–492.

47. Gram L. Tiagabine: a novel drug with a GABAergic mechanism of action. *Epilepsia* **35(Suppl. 5)** (1994) S85–S87.

48. Gregor, P., Nash, S. R., Caron, M. G., Seldin, M. F., and Warren, S. T. Assignment of the creatine transporter gene (SLC6A8) to human chromosome Xq28 telomeric to G6PD. *Genomics* **25** (1995) 332–333.

49. Guastella, J., Brecha, N., Weigmann, C., Lester, H. A., and Davidson, N. Cloning, expression, and localization of a rat brain high-affinity glycine transporter. *Proc. Natl. Acad. Sci. USA* **89** (1992) 7189–7193.

50. Guastella, J., Nelson, N., Nelson, H., Czyzyk, L., Keynan, S., Miedel, M. C., Davidson, N., Lester, H. A., and Kanner, B. I. Cloning and expression of a rat brain GABA transporter. *Science* **249** (1990) 1303–1306.

51. Guimbal, C. and Kilimann, M. W. A Na^+-dependent creatine transporter in rabbit brain, muscle, heart, and kidney: cDNA cloning and functional expression. *J. Biol. Chem.* **268** (1993) 8418–8421.

52. Guimbal, C. and Kilimann, M. W. A creatine transporter cDNA from *Torpedo* illustrates structure/function relationships in the GABA/noradrenaline transporter family. *J. Mol. Biol.* **241** (1994) 317–324.

53. Happe, H. K. and Murrin, L. C. In situ hybridization analysis of CHOT1, a creatine transporter, in the rat central nervous system. *J. Comp. Neurol.* **351** (1995) 94–103.

54. Henzi, V., Reichling, D. B., Helm, S. W., and Macdermott, A. B. L-Proline activates glutamate and glycine receptors in cultured rat dorsal horn neurons. *Mol. Pharmacol.* **41** (1992) 793–801.

55. Iversen, L. L. and Kelly, J. S. Uptake and metabolism of γ-aminobutyric acid by neurones and glial cells. *Biochem. Pharmacol.* **24** (1975) 933–938.

56. Iversen, L. L. and Neal, M. J. The uptake of [^{3}H]GABA by slices of rat cerebral cortex. *J. Neurochem.* **15** (1968) 1141–1149.

57. Jhiang, S. M., Fithian, L., Smanik, P., McGill, J., Tong, Q., and Mazzaferri, E. L. Cloning of the human taurine transporter and characterization of taurine uptake in thyroid cells. *FEBS Lett.* **318** (1993) 139–144.

58. Johnson, J. W. and Ascher, P. Glycine potentiates the NMDA response in cultured mouse brain neurons. *Nature* **325** (1987) 529–531.

59. Johnston, G. A. R. and Iversen, I. L. Glycine uptake in rat central nervous system slices and homogenates: evidence for different uptake systems in spinal cord and cerebral cortex. *J. Neurochem.* **18** (1971) 1951–1961.

60. Keshet, G. I., Bendahan, A., Su, H., Mager, S., Lester, H. A., and Kanner, B. I. Glutamate-101 is critical for the function of the sodium and chloride-coupled GABA transporter GAT-1. *FEBS Lett.* **371** (1995) 39–42.

61. Keynan, S., Suh, Y.- J., Kanner, B. I., and Rudnick, G. Expression of a cloned γ-aminobutyric acid transporter in mammalian cells. *Biochemistry* **31** (1992) 1974–1979.

62. Kim, K.-M., Kingsmore, S. F., Han, H., Yang-Feng, T. L., Godinot, N., Seldin, M. F., Caron, M. G., and Giros, B. Cloning of the human glycine transporter type 1: molecular and pharmacological characterization of novel isoform variants and chromosomal localization of the gene in the human and mouse genomes. *Mol. Pharmacol.* **45** (1995) 608–617.

63. Kitayama, S., Shimada, S., Xu, H., Markham, L., Donovan, D. M., and Uhl, G. R. Dopamine transporter site-directed mutations differentially alter substrate transport and cocaine binding. *Proc. Natl Acad. Sci USA* **89** (1992) 7782–7785.

64. Kleinberger-Doron, N. and Kanner, B. I. Identification of tryptophan residues critical for the function and targeting of the γ-aminobutyric acid transporter (subtype A). *J. Biol. Chem.* **269** (1994) 3063–3067.

65. Krogsgaard-Larsen, P., Falch, E., Larsson, O. M., and Schousboe, A. GABA uptake inhibitors: relevance to antiepileptic drug research. *Epil. Res.* **1** (1987) 77–93.

66. Ku, C.-P. and Passow, H. Creatine and creatinine transport in old and young human red blood cells. *Biochim. Biophys. Acta* **600** (1980) 212–227.

67. Kuhar, M. J. and Zarbin, M. A. Synaptosomal transport: a chloride dependence for choline, GABA, glycine and several other compounds. *J. Neurochem.* **31** (1978) 251–256.

68. Kulanthaivel, P., Cool, D. R., Ramamoorthy, S., Mahesh, V. B., Leibach, F. H., and Ganapathy, V. Transport of taurine and its regulation by protein kinase C in the JAR human placental choriocarcinoma cell line. *Biochem. J.* **277** (1991) 53–58.

69. Ladogana, A., Bouzamondo, E., Pocchiari, M., and Tsiang, H. Modification of tritiated γ-amino-n-butyric acid transport in rabies virus-infected primary cortical cultures. *J. Gen. Virol.* **75** (1994) 623–627.

70. Lewin, L., Mattsson, M.-O., and Sellström, A. Inhibition of transporter mediated γ-aminobutyric acid (GABA) release by SKF 89976-A, a GABA uptake inhibitor, studied in a primary neuronal culture from chicken. *Neurochem. Res.* **17** (1992) 577–584.

71. Liu, Q.-R., López-Corcuera, B., Mandiyan, S., Nelson, H., and Nelson, N. Cloning and expression of a spinal cord- and brain-specific glycine transporter with novel structural features. *J. Biol. Chem.* **268** (1993) 22,802–22,808.

72. Liu, Q.-R., López-Corcuera, B., Mandiyan, S., Nelson, H., and Nelson, N. Molecular characterization of four pharmacologically distinct γ-aminobutyric acid transporters in mouse brain. *J. Biol. Chem.* **268** (1993) 2106–2112.

73. Liu, Q.-R., López-Corcuera, B., Nelson, H., Mandiyan, S., and Nelson, N. Cloning and expression of a cDNA encoding the transporter of taurine and β-alanine in mouse brain. *Proc. Natl. Acad. Sci. USA* **89** (1992) 12,145–12,149.

74. Liu, Q. R., Madiyan, S., Nelson, H., and Nelson, N. A family of genes encoding neurotransmitter transporters. *Proc. Natl. Acad. Sci. USA* **89** (1992) 6639–6643.

75. Liu, Q.-R., Nelson, H., Mandiyan, S., López-Corcuera, B., and Nelson, N. Cloning and expression of a glycine transporter from mouse brain. *FEBS Lett.* **305** (1992) 110–114.

76. Logan, W. J. and Snyder, S. H. High affinity uptake systems for glycine, glutamic and aspartic acids in synaptosomes of rat central nervous tissues. *Brain Res.* **42** (1972) 413–431.

77. Loike, J. D., Somes, M., and Silverstein, S. C. Creatine uptake, metabolism, and efflux in human monocytes and macrophages. *Am. J. Physiol.* **251** (1986) C128–C135.

78. Loike, J. D., Zalutsky, D. L., Kaback, E., Miranda, A. F., and Silverstein, S. C. Extracellular creatine regulates creatine transport in rat and human muscle cells. *Proc. Natl. Acad. Sci. USA* **85** (1988) 807–811.

79. López-Corcuera, B., Alcántra, R., Vázquez, J., and Arabón, C. Hydrodynamic properties and immunological identification of the sodium- and chloride-coupled glycine transporter. *J. Biol. Chem.* **268** (1993) 2239–2243.

80. López-Corcuera, B., Liu, Q.-R., Mandiyan, S., Nelson, H., and Nelson, N. Expression of a mouse brain cDNA encoding novel γ-aminobutyric acid transporter. *J. Biol. Chem.* **267** (1992) 17,491–17,493.

81. Luque, J. M., Nelson, N., and Richards, J. G. Cellular expression of glycine transporter 2 messenger RNA exclusively in rat hindbrain and spinal cord. *Neuroscience* **64** (1995) 525–535.

82. Mabjeesh, N. J., Frese, M., Rauen, T., Jeserich, G., and Kanner, B. I. Neuronal and glial γ-aminobutyric acid transporters are distinct proteins. *FEBS Lett.* **299** (1992) 99–102.

83. Mabjeesh, N. J. and Kanner, B. I. Neither amino nor carboxyl termini are required for function of the sodium- and chloride-coupled γ-aminobutyric acid transporter from rat brain. *J. Biol. Chem.* **267** (1992) 2563–2568.

84. Mantz, J., Lecharny, J.-B., Laudenbach, V., Henzel, D., Peytavin, G., and Desmonts, J. -M. Anesthetics affect the uptake but not the depolarization-evoked release of GABA in rat striatal synaptosomes. *Anesthesiology* **82** (1995) 502–511.

85. Mbungu, D., Ross, L. S., and Gill, S. S. Cloning, functional expression, and pharmacology of a GABA transporter from *Manduca sexta. Arch. Biochem. Biophys.* **318** (1995) 489–497.

86. Minelli, A., Brecha, N. C., Karschin, C., DeBiasi, S., and Conti, F. GAT-1, a high affinity GABA plasma membrane transporter, is localized to neurons and astroglia in the cerebral cortex. *J. Neurosci.* **15** (1995) 7734–7746.

87. Minuk, G. Y. Gamma-aminobutyric acid and the liver. *Diges. Disord.* **11** (1993) 45–54.

88. Möller, A. and Hamprecht, B. Creatine transport in cultured cells of rat and mouse brain. *J. Neurochem.* **52** (1989) 544–550.

89. Nadler, J. V. Sodium-dependent proline uptake in the rat hippocampal formation: association with ipsilateral commissural projections of CA3 pyramidal cells. *J. Neurochem.* **49** (1987) 1155–1160.

90. Nadler, J. V., Bray, S. D., and Evenson, D. A. Autoradiographic localization of proline uptake in excitatory hippocampal pathways. *Hippocampus* **2** (1992) 269–78.

91. Nash, S. R., Giros, B., Kingsmore, S. F., Rochelle, J. M., Suter, S. T., Gregor, P., Seldin, M. F., and Caron, M. G. Cloning, pharmacological characterization, and genomic localization of the human creatine transporter. *Recept. Chan.* **2** (1994) 165–174.

92. Neal, M. J. and Iversen, L. L. Subcellular distribution of endogenous and [³H] γ-aminobutyric acid in rat cerebral cortex. *J. Neurochem.* **16** (1969) 1245–1252.

93. Neal, M. J. and Pickles, H. G. Uptake of ^{14}C-glycine by spinal cord. *Nature* **222** (1969) 679,680.

94. Nelson, H., Mandiyan, S., and Nelson N. Cloning of the human brain GABA transporter. *FEBS Lett.* **269** (1990) 181–184.

95. Nielsen, E. B. Anxiolytic effect of NO-328, a GABA uptake inhibitor. *Psychopharmacology* **96** (1988) P116 (abstract).

96. Nielsen, E. B., Suzdak, P. D., Andersen, K. E., Knutsen, L. J. S., Sonnewald, U., and Braestrup, C. Characterization of tiagabine (NO-328), a new potent and selective GABA uptake inhibitor. *Eur. J. Pharmacol.* **196** (1991) 257–266.

97. Norman, J. A., Ansell, J., Stone, G. A., Wennogle, L. P., and Wasley, J. W. F. CGS 9343 B, a novel, potent, and selective inhibitor of calmodulin activity. *Mol. Pharmacol.* **31** (1987) 535–540.

98. Núñez, E. and Aragón, C. Structural analysis and functional role of the carbohydrate component of glycine transporter. *J. Biol. Chem.* **269** (1994) 16,920–16,924.

99. Olivares, L., Aragón, C., Giménez, C., and Zafra, F. Carboxyl terminus of the glycine transporter GLYT1 is necessary for correct processing of the protein. *J. Biol. Chem.* **269** (1995) 28,400–28,404.

100. Olivares, L., Aragón, C., Giménez, C., and Zafra, F. The role of N-glycosylation in the targeting and activity of the GLYT1 glycine transporter. *J. Biol. Chem.* **270** (1995) 9437–9442.

101. Osawa, I., Saito, N., Koga, T., and Tanaka, C. Phorbol ester-induced inhibition of GABA uptake by synaptosomes and by *Xenopus* oocytes expressing GABA transporter (GAT-1). *Neurosci. Res.* **19** (1994) 287–293.

102. Pacholczyk, T., Blakely, R. D., and Amara, S. G. Expression cloning of a cocaine- and antidepressant-sensitive human noradrenaline transporter. *Nature* **350** (1991) 350–354.

103. Pantanowitz, S., Bendahan, A., and Kanner, B. I. Only one of the charged amino acids located in the transmembrane α-helices of the γ-aminobutyric acid transporter (subtype A) is essential for its activity. *J. Biol. Chem.* **268** (1993) 3222–3225.

104. Patel, A., Rochelle, J. M., Jones, J. M., Sumegi, J., Uhl, G. R., Seldin, M. F., Meisler, M. H., and Gregor, P. Mapping of the taurine transporter gene to mouse chromosome 6 and to the short arm of human chromosome 3. *Genomics* **25** (1995) 314–317.

105. Peterson, N. A. and Raghupathy, E. Characteristics of amino acid accumulation of synaptosomal particles isolated from rat brain. *J. Neurochem.* **19** (1972) 1423–1438.

106. Pierce, M. W., Suzdak, P. D., Guztavson, L. E., Mengel, H. B., McKelvy, J. F., and Mant, T. Tiagabine. *Epilepsy Res.* **12(Suppl. 3)** (1991) 157–160.

107. Pietrini, G., Suh, Y. J., Edelmann, L., Rudnick, G., and Caplan, M. J. The axonal γ-aminobutyric acid transporter GAT-1 is sorted to the apical membranes of polarized epithelial cells. *J. Biol. Chem.* **269** (1994) 4668–4674.

108. Radian, R., Bendahan, A., and Kanner, B. I. Purification and identification of the functional sodium- and chloride-coupled γ-aminobutyric acid transport glycoprotein from rat brain. *J. Biol. Chem.* **261** (1986) 15437–15441.

109. Radian, R., Ottersen, O. P., Storm-Mathisen, J., Castel, M., and Kanner, B. I. Immunocytochemical localization of the GABA transporter in rat brain. *J. Neurosci.* **10** (1990) 1319–1330.

110. Radulovic, L. L., Bockbrader, H. N., and Chang, T. Pharmacokinetics, mass balance, and induction potential of a novel GABA uptake inhibitor, CI-966 HCl, in laboratory animals. *Pharmaceut. Res.* **10** (1993) 1442–1445.

111. Ramamoorthy, S., Bauman, A. L., Moore, K. R., Han, H., Yang-Feng, T. L., Chang, A. S., Ganapathy, V., and Blakely, R. D. Antidepressant- and cocaine-sensitive human serotonin transporter: molecular cloning, expression, and chromosomal localization. *Proc. Natl. Acad. Sci. USA* **90** (1993) 2542–2546.

112. Ramamoorthy, S., Del Monte, M. A., Leibach, F. H., and Ganapathy, V. Molecular identity and camodulin-mediated regulation of the taurine transporter in a human retinal pigment epithelial cell line. *Curr. Eye Res.* **13** (1994) 523–529.

113. Ramamoorthy, S., Leibach, F. H., Mahesh, V. B., and Ganapathy, V. Selective impairment of taurine transport by cyclosporin A in a human placental cell line. *Pediatr. Res.* **32** (1992) 125–127.

114. Ramamoorthy, S., Leibach, F. H., Mahesh, V. B., Han, H., Yang-Feng, T., Blakely, R. D., and Ganapathy, V. Functional characterization and chromosomal localization of a cloned taurine transporter from human placenta. *Biochem. J.* **300** (1994) 893–900.

115. Rasola, A., Galietta, L. J. V., Barone, V., Romeo, G., and Bagnasco, S. Molecular cloning and functional characterization of a GABA/betaine transporter from human kidney. *FEBS Lett.* **373** (1995) 229–233.

116. Rhoads, D. E., Peterson, N. E., and Raghupathy, E. Selective inhibition of synaptosomal proline uptake by leucine and methionine enkephalins. *J. Biol. Chem.* **258** (1983) 12,233–12,237.

117. Richens, A., Chadwick, D., and Duncan, J. Safety and efficacy of tiagabine as adjunctive treatment for complex partial seizures. *Epilepsia* **33(Suppl. 3)** (1992) 119 (abstract).

118. Rowan, A. J., Ahmann, P., Wannamaker, B., Schacter, S., Rask, C., and Uthman, B. Safety and efficacy of three dose levels of tiagabine HCl versus placebo as adjunctive treatment for complex partial seizures. *Epilepsia* **34(Suppl. 2)** (1993) 157 (abstract).

119. Ruiz, M., Egal, H., Sarthy, V., Qian, X., and Sarkar, H. K. Cloning, expression, and localization of a mouse retinal γ-aminobutyric acid transporter. *Invest. Ophthalmol. Visual Sci.* **35** (1994) 4039–4048.

120. Sato, K., Adams, R., Betz, H., and Schloss, P. Modulation of a recombinant glycine transporter (GLYT1b) by activation of protein kinase C. *J. Neurochem.* **65** (1995) 1967–1973.

121. Schloss, P., Mayser, W., and Betz, H. The putative rat choline transporter CHOT1 transports creatine and is highly expressed in neural and muscle-rich tissues. *Biochem. Biophys. Res. Comm.* **198** (1994) 637–645.

122. Sheardown, M. J., Weis, J. U., Knutsen, L. I. S., et al. Analgesic effect of the GABA uptake inhibitor NO-328. *Soc. Neurosci. Abstracts* **15** (1989) 602 (abstract).

123. Shafqat, S., Velaz-Faircloth, M., Henzi, V., Yang-Feng, T., Seldin, M., and Fremeau, R. T., Jr. Human brain-specific L-proline transporter: molecular cloning, pharmacological characterization, and chromosomal localization of the gene in human and mouse genomes. *Mol. Pharmacol.* **48** (1995) 219–229.

124. Simpson, M. D. C., Slater, P., Royston, M. C., and Deakin, J. F. W. Regionally selective deficits in uptake sites for glutamate and gamma-aminobutyric acid in the basal ganglia in schizophrenia. *Psychiatry Res.* **42** (1992) 273–282

125. Smith, S. E. Kinetics of neutral amino acid transport in rat brain *in vitro*. *J. Neurochemistry* **14** (1967) 291–300.

126. Smith, K. E., Borden, L. A., Hartig, P. R., Branchek, T., and Weinshank, R. L. Cloning and expression of a glycine transporter reveal colocalizaion with NMDA receptors. *Neuron* **8** (1992) 927–935.

127. Smith, K. E., Borden, L. A., Wang, C.-H. D., Hartig, P. R., Branchek, T. A., and Weinshank, R. L. Cloning and expression of a high affinity taurine transporter from rat brain. *Mol. Pharmacol.* **42** (1992) 563–569.

128. Snow, H., Lowrie, M. B., and Bennett, J. P. A postsynaptic GABA transporter in rat spinal motor neurons. *Neurosci. Lett.* **143** (1992) 119–122.

129. Sora, I., Richman, J., Santoro, G., Wei, H., Wang, Y., Vaerah, T., Horvath, R., Nguyen, M., Waite, S., Roeske, W. R., and Yamamura, H. I. The cloning and expression of a human creatine transporter. *Biochem. Biophys. Res. Comm.* **204** (1994) 419–427.

130. Stevens, B. R., Kaunitz, J. D., and Wright, E. M. Intestinal transport of amino acids and sugars: advances using membrane vesicles. *Ann. Rev. Physiol.* **46** (1984) 417–433.

131. Strader, C. D., Sigal, I. S., and Dixon, R. A. Structural basis of beta-adrenergic receptor function. *FASEB J.* **3** (1989) 1825–1832.

132. Sturman, J. A. Taurine deficiency. *Prog. Clin. Biol. Res.* **351** (1990) 385–395.

133. Suzdak, P. D., Frederiksen, K., Andersen, K. E., Sørensen, P. O., Knutsen, L. J. S., and Nielsen, F. B. NNC-711, a novel potent and selective γ-aminobutyric acid uptake inhibitor: pharmacological characterization. *Eur. J. Pharmacol.* **224** (1992) 189–198.

134. Suzdak, P. D. and Jansen, J. A. A review of the preclinical pharmacology of tiagabine: a potent and selective anticonvulsant GABA uptake inhibitor. *Epilepsia* **36** (1995) 612–626.

135. Swan, M., Najlerahim, A., Watson, R. E. B., and Bennett, J. P. Distribution of mRNA for the GABA transporter GAT-1 in the rat brain: evidence that GABA uptake is not limited to presynaptic neurons. *J. Anat.* **185** (1994) 315–323.

136. Swanson, G. T., Umbach, J. A., and Gundersen, C. B. Glia of the cholinergic electromotor nucleus of *Torpedo* are the source of the cDNA encoding a GAT-1 GABA transporter. *J. Neurochem.* **63** (1994) 1–12.

137. Sweet, H. O. Clasper *(cla). Mouse News Lett.* **73** (1985) 18.

138. Swinyard, E. A., White, H. S., Wolf, H. H., and Bondinell, W. E. Anticonvulsant profiles of the potent and orally active GABA uptake inhibitors SK&F 89976-A and SK&F 100330-A and four prototype antiepileptic drugs in mice and rats. *Epilepsia* **32** (1991) 569–577.

139. Takenaka, M., Bagnasco, S. M., Preston, A. S., Uchida, S., Yamauchi, A., Kwon, H. M., and Handler, J. S. The canine betaine γ-amino-n-butyric acid transporter gene: diverse mRNA isoforms are regulated by hypertonicity and are expressed in a tissue-specific manner. *Proc. Natl. Acad. Sci. USA* **92** (1995) 1072–1076.

140. Takenaka, M., Preston, A. S., Kwon, H. M., and Handler, J. S. The tonicity-sensitive element that mediates increased transcription of the betaine transporter gene in response to hypertonic stress. *J. Biol. Chem.* **269** (1991) 29,379–29,381.

141. Tamura, S., Nelson, H., Tamura, A., and Nelson, N. Short external loops as potential substrate binding site of γ-aminobutyric acid transporters. *J. Biol. Chem.* **270** (1995) 28,712–28,715.

142. Taylor, C. P., Vartanian, M. G., Schwarz, R. D., Rock, D. M., Callahan, M. J., and Davis, M. D. Pharmacology of CI-966: a potent GABA uptake inhibitor, in vitro and in experimental animals. *Drug Dev. Res.* **21** (1990) 195–215.

143. Tian, Y., Kapatos, G., Granneman, J. G., and Bannon, M. J. Dopamine and γ-aminobutyric acid transporters: differential regulation by agents that promote phosphorylation. *Neurosci. Lett.* **173** (1994) 143–146.

144. Uchida, S., Kwon, H. M., Yamauchi, A., Preston, A. S., Maruma, E., and Handler, J. S. Molecular cloning of the cDNA for an MDCK cell Na^+- and Cl^--dependent taurine transporter that is regulated by hypertonicity. *Proc. Natl. Acad. Sci. USA* **89** (1992) 8230–8234.

145. Uchida, S., Kwon, H. M., Yamauchi, A., Preston, A. S., Maruma, F., and Handler, J. S. Correction to reference 12. *Proc. Natl. Acad. Sci USA.* **90** (1993) 7424.

146. Uchida, S., Yamauchi, A., Preston, A. S., Kwon, H. M., and Handler, J. S. Medium tonicity regulates expression of the Na^+- and Cl^--dependent betaine transporter in Madin-Darby canine kidney cells by increasing transcription of the transporter gene. *J. Clin. Invest.* **91** (1993) 1604–1607.

147. Varon, S., Weinstein, H., and Roberts, E. Exogenous and endogenous γ-aminobutyric acid of mouse brain particulates in a binding system *in vitro*. *Biochem. Pharmacol.* **13** (1964) 269–279.

148. Velaz-Faircloth, M., Guadano-Ferraz, A., Henzi, V., and Fremeau, R. T., Jr. Mammalian brain-specific L-proline transporter: neuronal localization of mRNA and enrichment of transporter protein in synaptic plasma membranes. *J. Biol. Chem.* **270** (1995) 15,755–15,761.

149. Waldmeier, P. C., Stöcklin, K., and Feldtrauer, J. -J. Weak effects of local and systemic administration of the GABA uptake inhibitor, SK&F 89976, on extracellular GABA in the rat striatum. *Naunyn-Schmiedeberg's Arch. Pharmacol.* **345** (1992) 544–547.

150. Wang, C. D., Buck, M. A., and Fraser, C. M. Site-directed mutagenesis of alpha 2A-adrenergic receptors: identification of amino acids involved in ligand binding and receptor activation by agonists. *Mol. Pharmacol.* **40** (1991) 168–179.

151. White, W. F. and Heller, A. H. Glycine receptor alteration in the mutant mouse *spastic*. *Nature* **298** (1982) 655–657.

152. Wong, P. T.-H. Interactions of indomethacin with central GABA systems. *Arch. Internat. Pharmacodynam.* **324** (1993) 5–16.

153. Wright, C. E., Tallan, H. H., Lin, Y. Y., and Gaull, G. E. Taurine: biological update. *Ann. Rev. Biochem.* **55** (1986) 427–453.

154. Yamauchi, A., Kwon, H. M., Uchida, S., Preston, A. S., and Handler, J. S. Myo-inositol and betaine transporters regulated by tonicity are basolateral in MDCK cells. *Am. J. Physiol.* **261(1 Pt 2)** (1991) F197–202.

155. Yamauchi, A., Uchida, S., Kwon, H. M., Preston, A. S., Robey, R. B., Garcia-Perez, A., Berg, M. B., and Handler, J. S. Cloning of a Na^+- and Cl^--dependent betaine transporter that is regulated by hypertonicity. *J. Biol. Chem.* **267** (1992) 649–652.

156. Yunger, L. M., Fowler, P. J., Zarevics, P., and Setler, P. E. Novel inhibitors of γ-aminobutyric acid (GABA) uptake: anticonvulsant actions in rats and mice. *J. Pharmacol. Exp. Ther.* **228** (1984) 109–115.

157. Zafra, F., Aragón, C., Olivares, L., Danbolt, N. C., Giménez, C., and Storm-Mathisen, J. Glycine transporters are differentially expressed among CNS cells. *J. Neurosci.* **15** (1995) 3952–3969.
158. Zafra, F. and Giménez, C. Characteristics and adaptive regulation of glycine transport in cultured glial cells. *Biochem. J.* **258** (1989) 403–408.
159. Zafra, F., Gomeza, J., Olivares, L., Aragón, C., and Giménez, C. Regional distribution and developmental variation of the glycine transporters GLYT1 and GLYT2 in the rat CNS. *Eur. J. Neurosci.* **7** (1995) 1342–1352.

CHAPTER 5

Sodium-Coupled GABA and Glutamate Transporters

Structure and Function

Baruch I. Kanner

Introduction

Sodium-coupled neurotransmitter transporters, located in the plasma membrane of nerve terminals and glial processes, serve to keep the extracellular transmitter levels below those which are neurotoxic. Moreover, they help, in conjunction with diffusion, to terminate its action in synaptic transmission. Such a termination mechanism operates with most transmitters, including γ-aminobutyric acid (GABA), L-glutamate, glycine, dopamine, serotonin, and norepinephrine. Another termination mechanism is observed with cholinergic transmission. After dissociation from its receptor, acetylcholine is hydrolyzed into choline and acetate. The choline moiety is then recovered by sodium-dependent transport as described. Since the concentration of the transmitters in the nerve terminals is typically as much as four orders of multitude higher than in the cleft, energy input is required. The transporters that are located in the plasma membranes of nerve endings and glial cells obtain this energy by coupling the flow of neurotransmitters to that of sodium. The $(Na^+ + K^+)$-ATPase generates an inwardly-directed electrochemical sodium gradient that is utilized by the transporters to drive uphill transport of the neurotransmitters (reviewed in refs. 30–32). Neurotransmitter uptake systems have been investigated in detail by using plasma membranes obtained on osmotic shock of synaptosomes. It appears that these transporters are coupled not

Neurotransmitter Transporters: Structure, Function, and Regulation
Ed.: M.E.A. Reith Humana Press Inc, Totowa, NJ

only to sodium, but also to additional ions like potassium or chloride (Table 1).

These transporters are of considerable medical interest. Since they function to regulate activity of neurotransmitters by removing them from the synaptic cleft, specific transporter inhibitors can potentially be used as novel drugs for treatment of neurological diseases. For instance, attenuation of GABA removal will prolong the effect of this inhibitory transporter, thereby potentiating its action. Consequently, inhibitors of GABA transport could represent a novel class of antiepileptic drugs. Well-known inhibitors that interfere with the functioning of biogenic amine transporters include antidepressant drugs and stimulants, such as amphetamines and cocaine. The neurotransmitter glutamate, at excessive local concentrations, causes cell death by activating N-methyl-D-aspartic acid (NMDA) receptors and subsequent calcium entry. The transmitter has been implicated in neuronal destruction during ischemia, epilepsy, stroke, amyotropic lateral sclerosis, and Huntington's disease. Neuronal and glial glutamate transporters may have a critical role in preventing glutamate from acting as an excitotoxin (28,56).

In the last few years, major advances have been made in the cloning of these neurotransmitter transporters. After the GABA transporter was purified (64), the ensuing protein sequence information was used to clone it (23). Subsequently, the expression cloning of a norepinephrine transporter (59) provided evidence that these two proteins are the first members of a novel superfamily of neurotransmitter transporters. Using polymerase chain reaction (PCR) and other technologies relying on sequence conservation, this result led to the isolation of a growing list of neurotransmitter transporters (reviewed in refs. 1,68,78). This list includes various subtypes of GABA transporters, as well as those for all the aforementioned neurotransmitters, except glutamate. All of the members of this superfamily that are dependent on sodium and chloride and, by analogy, with the GABA transporter (39) are likely to cotransport their transmitter with both sodium and chloride. Sodium-dependent glutamate transport is not chloride-dependent, but rather sodium and glutamate are countertransported with potassium (Table 1; [33,35]). A few years ago three distinct but highly related glutamate transporters were cloned (29,61,73). Very recently a fourth subtype was cloned, exhibiting a large chloride conductance (18). These transporters represent a distinct family of transporters. The following describes the current status on two prototypes of these distinct families: the GABA and glutamate transporters.

Table 1

Comparison of GABA and Glutamate Transporters

Property	GABA transporters	Glutamate transporters
Cosubstrates	Na^+, Cl^-	Na^+, K^+ (OH^- or H^+)
Electrogenicity	+	+
Localization	Neuronal, glial	Neuronal, glial
Sociology	Belong to large family of transporters for all neurotransmitters excluding glutamate	Belong to separate small family of glutamate transporters
Relationship to bacterial transporters	–	glt-P, glutamate transporter dct-A, dicarboxylic acid transporter
Predicted topology	12 TMs amino and carboxyl termini are cytoplasmic	6–10 TMs amino and carboxyl termini are cytoplasmatic
Glycosylation	+	+
Possible regulation	Protein kinase C	Protein kinase C arachidonic acid
Pore domain	Not yet identified	Confined to a short conserved stretch in the carboxyl terminal half of the transporter

Mechanism

The GABA transporter cotransports the neurotransmitter with sodium and chloride in an electrogenic fashion ([*30,39*]; Table 1; Fig. 1A). The available measurements include tracer fluxes (*39*) and electrophysiological approaches (*36,54*). The latter approach reveals that at very negative (inside) potentials, the chloride-dependency is not absolute (*54*). It is not now clear what the mechanistic interpretation of this result is. One possibility is that under these conditions, another anion, such as hydroxyl, may take over the role of chloride. In addition, a transient current is observed in the absence of GABA. This transient can be blocked by bulky GABA analogs, which can bind to the transporter, but are not translocated by it (*54*). It probably reflects a conformational change of the transporter occurring after the sodium has bound. These measurements also permit determination

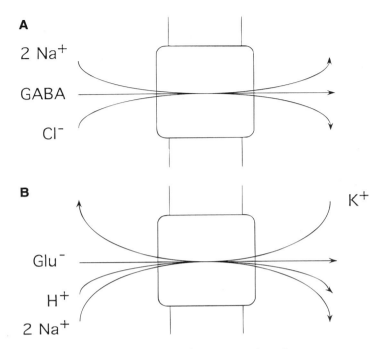

Fig. 1. Schematic representation of GABA and L-glutamate transport. The diagrams illustrate the coupled fluxes of GABA **(A)** and L-glutamate **(B)** with their cosubstrates. As indicated in the text, it is equally possible that an hydroxyl ion is countertransported, rather than the cotransport of a proton (or a hydronium ion).

of the turnover number of the transporter. These estimates of a few cycles per second (*54*) are in agreement with biochemical ones (*64*). It is of interest to note that, although both GABA and 5-HT transporters belong to the same transporter superfamily (Table 1), the latter one appears to exhibit quite distinct properties (*53*). It appears that the 5-HT transporter is electroneutral, but that a transporter-associated current can be detected. This is probably related to the observation that under some conditions this transporter may act as a channel. This transporter-channel appears to be less sodium-selective than the transporter mode that is carrying 5-HT in a coupled fashion (*53*).

The mechanism of sodium-dependent L-glutamate transport has been studied, initially using tracer flux studies employing radioactive glutamate. These studies indicated that the process is electrogenic, with positive charge moving in the direction of the glutamate (*35*). This observation suggested that it is possible to monitor L-glutamate transport electrically, using the whole-cell patch-clamp technique (*10*). In addition to L-glutamate, D- and L-aspartate are transportable substrates with affinities in the lower micromolar range. The system is stereospecific regarding glutamate, the D-isomer being a poor substrate. Glutamate uptake is driven by an inwardly directed sodium ion gradient and at the same time potassium is moving outwards. The potassium movement is not a passive movement in response to the charge carried by the transporter. Rather, it is an integral part of the translocation cycle catalyzed by the transporter. Its role is further described below. Recently, evidence has been presented that another ionic species (hydroxyl ions) is countertransported (in addition to potassium) (*9*).

The first-order dependence of the carrier current on internal potassium (*4*), together with the well-known first-order dependence on external L-glutamate and sigmoid dependence on external sodium, suggest a stoichiometry of $3Na^+:1K^+:1glutamate$ (*4,35*). This stoichiometry implies that one positive charge moves inward per glutamate anion entering the cell. If a hydroxyl anion is countertransported as well (*9*), the stoichiometry could be $2Na^+:1K^+:1glutamate:1OH^-$, and transport would still be electrogenic. However, the alternative, that a proton moves in, together with the sodium and the glutamate, is possible with an equal probability (Fig. 1B). A stoichiometry of $2Na^+:1glutamate$ is also favored by direct experimental evidence obtained by kinetic (*72*) and thermodynamic methods (*17*).

The study of the ion-dependence of partial reactions of the glutamate transporter has revealed that glutamate transport is an ordered process. First sodium and glutamate are translocated. After their release inside the cell, potassium binds and is translocated outward so that a new cycle can be initiated (*33,62*). Using electrophysiological methods, it has been possible to monitor binding of sodium to the glutamate transporter (*82*). The turnover number of the transporter (a few per second) is in the same order of that of the GABA transporter (*82,15*).

Reconstitution, Purification, and Localization

Using methodology that enables one to reconstitute many samples simultaneously and rapidly, one of the subtypes of the GABA (*64*) as well as of the L-glutamate transporter (*15*) has been purified to an apparent homogeneity. Both are glycoproteins and both have an apparent molecular mass of 70–80 kDa. The two transporters retain all the properties observed in membrane vesicles. They are distinct, not only because of their different functional properties, but also because antibodies generated against the GABA transporter (*64*) react (as detected by immunoblotting) only with fractions containing GABA transport activity, and not with those containing L-glutamate transport activity (*15*). The opposite is true for antibodies generated against the glutamate transporter (*16*). Recently, the glycine transporter has been purified and reconstituted as well. Interestingly, it appears to be a larger protein (approx 100 kDa) than the GABA and glutamate transporters (*50*). The serotonin transporter has also been purified, but these preparations, containing a band around 70 kDa, have been shown to be active only in the binding of [^{3}H]imipramine, but not in serotonin transport (*20,43*). Immunocytochemical localization studies of the GABA transporter revealed that in most brain areas it is located in the membranes of nerve terminals (*65*), although in some areas, such as substantia nigra, glial processes were labeled (Table 1).

Using the antibodies raised against the glutamate transporter, the immunocytochemical localization of the transporter was studied with light and electron microscopes in rat central nervous system. In all regions examined (including cerebral cortex, caudato-putamen, corpus callosum, hippocampus, cerebellum, and spinal cord) it was found to be located in glial cells rather than in neurons. In particular, fine astrocytic processes were strongly stained. Putative glutamatergic axon terminals appeared nonimmunoreactive (*16*). The uptake of glutamate by such terminals (for which there is strong previous evidence), therefore, may be caused by a subtype of glutamate transporter different from the glial transporter. Using a monoclonal antibody raised against this transporter, a similar glial localization of the transporter was found (*25*). Another glial transporter, as well as a neuronal one, has been identified (*see* Molecular Cloning and Predicted Structure of Glutamate Transporters).

The Large Superfamily of Na$^+$-Dependent Neurotransmitter Transporters

Partial sequencing of the purified GABA$_A$ transporter allowed the cloning of the first member of the new family of Na-dependent neurotransmitter transporters (*23*). After expression and cloning of the noradrenaline transporter (*59*), it became clear that it had significant homology with the GABA$_A$ transporter. The use of functional cDNA expression assays and amplification of related sequences by PCR resulted in the cloning of additional transporters that belong to this family, such as the dopamine (*40,70,79*) and serotonin (*7,26*) transporters, additional GABA transporters (*8,13,45,49*), transporters of glycine (*22,48,71*), proline (*19*), taurine (*47,77*), betaine (*83*), and orphan transporters, whose substrates are still unknown. In addition, another family member that was originally thought to be a choline transporter (*55*), probably is, in fact, a creatine transporter (*24*). A novel glycine transporter cDNA encoding for a 799 amino acid protein has recently been isolated (*46*). This is significantly longer than most members of the superfamily. If part of the mass of these transporters is constituted by sugar, it could encode for the 100 kDa glycine transporter that was purified and reconstituted (*49*).

The deduced amino acid sequences of these proteins reveal 30–65% identity between different members of the family. Based on these differences in homology, the family can be divided into four subgroups:

1. Transporters of biogenic amines (noradrenaline, dopamine, and serotonin);
2. Various GABA transporters, as well as transporters of taurine and creatine;
3. Transporters of proline and glycine; and
4. Orphan transporters.

These proteins share some features of a common secondary structure. Each transporter is composed of 12 hydrophobic putative transmembrane α-helices. The lack of a signal peptide suggests that both amino- and carboxy-termini face the cytoplasm. These regions contain putative phosphorylation sites that may be involved in regulation of the transport process (*see* Regulation of Neurotransmitter Transport). The second extracellular loop between helices 3 and 4 is the largest, and it contains putative glycosylation sites.

Alignment of the deduced amino acid sequences of 13 different members of this superfamily, whose substrates are known (subgroups 1–3) revealed that some segments within these proteins share a higher degree of homology than others. The most highly conserved regions (>50% homology) are helix 1, together with the extracellular loop connecting it with helix 2, and helix 5, together with a short intracellular loop connecting it with helix 4, and a larger extracellular loop connecting it with helix 6. These domains may be involved in stabilizing a tertiary structure that is essential for the function of all these transporters. Alternatively, they may be related to a common function of these transporters, such as the translocation of sodium ions. The region stretching on from helix 9 is far less conserved than the segment containing the first eight helices. Possibly, this domain contains some residues that are involved in translocating the different substrates. The least conserved segments are the amino- and carboxy-termini. As mentioned, these areas may be involved in regulation of the transport process. The orphan transporters differ from all other members of the family in three regions. They contain much larger extracellular loops between helices 7–8 and helices 11–12 and have a shorter extracellular loop connecting helices 3–4.

Molecular Cloning and Predicted Structure of Glutamate Transporters

Transporters for many neurotransmitters were cloned on the assumption that they are related to the GABA (*23*) and norepinephrine (*59*) transporters (*1,68,78*). This approach was unsuccessful for the glutamate transporter. Three different glutamate transporters were cloned by different approaches: GLAST (*73*), GLT-1 (*61*), and EAAC 1 (*29*). The former two appear to be of glial (*16,44,61,73*), the latter of neuronal, origin (*29,67*). It is not yet known whether the newly cloned EAAT-4 (*18*) is neuronal or glial. Indeed, the three transporters are not related to the above superfamily (*29,61,73*). On the other hand, they are very similar to each other, displaying ~50% identity and ~60% similarity. They also appear to be related to the proton-coupled glutamate transporter from *Escherichia coli* and other bacteria (glt-P, [*75*]) and the dicarboxylate transporter (dct-A, [*27*]) of *Rhizobium meliloti*. In these cases the identities are around 25–30%, so they form a distinct family. They contain between 500–600 amino acids. It has been shown that this family also encodes sodium-dependent transporters that do not use dicarboxylic acids as substrates, but rather neutral amino acids (*3,69*). Recently, the three human homologs of the rat brain glutamate transporters have been cloned (*2*), as well as a novel subtype that is characterized by a large substrate-induced chloride current (*18*). A similar but smaller current, which is not thermodynamically coupled to glutamate transport, has been observed in several of the other subtypes as well (*81*).

GLT-1, which encodes the glutamate transporter that was purified (*15,16,61*), has 573 amino acids and a relative molecular mass of 64 kDa, in good agreement with the value of 65 kDa of the purified and deglycosylated transporter (*16*). Hydropathy plots are relatively straightforward at the amino terminal side of the protein and the three different groups have predicted six transmembrane α-helices at very similar positions (29,61,73). On the other hand, there is much more ambiguity at the carboxyl side, where zero (73), two (61), or four (29) α-helices have been predicted. However, all three groups note uncertainty in assigning transmembrane α-helices in this part of the protein, taking into account alternative possibilities, including membrane-spanning β-sheets (73). It is clear that experimental approaches to delineate their topology are badly needed.

Regulation of Neurotransmitter Transport

It is conceivable that the reuptake process is subject to physiological regulation. However, our knowledge of this aspect of neurotransmitter function is rudimentary. It has been shown that arachidonic acid, which may be released via phospholipase A2, can inhibit several sodium-coupled uptake systems (66), including the uptake systems for glycine (84) and glutamate (5). Glutamate transport in rat brain membrane preparations is inhibited by arachidonate, and this compound also inhibits the purified and reconstituted glutamate transporter GLT-1 (76). However, the situation is more complex, because transport mediated by GLT-1 expressed in oocytes is stimulated by arachidonate, though the converse is true for another glutamate transporter (85). Nieoullon et al. (57) found that in vivo electrical stimulation (for 10 min) of frontal cortex increased high-affinity glutamate uptake in rat striatum. The increase was because of an increase in affinity. The uptake measurements were done in tissue samples dissected out 20 min after the cessation of stimulation. This increase from basal level could be inhibited by dopaminergic activity (37). The existence of putative phosphorylation sites (61) indicates that this glial glutamate transporter may be regulated by protein kinases and phosphatases. The finding that glutamate transport activity (V_{max}, but not K_m) is increased in cultured glial cells after incubation of the cells with phorbol esters (12), suggests that the putative phosphorylation sites are physiologically relevant. The author has provided evidence that this stimulation of glutamate transport by phorbol esters is caused by a direct phosphorylation of the transporter by protein kinase C. A single serine residue (serine 113), located in the loop connecting putative transmembrane helices 2 and 3, appears to be the major site of this phosphorylation (11).

In the case of the GABA transporter, modulation of GABA transport activity by phorbol esters has been reported. However, this phenomenon remains unclear because one group reported stimulation by the phorbol ester (14) and another group found preincubation of oocytes with this compound to be inhibiting (58).

Structure–Function Relationships in the Superfamily of Neurotransmitter Transporters

It has been shown that parts of amino- and carboxyl-termini of the $GABA_A$ transporter are not required for function (51). In order to define these domains, a series of deletion mutants was studied in the GABA transporter (6). Transporters truncated at either end until just a few amino-acids, distant from the beginning of helix 1 and the end of helix 12, retained their ability to catalyze sodium- and chloride-dependent GABA transport. These deleted segments did not contain any residues conserved among the different members of the super-family. Once the truncated segment included part of these conserved residues, the transporter's activity was severely reduced. However, the functional damage was not a result of impaired turnover or impaired targeting of the truncated proteins (6).

Fragments of the $(Na^+ + Cl^-)$-coupled $GABA_A$ transporter were produced by proteolysis of membrane vesicles and reconstituted preparations from rat brain (52). The former were digested with pronase, the latter with trypsin. Fragments with different apparent molecular masses were recognized by sequence-directed antibodies raised against this transporter. When GABA was present in the digestion medium, the generation of these fragments was almost entirely blocked (52). At the same time, the neurotransmitter largely prevented the loss of activity caused by the protease. The effect was specific for GABA; protection was not afforded by other neurotransmitters. It was only observed when the two cosubstrates, sodium and chloride, were present on the same side of the membrane as GABA (52). The results indicate that the transporter may exist in two conformations. In the absence of one or more of the substrates, multiple sites located throughout the transporter are accessible to the proteases. In the presence of all three substrates, a condition favoring the formation of the translocation complex, the conformation is changed so that these sites become inaccessible to protease action.

The author's group has investigated the role of the hydrophilic loops connecting the putative transmembrane α-helices connecting GAT-1. Deletions of randomly picked nonconserved single amino acids in the loops connecting helices 7 and 8 or 8 and 9 result in inactive transport on expression in Hela cells. However, transporters where these amino acids are replaced with glycine retain significant activity. The expression levels of the inactive mutant transporters were similar to that of the wild-type, but one of these, ΔVal-348, appears to be defectively targeted to the plasma membrane. The data are compatible with the idea that a minimal length of the loops is required, presumably to enable the transmembrane domains to interact optimally with each other (*34*).

The substrate translocation performed by the various members of the superfamily is sodium- and usually chloride-dependent. In addition, some of the substrates contain charged groups as well. Therefore, charged amino acids in the membrane domain of the transporters may be essential for their normal function. This was tested for the GABA transporter (*60*). Of five charged amino acids within its membrane domain, only one, arginine-69 in helix 1, is absolutely essential for activity (Fig. 2). It is not merely the positive charge that is important, since even its substitution to other positively charged amino acids does not restore activity. The functional damage is not caused by impaired turnover or impaired targeting of the mutated protein. The three other positively charged amino acids and the only negatively charged one are not critical (*60*). It is possible that the arginine-69 residue is involved in chloride binding.

The transporters of biogenic amines contain an additional negatively charged residue in helix 1:aspartate-79 (dopamine transporter numbering). Replacement of aspartate-79 in the dopamine transporter with alanine, glycine, or glutamate, significantly reduced the transport of dopamine, MPP$^+$, (Parkinsonism-inducing neurotoxin), and the binding of CFT (cocaine analog) without affecting B_{max}. Apparently, aspartate-79 in helix 1 interacts with dopamine's amine during the transport process. Serine-356 and serine-359 in helix 7 are also involved in dopamine binding and translocation, perhaps by interacting with the hydroxyls on the catechol (*41*).

Studies of other proteins indicate that in addition to charged amino acids, aromatic amino acids containing π-electrons are also involved in maintaining the structure and function of these proteins (*74*). Therefore, tryptophan residues in the membrane domain of the GABA transporter were mutated into serine as well as leucine (*42*). Mutations at the 68 and 222 position (in helix 1 and helix 4, respectively, Fig. 2) led to a decrease of over 90% of the GABA uptake. On the basis of the alignments of the transporters of the superfamily, it was postulated that tryptophan-222 is involved in the binding of the

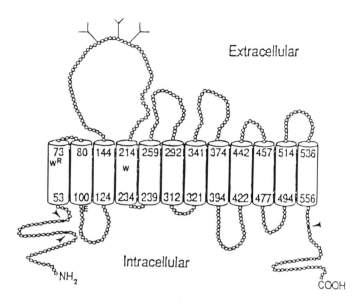

Fig. 2. Proposed topology for the GAT-1 transporter. Putative transmembrane α-helices are indicated as cylinders and individual amino acids as small circles. Also indicated are consensus sites for asparagine-linked glycosylation (Y) and protein kinase C phosphorylation (arrowheads). Amino acid residues critical for activity are indicated using the one letter code (*see* text).

amino group of GABA. The replacement of tryptophan-68 to leucine results in an increased affinity of the transporter for sodium (Mager, S., Kleinberger-Doron, N., Keshet, G., Davidson, N., Kanner, B. I., and Lester, H. A., unpublished experiments). This strongly suggests the involvement of this residue in sodium binding. Recently a glutamate residue, critical for GAT-1 function, has been identified (*38*).

Structure–Function Relationships for the Glutamate Transporters

In the case of the glutamate transporter GLT-1, in addition to the putative protein kinase C consensus sites, the conserved charged amino acids have been mutated and analyzed. These include a conserved lysine located in helix 5 and a histidine (histidine-326) (Fig. 3) in helix 6. The former is not critical, but the latter is (*86*). If, in fact, a proton and not an hydroxyl ion participates in the translocation cycle,

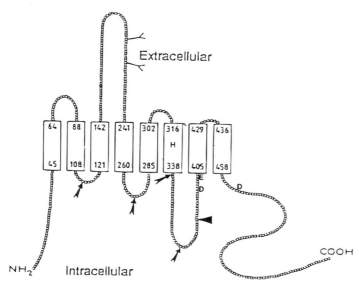

Fig. 3. Proposed topology for the GLT-1 transporter. Putative transmembrane α-helices are indicated as rectangles and individual amino acids as small circles. Also indicated are consensus sites for asparagine-linked glycosylation (Y) and for protein kinase C (arrows) and A (arrowhead) phosphorylation. Amino acid residues critical for activity are indicated using the one letter code (*see* text).

histidine-326 is an excellent candidate to serve as the proton binding site. Furthermore, five conserved negatively charged amino acids are clustered in the carboxy-terminal hydrophobic part of the transporter for which the hydrophaty plot is ambiguous. Three of these residues appear to be critical for the transporter's function (Fig. 3) and one of them, glutamate-404, appears to be involved in the substrate discrimination of the transporter (*63*). A mutation in this residue severely impairs transport of L-glutamate, but transport of D- and L-aspartate is almost unaffected. This suggests that the conserved stretch surrounding glutamate-404 may form the translocation pore of glutamate and aspartate. Evidence to support this comes from experiments in which the determinant of the binding of dihydrokainic acid, a glutamate analog, was found to be located within a stretch of 76 amino acids, in the middle of which is located residue glutamate 404 (*81*).

Substrate-induced conformational changes in the GLT-1 transporter have been detected, as revealed by the altered accessibility of trypsin-sensitive sites to the protease (21). These experiments indicate that lithium can occupy one of the sodium binding sites and also that there are at least two transporter-glutamate bound states (21).

Acknowledgments

I thank Beryl Levene for expert secretarial assistance and Michael P. Kavanaugh for information on important experimental studies prior to publication. The work from the author's laboratory was supported by the Bernard Katz Minerva Center for Cell Biophysics, and by grants from the US–Israel Binational Science Foundation, the Basic Research Foundation administered by the Israel Academy of Sciences and Humanities, the National Institutes of Health, and the Bundesministerium fur Forschung und Technologie.

References

1. Amara, S. G. and Kuhar, M. J. Neurotransmitter transporters: recent progress. *Ann. Rev. Neurosci.* **16** (1993) 73–93.
2. Arriza, J. L., Fairman, W. A., Wadiche, J. I., Murdoch, G. H., Kavanaugh, M. P., and Amara, S. G. Functional comparisons of three glutamate transporter subtypes cloned from human motor cortex. *J. Neurosci.* **14** (1994) 5559–5569.
3. Arriza, J. L., Kavanaugh, M. P., Fairman, W. A., Wu, Y.- N., Murdoch, G. H., North, R. A., and Amara, S. G. Cloning and expression of a human neutral amino acid transporter with structural similarity to the glutamate transporter gene family. *J. Biol. Chem.* **268** (1993) 15,329–15,332.
4. Barbour, B., Brew, H., and Atwell, D. Electrogenic glutamate uptake in glial cells is activated by intracellular potassium. *Nature* **335** (1988) 433–435.
5. Barbour, B., Szatkowski, M., Ingledew, N., and Atwell, D., Arachidonic acid induces a prolonged inhibition of glutamate in glial cells. *Nature* **342** (1989) 918–920.
6. Bendahan, A. and Kanner, B. I. Identification of domains of a cloned rat brain GABA transporter which are not required for its functional expression. *FEBS Lett.* **318** (1993) 41–44.
7. Blakely, R. D., Benson, H. E., Fremeau, R. T., Jr., Caron, M. G., Peek, M. M., Prince, H. K., and Bradley, C. C. Cloning and expression of a functional serotonin transporter from rat brain. *Nature* **353** (1991) 66–70.
8. Borden, L. A., Smith, K. E., Hartig, P. R., Branchek, T. A., and Weinshank, R. L. Molecular heterogeneity of the GABA transport system. *J. Biol. Chem.* **267** (1992) 21,098–21,104.
9. Bouvier, M., Szatkowski, M., Amato, A., and Atwell, D. The glial cell glutamate uptake carrier countertransports pH-changing anions. *Nature* **360** (1992) 471–484.
10. Brew, H. and Atwell, D. Electrogenic glutamate uptake is a major current carrier in the membrane of axolotl retinal glial cells. *Nature* **327** (1987) 707–709.

11. Casado, M., Bendahan, A., Zafra, F., Danbolt, N. C., Aragon, C., Gimenez, C., and Kanner, B. I. Phosphorylation and modulation of brain glutamate transporters by protein kinase C. *J. Biol. Chem.* **268** (1993) 27,313–27,317.

12. Casado, M., Zafra, F., Aragon, C., and Gimenez, C. Activation of high-affinity uptake of glutamate by phorbol esters in primary glial cell cultures. *J. Neurochem.* **57** (1991) 1185–1190.

13. Clark, J. A., Deutch, A. Y., Gallipoli, P. Z., and Amara, S. G. Functional expression and CNS distribution of a β-alanine-sensitive neuronal GABA transporter. *Neuron* **9** (1992) 337–348.

14. Corey, J. L., Davidson, N., Lester, H. A., Brecha, N., and Quick, M. W. Protein kinase C modulates the activity of a cloned γ-aminobutyric acid transporter expressed in *Xenopus* oocytes via a regulated subcellular redistribution of the transporter. *J. Biol. Chem.* **269** (1994) 14,759–14,767.

15. Danbolt, N. C., Pines, G., and Kanner, B. I. Purification and reconstitution of the sodium- and potassium-coupled glutamate transport glycoprotein from rat brain. *Biochemistry* **29** (1990) 6734–6740.

16. Danbolt, N. C., Storm-Mathisen, J., and Kanner, B. I. An [Na$^+$ + K$^+$] coupled L-transporter purified from rat brain is located in glial cell processes. *Neuroscience* **51** (1992) 295–310.

17. Erecinska, M., Wantorsky, D., and Wilson, D. F. Aspartate transport in synaptosomes from rat brain. *J. Biol. Chem.* **258** (1983) 9069–9077.

18. Fairman, W. A., Vandenberg, R. J., Arriza, J. L., Kavanaugh, M. P., and Amara, S. G. An excitatory amino-acid transporter with properties of a ligand-gated chloride channel. *Nature* **375** (1995) 599–603.

19. Fremeau, R. T., Jr., Caron, M. G., and Blakely, R. D. Molecular cloning and expression of a high affinity *l*-proline transporter expressed in putative glutamatergic pathways of rat brain. *Neuron* **8** (1992) 915–926.

20. Graham, D., Esnaud, H., and Langer, S. Z. Partial purification and characterization of the sodium-ion-coupled 5-hydroxytryptamine transporter of rat cerebral cortex. *Biochem. J.* **286** (1992) 801–805.

21. Grunewald, M. and Kanner, B. I. Conformational changes monitored on the glutamate transporter GLT-1 indicate the existence of two neurotransitter bound states. *J. Biol. Chem.* **270** (1995) 17,017–17,024.

22. Guastella, J., Brecha, N., Weigmann, C., and Lester, H. A. Cloning, expression, and localization of a rat brain high affinity glycine transporter. *Proc. Natl. Acad. Sci. USA* **89** (1992) 7189–7193.

23. Guastella, J., Nelson, N., Nelson, H., Czyzyk, L., Keynan, S., Miedel, M. C., Davidson, N., Lester, H., and Kanner, B. I. Cloning and expression of a rat brain GABA transporter. *Science* **249** (1990) 1303–1306.

24. Guimbal, C. and Kilimann, M. W. A Na$^+$-dependent creatine transporter in rabbit brain, muscle, heart and kidney. cDNA cloning and functional expression. *J. Biol. Chem.* **268** (1993) 8418–8421.

25. Hees, B., Danbolt, N. C., Kanner, B. I., Haase, W., Heitmann, K., and Koepsell, H. A monoclonal antibody against a Na$^+$-L-glutamate cotransporter from rat brain. *J. Biol. Chem.* **267** (1992) 23,275–23,281.

26. Hoffman, B. J., Mezey, E., and Brownstein, M. J. Cloning of a serotonin transporter affected by antidepressants. *Science* **254** (1991) 579–580.

27. Jiang, J., Gu, B., Albright, L. M., and Nixon, B. T. Conservation between coding and regulatory elements of *Rhizobium meliloti* and *Rhizobium leguminosarum* dct genes. *J. Bacteriol.* **171** (1989) 5244–5253.

28. Johnston, G. A. R. In Roberts, P. J., Storm-Mathisen, J., and Johnston, G. A. R. (eds.), *Glutamate: Transmitter in the Central Nervous System,* Wiley, Chichester, UK (1981) pp. 77–87.

29. Kanai, Y. and Hediger, M. A. Primary structure and functional characterization of a high affinity glutamate transporter. *Nature* **360** (1992) 467–471.

30. Kanner, B. I. Bioenergetics of neurotransmitter transport. *Biochim. Biophys. Acta* **726** (1983) 293–316.

31. Kanner, B. I. Ion-coupled neurotransmitter transport. *Curr. Opin. Cell Biol.* **1** (1989) 735–738.

32. Kanner, B. I. and Schuldiner, S. Mechanism of transport and storage of neurotransmitters. *CRC Crit. Rev. Biochem.* **22** (1987) 1–39.

33. Kanner, B. I. and Bendahan, A. Binding order of substrates to the sodium and potassium ion coupled L-glutamate transporter from rat brain. *Biochemistry* **21** (1982) 6327–6330.

34. Kanner, B. I., Bendahan, A., Pantanowitz, S., and Su, H. The number of amino acid residues in hydrophillic loops connecting transmembrane domains of the GABA transporter GAT-1 is critical for its function. *FEBS Lett.* **356** (1994) 192–194.

35. Kanner, B. I. and Sharon, I. Active transport of L-glutamate by membrane vesicles isolated from rat brain. *Biochemistry* **17** (1978) 3949–3953.

36. Kavanaugh, M. P., Arriza, J. L., North, R. A., and Amara, S. G. Electrogenic uptake of γ-aminobutyric acid by a cloned transporter expressed in oocytes. *J. Biol. Chem.* **267** (1992) 22,007–22,009.

37. Kerkerian, L., Dusticier, N., and Nieoullon, A. Modulatory effect of dopamine on high-affinity glutamate uptake in the rat striatum. *J. Neurochem.* **48** (1987) 1301–1306.

38. Keshet, G. I., Bendahan, A., Su, H., Mager, S., Lester, H. A., and Kanner, B. I. Glutamate 101 is critical for the function of the sodium and chloride-coupled GABA transporter GAT-1. *FEBS Lett.* **371** (1995) 39–42.

39. Keynan, S. and Kanner, B. I. Gamma-aminobutyric acid transport in reconstituted preparations from rat brain: coupled sodium and chloride fluxes. *Biochemistry* **27** (1988) 12–17.

40. Kilty, J. E., Lorang, D., and Amara, S. G. Cloning and expression of a cocaine-sensitive rat dopamine transporter. *Science* **254** (1991) 578–579.

41. Kitayama, S., Shimada, S., Xu, H., Markham, L., Donovan, D. M., and Uhl, G. R. Dopamine transporter site-directed mutations differentially alter substrate transport and cocaine binding. *Proc. Natl. Acad. Sci. USA* **89** (1992) 7782–7785.

42. Kleinberger-Doron, N. and Kanner, B. I. Identification of tryptophan residues critical for the function and targeting of the γ-aminobutyric acid transporter (subtype A). *J. Biol. Chem.* **269** (1994) 3063–3067.

43. Launay, J. M., Geoffroy, C., Mutel, V., Buckle, M., Cesura, A., Alouf, J. E., and Da-Prada, M. One-step purification of the serotonin transporter located at the human platelet plasma membrane. *J. Biol. Chem.* **267** (1992) 11,344–11,351.

44. Lehre, K. P., Levy, L. M., Ottersen, O. P., Storm-Mathisen, J., and Danbolt, N. C. Differential expression of two glial glutamate transporters in the rat brain: quantitative and immunocytochemical observations. *J. Neurosci.* **15** (1995) 1835–1853.

45. Liu, Q. R., Lopez-Corcuera, B., Mandiyan, S., Nelson, H., and Nelson, N. Molecular characterization of four pharmacology distinct γ-amino-butyric acid transporters in mouse brain. *J. Biol. Chem.* **268** (1993) 2104–2112.

46. Liu, Q. R., Lopez-Corcuera, B., Mandiyan, S., Nelson, H., and Nelson, N. A rat brain cDNA encoding the neurotransmitter transporter with an unusual structure. *J. Biol. Chem.* **268** (1993) 22,802–22,808.

47. Liu, Q. R., Lopez-Corcuera, B., Nelson, H., Mandiyan, S., and Nelson, N. Cloning and expression of a cDNA encoding the transporter of taurine and β-alanine in mouse brain. *Proc. Natl. Acad. Sci. USA* **89** (1992) 12,145–12,149.

48. Liu, Q. R., Nelson, H., Mandiyan, S., Lopez-Corcuera, B., and Nelson, N. Cloning and expression of a glycine transporter from mouse brain. *FEBS Lett.* **305** (1992) 110–114.

49. Lopez-Corcuera, B., Liu, Q. R., Mandiyan, S., Nelson, H., and Nelson, N. Expression of a mouse brain cDNA encoding novel γ-amino-butyric acid transporter. *J. Biol. Chem.* **267** (1992) 17491–17493.

50. Lopez-Corcuera, B., Vazquez, J., and Aragon, C. Purification of the sodium- and chloride-coupled glycine transporter from central nervous system. *J. Biol. Chem.* **266** (1991) 24,809–24,814.

51. Mabjeesh, N. J. and Kanner, B. I. Neither amino nor carboxyl termini are required for function of the sodium- and chloride-coupled gamma-aminobutyric acid transporter from rat brain. *J. Biol. Chem.* **267** (1992) 2563–2568.

52. Mabjeesh, N. J. and Kanner, B. I. The substrates of a sodium- and chloride-coupled γ-aminobutyric acid transporter protect multiple sites throughout the protein against proteolytic cleavage. *Biochemistry* **32** (1993) 8540–8546.

53. Mager, S., Min, C., Henry, D. J., Chavkin, L., Hoffman, B. J., Davidson, N., and Lester, H. A. Conducting states of a mammalian serotonin transporter. *Neuron* **12** (1994) 845–859.

54. Mager, S. J., Naeve, J., Quick, M., Guastella, J., Davidson, N., and Lester, H. A. Steady states, charge movements, and rates for a cloned GABA transporter expressed in *Xenopus* oocytes. *Neuron* **10** (1993) 177–188.

55. Mayser, W., Schloss, P., and Betz, H. Primary structure and functional expression of a choline transporter expressed in the rat nervous system. *FEBS Lett.* **305** (1992) 31–36.

56. McBean, G. J. and Roberts, P. J. Neurotoxicity of glutamate and DL-*threo*-hydroxyaspartate in the rat striatum. *J. Neurochem.* **44** (1985) 247–254.

57. Nieoullon, A., Kerkerian, L., and Dusticier, N. Presynaptic dopaminergic control of high affinity glutamate uptake in the striatum. *Neurosci. Lett.* **43** (1983) 191–196.

58. Osawa, I., Saito, N., Koga, T., and Tanaka, C. Phorbol ester-induced inhibition of GABA uptake by synaptosomes and by *Xenopus* oocytes expressing GABA transporter (GAT1). *Neurosci. Res.* **19** (1994) 287–293.

59. Pacholczyk, T., Blakely, R. D., and Amara, S. G. Expression cloning of a cocaine- and antidepressant-sensitive human noradrenaline transporter. *Nature* **350** (1991) 350–353.

60. Pantanowitz, S., Bendahan, A., and Kanner, B. I. Only one of the charged amino acids located in the transmembrane α-helices of the γ-aminobutyric acid transporter (subtype A) is essential for its activity. *J. Biol. Chem.* **268** (1993) 3222–3225.

61. Pines, G., Danbolt, N. C., Bjoras, M., Zhang, Y., Bendahan, A., Eide, L., Koepsell, H., Storm-Mathisen, J., Seeberg, E., and Kanner, B. I. Cloning and expression of a rat brain L-glutamate transporter. *Nature* **360** (1992) 464–467.

62. Pines, G. and Kanner, B. I. Counterflow of L-glutamate in plasma membrane vesicles and reconstituted preparations from rat brain. *Biochemistry* **29** (1990) 11,209–11,214.

63. Pines, G., Zhang, Y., and Kanner, B. I. Glutamate 404 is involved in the substrate discrimination of GLT-1, a ($Na^+ + K^+$)-coupled glutamate transporter from rat brain. *J. Biol. Chem.* **270** (1995) 17,093–17,097.

64. Radian, R., Bendahan, A., and Kanner, B. I. Purification and identification of the functional sodium- and chloride-coupled gamma-aminobutyric acid transport glycoprotein from rat brain. *J. Biol. Chem.* **261** (1986) 15,437–15,441.

65. Radian, R., Ottersen, O. L., Storm-Mathisen, J., Castel, M., and Kanner, B. I. Immunocytochemical localization of the GABA transporter in rat brain. *J. Neurosci.* **10** (1990) 1319–1330.

66. Rhoads, D. E., Ockner, B. K., Peterson, N. A., and Raghupathy, E. Modulation of membrane transport by free fatty acids: inhibition of synaptosomal sodium-dependent amino acid uptake. *Biochemistry* **22** (1983) 1965–1970.

67. Rothstein, J. D., Martin, L., Levey, A. I., Dykes-Hoberg, M., Jun, L., Wu, D., Nash, N., and Kuncl, R. W. Localization of neuronal and glial glutamate transporters. *Neuron* **13** (1994) 713–725.

68. Schloss, P., Mayser, W., and Betz, H. Neurotransmitter transporters. A novel family of integral plasma membrane proteins. *FEBS Lett.* **307** (1992) 76–78.

69. Shafqat, S., Tamarappoo, B. K., Kilberg, M. S., Puranam, R. S., McNamara, J. O., Guadaño-Ferraz, A., and Fremeau, R. T. Cloning and expression of a novel Na^+-dependent neutral amino acid transporter structurally related to mammalian Na/glutamate cotransporters. *J. Biol. Chem.* **268** (1993) 15,351–15,355.

70. Shimada, S., Kitayama, S., Lin, C. L., Patel, A., Nanthakumar, E., Gregor, P., Kuhar, M., and Uhl, G. Cloning and expression of a cocaine-sensitive dopamine transporter complementary DNA. *Science* **254** (1991) 576–578.

71. Smith, K. E., Borden, L. A., Hartig, P. A., Branchek, T., and Weinshank, R. L. Cloning and expression of a glycine transporter reveal colocalization with NMDA receptors. *Neuron* **8** (1992) 927–935.

72. Stallcup, W. B., Bullock, K., and Baetge, E. E. Coupled transport of glutamate and sodium in a cerebellar nerve cell line. *J. Neurochem.* **32** (1979) 57–65.

73. Storck, T., Schulte, S., Hofmann, K., and Stoffel, W. Structure, expression, and functional analysis of a Na^+-dependent glutamate/aspartate transporter from rat brain. *Proc. Natl. Acad. Sci. USA* **89** (1992) 10,955–10,959.

74. Sussman, J. L. and Silman, I. Acetylcholinesterase: structure and use as a model for specific cation-protein interactions. *Curr. Opin. Struc. Biol.* **2** (1992) 721–729.

75. Tolner, B., Poolman, B., Wallace, B., and Konings, W. N. Revised nucleotide sequence of the gltP gene, which encodes the proton-glutamate-aspartate transport protein of *Escherichia coli* K-12. *J. Bacteriol* **174** (1992) 2391–2393.

76. Trotti, D., Volterra, A., Lehre, K. P., Rossi, D., Gjesdal, O., Racagni, G., and Danbolt, N. C. Arachidonic acid inhibits a purified and reconstituted glutamate transporter directly from the water phase and not via the phosholipid membrane. *J. Biol. Chem.* **270** (1995) 9890–9895.

77. Uchida, S., Kwon, H. M., Yamauchi, A., Preston, A. S., Marumo, F., and Handler, J. S. Molecular cloning of the cDNA for an MDCK cell Na$^+$- and Cl$^-$-dependent taurine transporter that is regulated by hypertonicity. *Proc. Natl. Acad. Sci. USA* **89** (1992) 8230–8234.

78. Uhl, G. R. Neurotransmitter transporters (plus): A promising new gene family. *Trends Neurosci.* **15** (1992) 265–268.

79. Usdin, T. B., Mezey, E., Chen, C., Brownstein, M. J., and Hoffman, B. J. Cloning of the cocaine-sensitive bovine dopamine transporter. *Proc. Natl. Acad. Sci. USA* **88** (1991) 11,168–11,171.

80. Wadiche, J. I., Arriza, J. L., Amara, S. G., and Kavanaugh, M. P. Kinetics of a human glutamate transporter. *Neuron* **14** (1995) 1019–1027.

81. Vandenberg, R. J., Arriza, J. L., Amara, S. G., and Kavanaugh, M. P. Constitutive ion fluxes and substrate binding domains of human glutamate transporters. *J. Biol. Chem.* **270** (1995) 17,668–17,671.

82. Wadiche, J. I., Amara, S. G., and Kavanaugh, M. P. Ion fluxes associated with excitatory amino acid transport. *Neuron* **15** (1995) 721–728.

83. Yamauchi, A., Uchida, S., Kwon, H. M., Preston, A. S., Robey, R. B., Garcia-Perez, A., Burg, M. B., and Handler, J. S. Cloning of a Na$^+$- and Cl$^-$-dependent betaine transporter that is regulated by hypertonicity. *J. Biol. Chem.* **267** (1992) 649–652.

84. Zafra, F., Alcantara, R., Gomeza, J., Aragon, C., and Gimenez, E. Arachidonic acid inhibits glycine transport in cultured glial cells. *Biochem. J.* **271** (1990) 237–242.

85. Zerangue, N., Arriza, J. L., Amara, S. G., and Kavanaugh, M. P. Differential modulation of human glutamate transporter subtypes by arachidonic acid. *J. Biol. Chem.* **270** (1995) 6433–6435.

86. Zhang, Y., Pines, G., and Kanner, B. I. Histidine 326 is critical for the function of GLT-1, a (Na$^+$ + K$^+$)-coupled glutamate transporter from rat brain. *J. Biol. Chem.* **269** (1994) 19,573–19,577.

CHAPTER 6

The High-Affinity Glutamate Transporter Family

Structure, Function, and Physiological Relevance

Yoshikatsu Kanai, Davide Trotti, Stephan Nussberger, and Matthias A. Hediger

Introduction

Extensive studies of glutamate uptake in neurons, glial cells, and epithelial cells, using a variety of preparations, revealed the existence of several transporter subtypes with distinct tissue distributions and kinetic and pharmacologic properties. High-affinity ($K_{0.5} = 1–50\ \mu M$) and low-affinity ($K_{0.5} > 100\ \mu M$) Na^+- and K^+-dependent glutamate transporters were identified in brain, kidney, and intestine (17,19,25,26,50,58,77,82,98). Similar systems were also described in epithelial cells of kidney and intestine. Despite the far-reaching physiologic importance of these excitatory neurotransmitter transporters, progress in this field has been slow until recently, and there was limited information available about the molecular properties and physiological roles of these proteins. The focus of this chapter is on the recent insights into the structure, in vivo functional roles, and pathological implications of high-affinity Na^+- and K^+-dependent glutamate transporters in the central nervous system. We also discuss hypothetical kinetic models addressing the complex transport mechanisms of glutamate transporters that are coupled to the cotransport of Na^+ and H^+, and the countertransport of K^+. We furthermore review recent advances in cloning and characterizing a new group of neutral amino acid transporters that are structurally related to glutamate transporters.

Neurotransmitter Transporters: Structure, Function, and Regulation
Ed. M. E. A. Reith Humana Press Inc., Totowa, NJ

Molecular Cloning of Na⁺- and K⁺-Dependent Glutamate and Neutral Amino Acid Transporters

Four high-affinity glutamate transporters and two neutral amino acid transporters were recently cloned by different approaches. Kanai and Hediger (*38*) isolated a cDNA encoding the neuronal and epithelial high-affinity glutamate transporter EAAC1 (excitatory amino acid carrier 1), using a *Xenopus laevis* oocytes expression cloning approach. This approach relied on the capacity of cDNA clones to induce transport function in oocytes (*32*). To isolate a glutamate transporter cDNA, they began their search in the intestine, because injection of poly(A)⁺RNA extracted from rabbit jejunum into oocytes induced a large increase in the uptake of Na⁺-dependent ¹⁴C-labeled L-glutamate uptake. Size-fractionation of poly(A)⁺RNA using preparative gel electrophoresis resulted in the identification of a 2.4–4.4-kb fraction that showed peak stimulation of L-glutamate uptake. The fraction was used to prepare a cDNA library and the library was screened by injecting in vitro transcribed cDNA into oocytes and measuring the uptake of ¹⁴C-L-glutamate. A cDNA was isolated which encodes a 524-residue protein (EAAC1). The cDNA induced Na⁺-dependent L-glutamate uptake 1300-fold above that of water-injected control oocytes. High-stringency Northern analysis revealed that EAAC1 is expressed strongly in both neuronal and epithelial tissues.

Danbolt et al. (*20*) purified a 73-kDa glycoprotein (GLT-1) (glutamate transporter 1) from crude synaptosome fraction P_2 that, when reconstituted into liposomes, exhibited high-affinity glutamate transport activity. An antibody was then raised against the purified protein and used to isolate a clone from a rat brain cDNA library that encodes a 543-residue protein (*62*). Expression studies in HeLa cells confirmed that it is a high-affinity glutamate transporter.

Storck et al. (*84*) copurified a 66-kDa hydrophobic glycoprotein (GLAST) (glutamate/aspartate transporter) during the isolation of UDPgalactose:ceramide galactosyltransferase. Part of the protein was sequenced by Edman degradation and, based on this sequence, degenerative oligonucleotides were designed to the C-terminus of the protein. These were used as a probe to screen a rat brain cDNA library, and subsequently a cDNA clone was isolated that encoded a 573-residues protein. Expression in *X. laevis* oocytes led to the demonstration that the GLAST is a high-affinity glutamate transporter.

Using a cloning approach that was based on the polymerase chain reaction (PCR)-amplification of cDNA using degenerate oligonucleotide primers, Fairman et al. (22) subsequently isolated a cDNA from a human motor cortex that encodes the glutamate transporter subtype EAAT4 (excitatory amino acid transporter 4). The PCR primers they used corresponded to the conserved regions of EAAC1, GLT-1, and GLAST just N-terminal to the fourth putative transmembrane domain, and within the eighth putative transmembrane domain (*see* Figs. 1 and 2). EAAT4 exhibits 58, 39, and 51% amino acid sequence identity to the human glutamate transporters GLAST, GLT-1, and EAAC1, respectively.

The neutral amino acid transporter ASCT1 was independently isolated by two different laboratories. One laboratory used PCR primers, corresponding to a previously described human hippocampal-expressed sequence tag, to amplify the cDNA encoding the transporter (*78*). The other laboratory screened a human cortex cDNA library using a ^{32}P labeled, 128-fold degenerate oligonucleotide, corresponding to the conserved eighth putative transmembrane domain (*see* Fig. 2; residues 363–383 in Fig. 1) (*2*). Both cDNAs encode the same transporter (ASCT1), which has properties reminiscent of the ASC system (Ala, Ser, and Cys preferring system).

Kanai and coworkers (*92*) recently isolated a second neutral amino acid transporter, ASCT2, from mouse testis. The cDNA encoding this transporter was obtained using degenerative oligonucleotide primers corresponding to the well-conserved region located at the end of the tenth putative membrane domain (*see* Fig. 2). Using the resulting PCR product as a probe, a full-length cDNA was isolated from a mouse testis cDNA library. Based on *Xenopus* oocyte expression studies, ASCT2 also has properties reminiscent of system ASC, yet its functional properties and tissue distribution are distinct from those of ASCT1 (*see* ref. *92* and section on Function Comparison of High-Affinity Transporters).

Molecular Characteristics, Evolutionary Aspects, and Chromosomal Assignments of High-Affinity Glutamate Transporters

The four high-affinity glutamate transporters, EAAC1, GLT-1, GLAST, and EAAT4, are part of a large protein family of prokaryotic and eukaryotic Na$^+$-coupled organic solute transporters. The characteristics of these transporters are summarized in Table 1. EAAC1, GLT-1, GLAST, and EAAT4 exhibit 39–55% amino acid sequence identities with each other (51–55% identity between EAAC1, GLT-1,

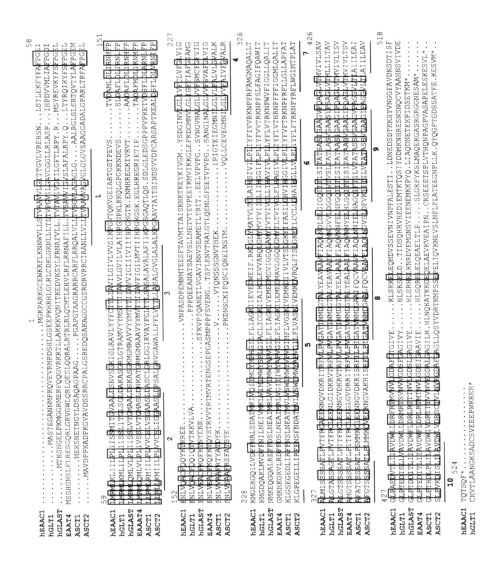

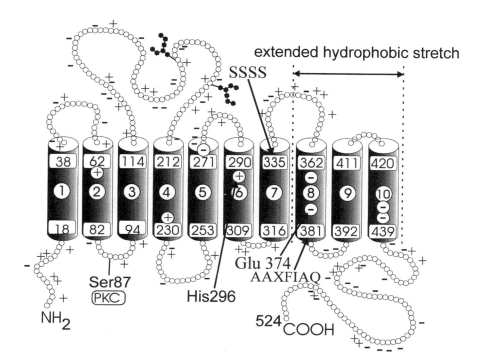

Fig. 2. A structural model for human EAACI. Predicted membrane-spanning regions are indicated (*see* ref. *40*). The exact number of membrane-spanning domains in the highly conserved extended hydrophobic stretch are not known. GLT-1, GLAST, EAAT4, ASCT1, and ASCT2 are predicted to have the same topology. The putative PKC-dependent phosphorylation site PKC at Ser 87 of EAAC1 is marked, as well as potential N-glycosylation sites (N-X-S/T). SSSS indicates the serine-rich motif, AAXFIAQ the conserved motif.

Fig. 1. (*previous page*) Alignment of the human glutamate transporters EAAC1, GLAST, and GLT-1, the human neutral amino acid transporter ASCT1, and the mouse neutral amino acid transporter ASCT2. Residues identical between all sequences are framed. Predicted membrane spanning regions of human EAAC1 are shown by lines below the sequences. Numbers above the sequences refer to the amino acid sequence of human EAAC1 (*41*). In ref. *1*, the human glutamate transporters EAAC1, GLAST, and GLT-1 are referred to as EAAT3, EAAT1, and EAAT2, respectively.

Table 1
Charateristics of High-Affinity Glutamate Transporters

Name of protein	EAAC 1	GLT-1	GLAST	EAAT4
Human gene/ chromosomal loc.	SLC1A1/9p21	SLC1A2/ 11p	SLC1A3/5p13	ND
Tissue origin	Rabbit small intestine	Rat brain	Rat brain	Human cerebellum
Size (amino acids)	524	543	573	564
% Identity to EAAC1	100%	55%	51%	48%
Tissue distribution	Brain, intestine, kidney, liver, heart	Brain, liver	Brain (in particular cerebellum) heart, lung, skeletal muscle, placenta	Cerebellum, placenta
Cellular localization	Neurons, throughout CNS; epithelia	Astrocytes, through-out CNS	Astrocytes, throughout CNS	Purkinje cells
K_m for L-glutamate (X. *oocytes*)	30 μM (human)	18 μM (human)	20 μM (human)	2.5 μM (human)
Sensitivity to uptake inhibitors	THA>PDC>SOS>> AAD>>DHK	PDC>THA>DHK> KA>>SOS	THA>PDC>SOS>>DHK	PDC>AAD>>KA

and GLAST). The neutral amino acid transporters ASCT1 and ASCT2 are 57% identical to each other and show 40–44% sequence identity to the cloned glutamate transporters. An alignment of the glutamate and neutral amino acid transporters is presented in Fig. 1. All these transporters also have significant homology to the H^+-coupled GLTP glutamate transporters of *Escherichia coli, B. stearothermophilus*, and *B. caldotenax*, and to the DCTA dicarboxylate transporter of *Rhizobiurn meliloti*, with sequence identities ranging from 27–32% (*see* ref. *40* for review). There is no significant homology with other Na^+-coupled transporters, such as members of the Na^+- and Cl^--dependent GABA/neurotransmitter transporter family (*see* Chapters 1, 4, and 5) or members of the Na^+/glucose cotransporter family (*32*).

All eukaryotic and prokaryotic high-affinity glutamate transporter family members appear to have the same topology in the membrane, with approx 10 transmembrane domains (Fig. 2). The presence of a large hydrophobic stretch near the C-terminus (residues 356–438) (Fig. 2) is unique and suggests that a major portion of this region is embedded in the membrane. Since it is difficult to predict the exact number of transmembrane domains for this region, alternative models with fewer membrane-spanning domains can be predicted.

According to the nomenclature of the Human Genome Database, the names for the human EAAC1, GLT-1, GLAST, and EAAT4 genes are SLC1A1, SLC1A2, SLC1A3, and SLC1A4, respectively. SLC1 refers to solute carrier family number 1 and A1 to family member number 1. Fluorescence *in situ* hybridization studies of human metaphase chromosome spreads revealed that SLC1A1 resides on chromosome 9p21 (*81*), SLC1A2 on the short arm of human chromosome 11 (*48*), and SLC1A3 on chromosome 5p13 (*44*) (Table 1). These gene loci have not yet been linked to diseases.

Functional and Kinetic Properties of High-Affinity Glutamate Transporters

Stoichiometry of High-Affinity Glutamate Transporters

High-affinity glutamate transporters are coupled to the inwardly directed electrochemical potential gradients of Na^+, K^+ and H^+ (or, alternatively, OH^-). This unique coupling stoichiometry allows efficient removal of glutamate from extracellular fluids, such as the cerebrospinal fluid (CSF), the intestinal lumen, and the lumen of renal proximal tubules. Knowledge of the precise coupling stoichiometry is therefore important, because it determines the concentrating capacity of these transporters. In addition, the ion-dependence and the voltage-dependence of glutamate uptake is predicted to have direct pathological implications. For example, during brain ischemia after a stroke, when extracellular K^+ rises, extracellular Na^+ decreases, and the membrane depolarizes, the electrochemical gradients for these ions fail to drive removal of extracellular glutamate from the CSF, resulting in accumulation of extracellular glutamate to neurotoxic levels (*see* Glutamate Transporters and Ischemia).

Coupling Stoichiometry of High-Affinity Glutamate Transporters in Neuronal, Glial, and Epithelial Cells

In the past decade, the stoichiometries of high-affinity glutamate transporters were estimated using a variety of preparations, including a neuronal cell line from mouse cerebellum (*83*), salamander retinal glial cells (*4,10,75*), rabbit glial cells (*43*), kidney brush-border membrane vesicles (*26,33,57*), proteoliposomes containing partially purified renal brush-border membrane glutamate transporters (*46*), and eel intestinal brush-border membrane vesicles (*68*). The Na^+, K^+, and glutamate stoichiometries were investigated, based on Hill analysis of the ion-dependence of glutamate uptake or the glutamate-evoked currents, and based on direct comparison of the ion and glutamate fluxes. Studies of glutamate transport in glial cells from salamander retina (*4,10,75*) and rabbit brain (*43*) suggested a Na^+ to glutamate coupling ratio of 2:1. Glutamate uptake in salamander retinal glial cells was not chloride-dependent (*5*).

To study whether K^+ is involved in glutamate transport, Attwell and colleagues (*4,75*) used whole-cell voltage-clamp analysis of salamander retinal glial cells (*5*). By changing the intracellular K^+ concentration, these investigators showed a strong dependence of glutamate-evoked currents on intracellular K^+, indicating that glutamate uptake is coupled to the countertransport of K^+.

A similar approach was used to study the pH dependence of retinal glial glutamate uptake. The studies suggested that the transport of glutamate is coupled to the countertransport OH^- ions, rather than to the cotransport of H^+. This conclusion was based on the observation that anion efflux accounted for intracellular acidification. The data showed that the OH^- anion on the intracellular membrane surface can be replaced by other small anions, such as NO_3^-, HCO_3^-, and ClO_4^- (*8,9*), and that glutamate uptake resulted in the exit of these ions. Recent studies, however, indicated that high-affinity glutamate transporters, in particular GLAST and EAAT4, exhibit glutamate-gated anion conductances (*see* Electrogenic Properties of Glutamate Transporters and Fig. 4). It is possible that the observed countertransport of NO_3^-, HCO_3^- and ClO_4^- in salamander retinal glia is related to this anion conductance. Additional studies will be required to determine whether high-affinity glutamate transporters are coupled to the cotransport of H^+ or the countertransport of OH^-.

Although the individual studies described did not provide unambiguous overall stoichiometries, their combined information provided convincing evidence that high-affinity glutamate transporters link uphill glutamate transport to the cotransport of 2 Na^+ ions (*10*), the countertransport of 1 K^+ ion (*4,75*), and either the cotransport of 1 H^+ ion or the countertransport of 1 OH^- ion (*9*).

Coupling Stoichiometry of a Cloned Glutamate Transporter (EAAC1)

To test this proposed stoichiometry, Kanai et al. (*39*) performed a detailed ion-coupling analysis of the glutamate transport induced by the recently cloned high-affinity glutamate transporter EAAC1 expressed in *Xenopus* oocytes. The stoichiometry was studied by comparing the charge flux, the H^+ or OH^- flux, and the initial rates of the $^{22}Na^+$- and ^{14}C-glutamate uptakes. Two electrode voltage-clamp analyses of glutamate-evoked currents gave a first-order dependence of the current on extracellular glutamate concentration, indicating that one glutamate molecule is translocated during each transport cycle. Hill analysis of the Na^+-dependence of the glutamate-evoked currents in oocytes gave Hill coefficients for Na^+ that were strongly dependent on extracellular glutamate concentration. The Hill coefficient was ~1.2 at 1 mM glutamate, 2 at 200 µM glutamate, and >2 at glutamate <40 µM. Since the Hill coefficient is generally considered to be an indicator of the coupling stoichiometry, this would suggest that the Na^+ to glutamate coupling ratio depends on extracellular glutamate concentration. However, flux measurements using $^{22}Na^+$- and ^{14}C-glutamate gave a constant Na^+ to glutamate coupling ratio of 2:1, independent of extracellular glutamate concentration. It was therefore concluded that EAAC1-mediated glutamate uptake is coupled to the cotransport of 2 Na^+-ions. The unexpected result from Hill plot analysis is probably caused by complex cooperativity between the Na^+ and glutamate binding sites (*39*).

To test whether transport mediated by EAAC1 is coupled to the cotransport of H^+ (or the countertransport of OH^-), the intracellular pH in oocytes was measured using pH-sensitive microelectrodes impaled into oocytes. The studies revealed that EAAC1-mediated transport is associated with an intracellular acidification. The H^+ (or OH^-) to charge coupling ratio was estimated from the rate of the pH decrease and the depolarization and gave approximately a 1:1 coupling ratio. Transport mediated by EAAC1 was also shown to be linked with countertransport of K^+ (*see* next section). These data give an overall stoichiometry for EAAC1-mediated glutamate transport of 1 glutamate to 2 Na^+ to 1 H^+ (or OH^-) to 1 K^+.

Examination of the K^+-Coupling of EAAC1 by Capillary Zone Electrophoresis

Nussberger et al. (*59*) recently reported a new approach based on capillary zone electrophoresis (CZE) to monitor solute transport into oocytes at the level of a single cell. This technique allowed the simultaneous detection of changes of intracellular Na^+ and K^+ concentrations in response to EAAC1-mediated Na^+ cotransport and K^+ countertransport. The studies on the Na^+- and K^+-coupled glutamate transporter EAAC1 expressed in *Xenopus* oocytes demonstrated that transport of the Na^+ and K^+ ions can be monitored by measuring intracellular ion concentrations by CZE using indirect on-column UV-detection (Fig. 3). This detection mode takes advantage of the displacement of an organic UV-absorbing compound, such as imidazole, by the inorganic ion. Based on CZE analysis, these investigators confirmed that EAAC1-mediated uptake of glutamate results in an increase of intracellular Na^+ ions (Fig. 3). In response to glutamate application, intracellular K^+ levels decreased, consistent with the model that glutamate uptake is countertransported by K^+ ions. Water- or noninjected oocytes did not show significant changes of the intracellular Na^+ and K^+ concentrations in response to application of L-glutamate.

The exact amount of Na^+ and K^+ ions transported across the oocyte plasma membranes in response to EAAC1-mediated glutamate uptake was estimated using Rb^+ as an internal standard and using Na^+ and K^+ calibration solutions (Fig. 3). Based on the CZE analysis, EAAC1-mediated uptake of glutamate resulted in an increase in intracellular Na^+ by roughly 3500 pmol/1 h in the presence of 1 mM L-glutamate. This result was entirely consistent with previous [22]Na^+ uptake experiments (*39*). The K^+ efflux was roughly equal to that of Na^+ (Fig. 3C), which appears to be inconsistent with the proposed Na^+ to K^+ ratio of 2:1. However, since the studies were performed under nonvoltage-clamp conditions, the reason for this difference is probably because of the exit of charge in the form of K^+ ions through K^+ channels. For each positive

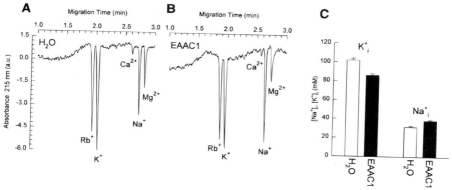

Fig. 3. Na$^+$/K$^+$-coupled glutamate transport mediated by human EAAC1. Electropherograms of water **(A)** and cRNA **(B)** injected oocytes incubated during 60 min in 1 mM L-glutamate in ND96 uptake solution (96 mM NaCl, 2 mM KCl, 1.8 mM CaCl$_2$ 1 mM MgCl$_2$ and 5 mM HEPES, pH 7.4). Ouabain, amiloride, and bumetanide were added to inhibit endogenous Na$^+$ and K$^+$ transport. After the uptake experiment, each oocyte was dissolved in 100 µL deionized water. Following centrifugation, an aliquot of the supernatant was mixed with an equal vol of RbCl solution (500 µM), used as internal standard to correct for injection volume errors. The peak areas of Rb$^+$ therefore correspond to 250 µM Rb$^+$. The electropherograms show representative results obtained from single oocytes. Oocytes expressing EAAC1 gave large glutamate-induced Na$^+$ uptakes. Comparison of the Na$^+$ and K$^+$ peaks of water and EAAC1 injected oocytes shows that EAAC1-mediated glutamate transport is coupled to the cotransport of Na$^+$ ions and the countertransport of K$^+$ ions. **(C)** The intracellular ion concentrations were calculated from the corresponding peak areas of the electropherograms, using the peak of Rb$^+$ as a reference. Application of 1 mM glutamate increased the intracellular Na$^+$ concentration in oocytes from 29–40 mM, and decreased the extracellular K$^+$ concentration from 100–86 mM (*see* text).

charge that is associated with the uptake of one glutamate molecule, one additional K$^+$ ion is predicted to leave the cell. Thus, the capillary electrophoresis data completely agree with the model that high-affinity glutamate uptake is coupled to the countertransport of one K$^+$ ion.

Electrogenic Properties of Glutamate Transporters

As predicted from the coupling stoichiometry of high-affinity glutamate transporters, these transporters are electrogenic. As a consequence, transport substrates, such as L-glutamate and D- and L-aspartate, induced inward currents when the transporters were expressed in *Xenopus* oocytes or cultured mammalian cells (*1,22,37,39,41,45,97*). The detailed analysis of the presteady-state and steady-state currents displayed by these transporters, in response to step changes of the membrane potential, provided important information on their dynamics (i.e., the kinetics of the transitions between the empty transporters and the transporter–substrate complexes) and on their structures (i.e., whether the substrate binding sites are within or outside the membrane electric field) (52,53,97). Such approaches were particularly successful for the determination of the kinetic properties of individual transport steps and to estimate the turnover rates of the Na^+/glucose cotransporter and the GABA transporter (52,53). In response to sudden changes of the membrane potential, two components of electric currents were usually observed in oocytes expressing the transporters, the transient presteady-state currents and the steady-state currents. With glutamate transporters, such as EAAC1, the accurate determination of presteady-state currents has been difficult, because they are much smaller than those of the Na^+/glucose cotransporter and the GABA transporter, and because useful inhibitors that freeze the transporter–inhibitor complex in a nontransporting form are not available for EAAC1 and GLAST (39,41,52,53,97). Recently, Wadiche et al. (97) used kainate, which is a nontransported inhibitor of GLT-1, to isolate presteady-state currents for human GLT-1 (EAAT2) The presteady currents had the properties of a nonlinear capacitive current and the total charge transfer was obtained as the time integral of the current fit to the Boltzmann distribution. The charge transfer is therefore analogous in its properties to those obtained for the Na^+/glucose cotransporter and the GABA transporter. Based on the Na^+-dependence of the presteady-state currents, the investigators concluded that the currents reflect the voltage-dependent binding and unbinding of Na^+ near the extracellular surface of the transporter. In contrast, the presteady-state transient currents of the Na^+/glucose cotransporter were thought to reflect the voltage-driven rapid shift of the negatively charged empty carrier after unbinding of Na^+ (52). The presteady-state currents of GLT-1 did not appear to reflect conformational changes of the transporter molecule (97). This is in agreement with the idea that the empty carrier is electroneutral (33).

Given the electroneutral behavior of the empty carrier within the membrane, the fully loaded carrier, which carries one glutamate anion, two Na^+ ions, and possibly one H^+, has one or two positive charges overall, and its translocation is therefore electrogenic. Consistent with this, the current–voltage relationships of glutamate-induced steady-state currents of EAAC1, GLT-1, and GLAST exhib-

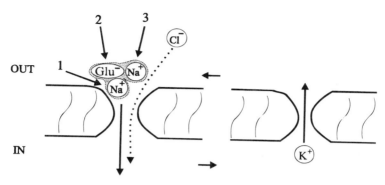

Fig. 4. Hypothetical kinetic transport model of high affinity-glutamate transporters. The model predicts that the kinetics of transport are ordered. Loading of the carrier at the extracellular surface is predicted to involve binding of a Na^+ ion, followed by binding of glutamate and then of a second Na^+ ion. The complex then translocates to the inside. Under normal conditions, this translocation process is predicted to be rate-limiting (*41*). The relocation step is predicted to be coupled to the countertransport of one K^+ ion and possibly also one OH^- ion (not shown) (*39*). It is also possible that high-affinity glutamate transporters are coupled to the cotransport of H^+ instead of to the countertransport of OH^-. The exact role of H^+ or OH^- in the transport process is unknown (*see* text for discussion). The diagram also indicates the glutamate-gated Cl^- channel feature displayed to various extents by high-affinity glutamate transporters. The figure is consistent with the proposal of Wadiche et al. (*97*) that a potential mechanism that may affect the channel selectivity is that bound glutamate itself constitutes a critical part of the ion channel selectivity, e.g., by contributing a positively charged α-amino group with which the anion could interact in transit. Alternatively, Na^+ ions may be involved in the ion permeation pathway.

ited strong voltage dependencies (*22,39,41,45,97*). At saturating glutamate concentration, the glutamate-induced currents of EAAC1 increased with hyperpolarization of the membrane (*39*). For that reason, a specific voltage-dependent step must be rate-limiting for the glutamate translocation process. This step was referred to as the voltage-dependent charge translocation step of the fully loaded carrier (*39,41*). The countertransport of K^+ appears to facilitate the relocation of the empty carrier, so that the relocation step is faster than the charge translocation step (*39,41*). The role of H^+ or OH^- in the transport process is not yet clear. H^+ or OH^- are either involved in the relocation or in the charge translocation step (Fig. 4).

The functional characterization of EAAT4 has led to the identification of an additional property displayed by high-affinity glutamate transporters (22). Although the current–voltage relationship of the other glutamate transporter isoforms, such as EAAC1 (41), apparently exhibited inward rectification without significant current reversals at potentials of up to +50 mV, the current mediated by EAAT4 expressed in *Xenopus* oocytes was linearly dependent on membrane potential and reversed at around –20 mV. The substrate-induced current in EAAT4 was composed of two components, a transporter current, reflecting translocation of substrates across the membrane, and a Cl^- current. The latter component had the characteristics of a substrate-gated chloride channel. The anion selectivity of the channel was $NO_3^- > I^- > Br^- > Cl^- > F^-$. The Cl^- was only translocated in the presence of glutamate or related substrates and its movement was not thermodynamically coupled to the substrate transport; therefore, Cl^- is not necessary for substrate translocation. Although the possibility that EAAT4 couples to an endogenous oocyte Cl^- channel cannot be completely ruled out, the results from Fairman et al. (22) strongly indicate that EAAT4 itself functions as a Cl^- channel. One possible explanation of this phenomenon is that the conformation of EAAT4, when transporting glutamate or aspartate, may have a loose structure in which a path for Cl^- is accidentally created (*see* Fig. 4). Consistent with this hypothesis is the observation that the Cl^- conductance is larger when aspartate is transported instead of glutamate, because aspartate is smaller than glutamate (22). Wadiche et al. (97) also observed that the other glutamate transporter isoforms, GLAST in particular, exhibit current reversals to various degrees when the membrane potential was shifted to more positive potentials. Thus glutamate transporters appear to possess structures that can function as chloride channels.

Functional Comparison of High-Affinity Glutamate Transporters and Na⁺-Dependent Neutral Amino Acid Transporters

As discussed, the glutamate transporter family includes Na^+-dependent neutral amino acid transporters, which have properties of the classically characterized Na^+-dependent neutral amino acid transport system (ASC) (2,40,78,92) Glutamate transporters transport L-glutamate and D- and L-aspartate and do not accept neutral amino acids. On the other hand, ASC transporters have a high-affinity for alanine, serine, threonine, and cysteine, and the preferred substrates are amino acids without highly branched or bulky side chains (2,17,78,92). The two ASC transporters ASCT1 and ASCT2 exhibit distinct substrate selectivities (2,78,92). In addition to the common substrates of ASC transporters, ASCT2 also accepts glutamine and asparagine as high-affinity substrates; and methionine, leucine, and glycine as low-affinity substrates, in contrast ASCT1 does not accept these substrates. ASCT2 also has a low affinity for the acidic amino acid glutamate, suggesting that ASCT2 has a binding site that has a spacial configuration similar to those of high-affinity glutamate transporters (92).

The detailed functional analysis of ASCT2 expressed in *Xenopus* oocytes revealed additional interesting transport properties. ASCT2-mediated transport was not electrogenic, although glutamate transporters and the other ASC transporter isoform ASCT1 are electrogenic. This suggests that ASCT2 has a different stoichiometry compared to other members of the family (2,92). The Na^+-dependence of ASCT2-mediated alanine uptake fits well the Michaelis-Menten equation (Hill coefficient almost 1) (92). This suggests that ASCT2 couples the uptake of neutral amino acids to the cotransport of a single Na^+ ion. For ASCT2-mediated neutral amino acid transport to be electroneutral, transport must be coupled to either the countertransport of a cation or the cotransport of an anion. Given that alanine uptake was not dependent on extracellular Cl^- and that it was inhibited with increasing the extracellular K^+ concentration, it is likely that transport by ASCT2 is coupled to the countertransport of a K^+ ion, analogous to the high-affinity glutamate transporters (92). ASCT2-mediated glutamate transport increased when the extracellular pH was reduced, but transport of neutral amino acids did not exhibit such a pH dependence (92). This suggests that glutamate is transported in the protonated form, consistent with the observation that transport of both glutamate and neutral amino acids was electroneutral in ASCT2. Thus, ASCT2 appears to have a substrate binding site that accepts both neutral amino acids and protonated acidic amino acids.

Structure–Function Relationships of Glutamate Transporters

Since high-affinity glutamate transporters have a unique, highly conserved long hydrophobic stretch near the C-terminus (*see* Figs. 1 and 2; putative transmembrane domains 8, 9, and 10), it is reasonable to predict that this region is responsible for binding and translocation of the substrates (*40*). Although the structure–function relationship of glutamate transporters has not yet been studied in great detail, several pieces of information are now available from site-directed mutagenesis and pharmacological studies. In support of this proposal, mutagenesis studies of GLT-1 by Pines et al. (*63*) suggested that Glu 404 is located in the vicinity of the glutamate–aspartate permeation pathway. This residue corresponds to Glu 374 in EAAC1 and resides in the eighth putative transmembrane domain within the conserved C-terminal hydrophobic stretch (Fig. 2). The residue is also conserved in GLAST and EAAT4, but not in the neutral amino acid transporters ASCT1 and ASCT2 (Fig. 1), where there is a glutamine in this position.

The conserved motif AAXFIAQ (residues 376–382 in EAAC1, Fig. 2) is also part of this hydrophobic region and may be of particular functional importance. In addition, a unique sequence located in this region, which consists of several consecutive serine residues (SSSS in EAAC1 and GLAST and ASSA in GLT-1, Fig. 2), is reminiscent of three consecutive serine residues in the mGluRl metabotropic glutamate receptor, which were suggested to be involved in hydrogen bonding to glutamate (*60*). Given that this motif is common to all prokaryotic and eukaryotic glutamate transporter family members, it is likely that it represents part of the substrate binding and translocation sites of glutamate transporters.

A challenging task is the identification of the residues of high-affinity glutamate transporters involved in Na^+, K^+, and H^+ or OH^- coupling, or in the glutamate-gated Cl^- conductance. To this end, Zhang et al. (*101*) demonstrated that His 326 of GLT-1, which is present in the center of the predicted sixth transmembrane domain, is critical for glutamate transporter function. This residue is conserved in the other glutamate transporter family members and corresponds to His 296 in EAAC1 (Fig. 2). Histidine residues have been found to be important also in other H^+-coupled transporters, such as the *E. coli* Na^+/H^+ antiporter (*28*), the lactoses permease (*66,67*), and the melibiose transporter (*65*).

Additional information on the structure–function relationship of glutamate transporters was obtained from studies addressing the phosphorylation sites. GLT-1-mediated glutamate transport is enhanced by protein kinase C (PKC)-dependent phosphorylation with an increase in V_{max} and no change in K_m (*13*). The PKC-dependent phosphorylation site in GLT-1 is Ser 113, located in the intracellular loop between transmembrane domains 2 and 3. This site is conserved in EAAC1 and GLAST and corresponds to Ser 87 in EAAC1 (Fig. 2).

The cloned glutamate transporters are also sensitive to sulfhydryl-specific reagents. Glutamate transport was inhibited by Hg^{2+} and PCMB, and it was suggested that cysteine residues are critical for glutamate transporter activity (1).

Distribution of Expression of Glummate Transporters

Cellular and Subcellular Localization of GLT-1 and GLAST in Brain

The high-affinity glutamate transporter GLT-1 was localized immunocytochemically in rat brain using polyclonal antibodies (20), a monoclonal antibody-recognizing GLT-1 amino acid residues 518–525 (51), and antibodies against peptides corresponding to GLT-1 amino acid residues 12–26, 493–508 (49), and 559–573 (71). Based on these studies, GLT-1 is exclusively expressed in glial cells (see Fig. 9). GLT-1 was detected throughout the brain (Fig. 5A); expression levels were particularly strong in the forebrain, hippocampus, cerebral cortex, and striatum.

The distribution of the high-affinity glutamate transporter GLAST was also shown by immunocytochemistry (49,71), using antibodies raised against peptides corresponding to GLAST amino acids residues 522–541 (49) and 504–518 (71). The results demonstrated that expression of GLAST is restricted to glial cells as well. However, in contrast to GLT-1, GLAST is preferentially expressed in the molecular layer of the cerebellum, which appears to correspond to the staining of processes of Bergman glia (Fig. 6), and in the olfactory bulb. At low levels, GLAST was also present throughout the brain (Fig. 5B) (49,71). The same regional labeling was observed by *in situ* hybridization (84,88).

Both GLT-1 and GLAST exhibit a gradual decline in the rostro-caudal direction (Fig. 5). A more detailed study, using immunogold labeling on ultrathin sections of rat brain tissue (14), showed that GLT-1 and GLAST are not only exclusively localized to glial cell plasma membranes, but that some glial cells also express both transporters in different proportions.

Cellular and Subcellular Localization of EAACl in Brain and Spinal Cord

The expression of EAAC1 was studied in rat brain and spinal cord by *in situ* hybridization (36) and immunocytochemistry, using polyclonal antibodies against a C-terminal peptide (residues 510–523) of

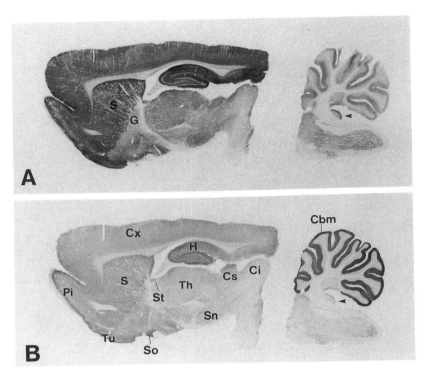

Fig. 5. Regional distribution of GLT-1 and GLAST in rat brain based on immunocytochemistry. The figure shows the immunocytochemical localization of GLT-1 **(A)** and GLAST **(B)** in closely spaced parasagittal sections incubated with antibodies to peptides 12–26 (KQVEVRMHDSHLSSE) of GLT-1 and 522–541 (PYQLIAQDNEPEKPVADSET) of GLAST (*see* ref. *49*). Note that GLT-1 and GLAST occur in all regions, but at varying concentrations. GLAST is concentrated in the cerebellar molecular layer (Cbm), and less so in a few forebrain regions (So, Pi). GLT-1 is high in telencephalic areas (H, Cx, Pi, Tu, S). Abbreviations: Cbm, cerebellar molecular layer; Ci and Cs, inferior and superior colliculi; Cx, cerebral cortex; G, globus pallidus; H, hippocampal formation; Pi, piriform cortex; S, corpus striatum; Sn, substantia nigra; So, supraoptic nucleus; St, stria terminalis; Th, thalamus; Tu, olfactory tubercle. Arrowhead: Molecular layer of dorsal cochlear nucleus. Perfusion fixation was performed with a mixture of 4% formaldehyde, 0.2% picric acid, 0.05% glutaraldehyde. Sections were processed with antibodies in the presence of Triton X-100. The antibody concentrations (0.1 µg/mL) were chosen to give similar maximum staining intenstities for GLT-1 and GLAST. (Reproduced with permission from Lehre et al. [*49*].)

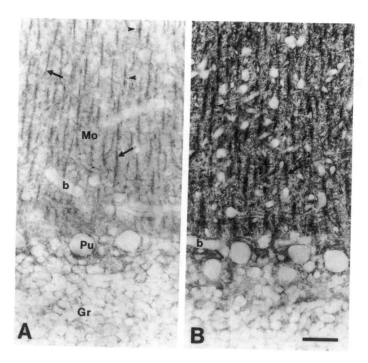

Fig. 6. Expression of GLT-1 and GLAST in rat cerebellum. Parasagittal sections of rat cerebellum, processed at antibody concentrations giving similar staining intensities for GLT-1 **(A)** and GLAST **(B)**. Note that the signal for GLAST is much stronger in the molecular layer than for GLT-1. The difference is restricted to the molecular layer, which contains the stained Bergmann glial fibers (arrows) and fine processes (arrowheads). Blood vessels (b) are unstained. Mo, Pu, and Gr, molecular Purkinje cell, and granular layers. The antibodies were the same as those used in Fig. 5. Scale bars, 30 μm. (Reproduced with permission from Lehre et al. [49].)

EAAC1 (71). Based on *in situ* hybridization, EAAC1 mRNA expression was heterogeneous throughout the CNS (Fig. 7A,C,E,G and Table 2). High levels of EAAC1 mRNA were also present in the retina (Table 2, ref. 36). The conclusion that EAAC1 is a neuron-specific glutamate transporter in the central nervous system (CNS) is based on the following observations. First the hybridization signal for EAAC1 mRNA was strong in the gray matter and at background levels in the white matter in both brain and spinal cord (Table 2, p. 192). Second, the morphological characteristics, such as cell body size and presence of proximal dendrites of cells expressing EAAC1 mRNA, was characteristic of neurons but not of glia.

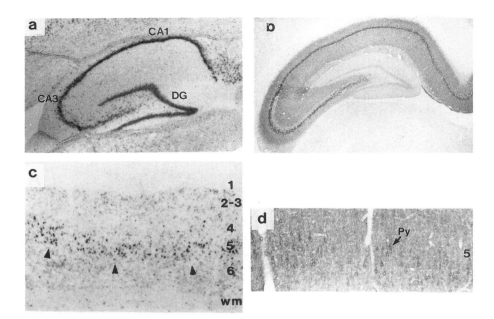

Fig. 7. Distribution of EAAC1 mRNA (A,C,E,G) and protein (B,D,F,H) in rat brain and spinal cord, based on *in situ* hybridization and immunocytochemistry. *In situ* hybridization was performed after perfusion fixation with 4% paraformaldehyde, using 14-μm thick parasaggital or cross cryosections, and ³⁵S-labeled antisense cRNA probes. Immunocytochemistry was performed using polyclonal antibodies (*71*) against a peptide corresponding to the C-terminal residues 510–523 of rat EAACI (DKSDTISFTQTSQF) (*see* ref. *36*). The figure shows the expression of EAAC1 mRNA and protein in the hippocampal formation (regions CA1–CA3) and the granular layer of the dentate gyrus (DG) **(A,B)**. In the cerebral cortex, EAACI mRNA and protein were expressed in layers 2–6, in particular, in pyramidal cells (Py) of layer 5 **(C,D)**, but the signals were absent in layer 1. In the cerebellum, expression of EAAC1 mRNA was observed in Purkinje cells (Pu) and cells of the deep cerebellar nuclei (dcn) **(E).**

Although EAAC1 was originally thought to be a presynaptic uptake carrier (*see* ref. *42*), immunocytochemical data by Rothstein et al. (*71*) suggested that EAAC1 is a postsynaptic transporter. In particular, these investigators observed that there is strong EAAC1 immunoreactivity in postsynaptic elements, such as dendritic shafts and spines, but presynaptic glutamatergic elements, such as corticostriatal terminals in the caudate putamen, appeared to be devoid of EAAC1 immunoreactivity. Therefore, in Fig. 9, EAAC1 is shown on dendritic spines and shafts.

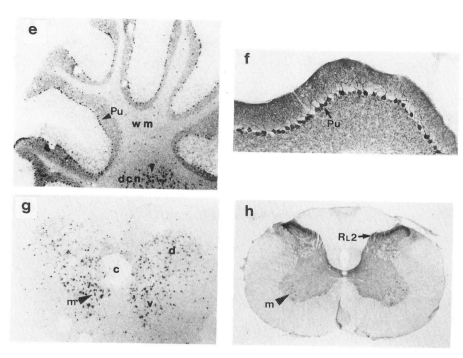

Fig. 7. *(continued)* Expression of EAAC1 protein was enriched in Purkinje cell somata **(F)**. In deep cerebellar nuclei, presynaptic boutons that surrounded deep cerebellar neurons were EAAC1 immunopositive (not shown) (71). In spinal cord, EAAC1 mRNA was detected diffusely throughout the gray matter **(G)** and was particularly strong (arrowhead) over large cells in the ventral horn (v) that probably correspond to α-motor neurons (m). Based on immunocytochemistry of spinal cord **(H)**, small neurons and the neuropil in Rexed layer 2 (RL2) were strongly EAAC1 immunoreactive, whereas α-motor neurons displayed moderate immunoreactivity. wm, white matter; c, central canal of the spinal cord; d, dorsal horn of the spinal cord. The immunocytochemistry data were provided by Jeffrey Rothstein.

If EAAC1 is indeed not expressed in presynaptic terminals, the *in situ* mRNA hybridization and immunocytochemistry signals should reveal similar patterns of expression throughout the CNS. Comparison of the data obtained for EAAC1 in different parts of the CNS, using *in situ* hybridization and immunocytochemistry, revealed that this prediction is generally correct, but there were a few exeptions to this rule, as discussed in the following sections.

Table 2
Intensity of the EAACI *In Situ* Hybridization
Signal in the Rat CNS[a]

Cerebral cortex	
Layers 2, 3, 4 and 6	++
Layer 5	++++
Corpus callosum	+
Caudate-putamen	++
Olfactory bulb	
Mitral cell layer	+++++
Olfactory tubercle	++++
Nucleus accumbens	+
Diagonal band of Broca	+++
Septum	
Dorso-lateral	++++
Lateral and medial	+++
Thalamus	
Ventrolateral	+++++
Medial and dorsolateral	+++
Hypothalamus	+
Hippocampus, dantate gyrus	
Pyramidal cell layer	+++++
Granule cell layer	+++++
Superior colliculus	
Intermediate gray	+++++
Cerebellum	
Purkinje cell layer	++
Deep cerebellar nuclei	++++
Granule cell layer	+
Brain stem nuclei	+++
Spinal cord	
Dorsal gray	+
Ventral gray (α motor neurons)	++++
Retina	
Ganglion cell layer	++++
Inner nuclear layer	+++++

*Only those CNS regions in which the level of hybridization was above the background levels are included. The level of hybridization is based on visual evaluation of the hybridization signal. +, just above background; +++++, maximum intensity of labeling; ++, +++, and ++++, intermediate levels of labeling.

Expression in the Hippocampal Formation

Based on *in situ* hybridization, a robust signal was seen in the pyramidal layer of the hippocampus from CA1 to CA4 (Fig. 7A). An equally strong signal was present in the granular layer of the dentate gyrus (Fig. 7A). The immunocytochemistry data were consistent with these observations (Fig. 7B), except that the dentate gyrus showed a weak immunoreactivity that did not correlate with the strong mRNA hybridization signal. A possible explanation for this difference is that expression of EAAC1 is regulated at the translational level in this region.

Expression in the Cerebral Cortex

A moderate to strong *in situ* hybridization signal was present in the cerebral cortex in layers 2–6 at all rostrocaudal levels, but the signal was absent in layer 1 and in the subcortical white matter. The signal was particularly dense over cells in layer 5 (Fig. 7C). Although it was difficult to identify the labeled cells as granule or pyramidal neurons, both cell types appeared to express EAAC1 mRNA. The immunocytochemistry data for cerebral cortex were entirely consistent with the results from *in situ* hybridization (Fig. 7D).

Expression in Cerebellum and Potential Role in GABA Synthesis

Based on *in situ* hybridization, moderate levels of hybridization were seen in cerebellar Purkinje cells (Fig. 7E). Immunocytochemistry also showed strong reactivity on cell bodies of Purkinje cells. Rothstein et al. (71) detected abundant staining of presynaptic boutons in deep cerebellar nuclei, which are thought to contain terminals of Purkinje cells. The staining was diffusely distributed over presynaptic boutons. The signal did not appear to be particularly restricted to presynaptic membranes. It presumably resides at or near GABA-ergic terminals where GABA is synthesized. In GABA-ergic neurons, GABA is predominantly formed from L-glutamate by α-decarboxylation, a reaction catalyzed by glutamic acid decarboxylase. EAAC1 in axon terminals of Purkinje cells may therefore provide these neurons with large amounts of glutamate to maintain their GABA transmitter pool.

In situ hybridization also gave a signal in neurons in the deep cerebellar nuclei cells (Fig. 7E). These neurons did not appear to be immunopositive for EAAC1 (71). Only pre-synaptic preboutons from Purkinje cells were reported to be immunoreactive in this region.

Spinal Cord

In situ hybridization of the spinal cord revealed diffuse EAAC1 mRNA expression in neurons throughout the gray matter. In addition, a prominent signal was present over large cells of the ventral horn that probably correspond to α motor neurons (Fig. 7G). This result did not correlate with the result from immunocytochemistry, which showed a strong immunoreactivity in the dorsal horn and relatively weak labeling in the ventral horn (Fig. 7H). Small neurons (possibly dorsal horn sensory neurons) and the neuropil in Rexed layer 2 were strongly EAAC1 immunoreactive; in contrast, motor neurons displayed moderate immunoreactivity. A possible explanation for this discrepancy is that sensory neuron nerve endings that make synaptic contact in layer 2 express EAAC1 protein. In this case, EAAC1 mRNA would be expected to be located in the dorsal root ganglia, which have not yet been examined by *in situ* hybridization.

Expression of GLT-1 and GLAST in Spinal Cord

Based on immunocytochemistry using antibodies against GLT-1 and GLAST (49), highest signals were observed in areas receiving primary afferents (Fig. 8). The distribution of GLAST was highly concentrated in the dorsal horn (laminae 1 and 2 [= Rexed layer 1 and 2]) and in a region close to the central canal (Fig. 8B). Staining of GLT-1 is high also in the deep parts of the dorsal horn and in neuropils surrounding α-motor neurons in the ventral horn (Fig. 8A).

Distribution of Expression of EAAT4

Limited information is also available on the localization of EAAT4. Northern analysis indicated that EAAT4 mRNA is most abundant in human cerebellum (21). Based on *in situ* hybridization, EAAT4 mRNA is prominently expressed in Purkinje cells (23). Immunocytochemistry showed staining in cell soma and dendritic trees of Purkinje cells (23).

Glutamate Transporter Development

Based on studies of Shibata et al. (79) targeting embryonic and neonatal mouse brain, GLAST is primarily involved in the early stage of the brain development. GLAST mRNA was found to be prominently expressed in the ventricular (proliferative) zone throughout the brain during embryonic stages. In late embryonic and early postnatal development, expression in the ventricular zone gradually diminished and disappeared, but expression in the mantel zone increased progressively. The increase in expression of GLAST was particularly evident in Bergmann glia. The expression of GLAST in the proliferating zone suggests that it may be required for nutritional purposes of

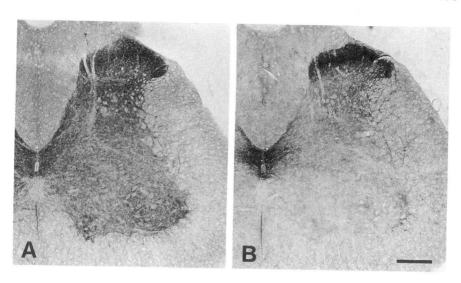

Fig. 8. Localization of GLT-1 and GLAST in rat spinal cord based on immuno-cytochemistry. Peptide-specific polyclonal antibodies against the following regions of GLT-1 and GLAST were used: GLT-1 residues 493–508 (YHLSKSELDTIDSQHR) and GLAST residues 522–541 (PYQLIAQDNEPEKP-VADSET) (*see* ref. *49*). GLT-1 and GLAST have similar staining intensities in the substantia gelatinosa of the dorsal horn and close to the central canal, but in other areas they exhibit different staining intensities. Staining of GLT-1 is also high in the deep parts of the dorsal horn, and in cells of the ventral horn that surround α-motor neurons expressing EAAC 1 (*see* Fig. 7G,H). Scale bar, 300 μm. (Reproduced with permission from Lehre et al. [49].)

highly proliferating cells, such as neuroblast and glioblast. In contrast to GLAST, GLT-1 mRNA suddenly became evident during the second postnatal week. The expression level was augmented prominently in the telencephalon, including the cerebral cortex, hippocampal CA3, and septum. This onset of GLT-1 expression appears to coincide with the development of the glutamatergic transmission. EAAC1 message was not evident in the early development. The signals for the EAAC1 mRNA increased gradually over the brain gray matter, with higher levels in the hippocampal CA1 region and dentate gyrus. EAAC1 immunoreactivity in embryonic hippocampal neurons in culture was localized at the somato-dendritic level. At the dendritic level, EAAC1 staining did not appear to coincide exactly with the postsynaptic sites on spines, but was generally slightly away on dendritic shafts (*54*) (*see* Fig. 9), suggesting a role of EAAC1 in the later stage of brain develop-

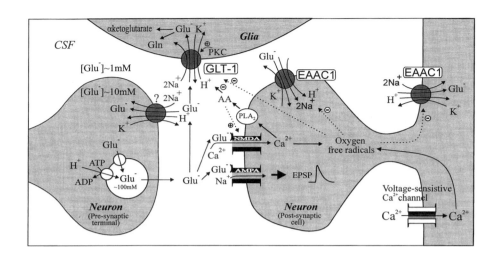

Fig. 9. Glutamate transporters at glutamatergic synapses. The excitatory neuro-transmitter L-glutamate is stored in synaptic vesicles at presynaptic terminals and released into the synaptic cleft to act on glutamate receptors. The AMPA receptors mediate fast excitatory postsynaptic potentials (EPSP); in contrast, the NMDA receptors possess a cation channel that is permeable to Ca^{2+}. High-affinity gluta-mate transporters play important roles in removing released glutamate from the synaptic cleft. These transporters are also crucial for maintaining the extracellular glutamate concentration of the CSF below neurotoxic levels. The high accumula-tive power of glutamate transporters is provided by the coupling transport to the co- or countertransport of the ions Na^+, K^+, and OH^- or H^+. The figure shows the glial glutamate transporter GLT-1 and the neuronal glutamate transporter EAAC1. Although EAAC1 was originally thought to be a presynaptic uptake carrier, recent immunocytochemical data suggest that it is expressed in postsynaptic elements, such as dendritic shafts and spines, but that there is no detectable immunostaining at glutamatergic terminals (71). At present, it is not clear whether glutamatergic terminals also possess a specialized presynaptic glutamate transporter.

Glutamate taken up into glial cells via GLT-1 or GLAST is metabolized to glu-tamine by glutamine synthase (with hydrolysis of ATP) and to α-ketoglutarate by glutamate dehydrogenase or glutamate oxaloacetate transaminase. Glia in turn supply the nerve terminal with glutamine and α-ketoglutarate, which can serve as precursors of glutamate synthesis.

Arachidonic acid (AA) and reactive oxygen species are both liberated in response to glutamate receptor activation. Moreover, certain forms of familial ALS are caused by genetic defects of the cytosolic superoxide dismutase (SOD1). The pathogenesis of motor neuron degeneration is thought to involve stimulation, over a lifetime, of non-NMDA receptors and activation of voltage-dependent Ca^{2+} channels, leading to the production of oxygen free radicals through activation of xanthine oxidase, and because of the decreased SOD1 oxygen free radical scavenging capacity, to neu-ronal death. Arachidonic acid and reactive oxygen species were shown to inhibit or modulate the function of high-affinity glutamate transporters, which can lead to the elevation of extracellular glutamate to neurotoxic levels. PLA, phospholipase A.

ment, such as during the synaptic formation. Taken together, these findings suggest that GLAST, GLT-1, and EAAC1 play important roles in brain development and that each transporter subtype plays a distinct role in this process.

Physiological Significance of Glutamate Transporters

Role of Glutamate Transporters in Glutamatergic Transmission

Glutamate transporters are thought to play important roles in the termination of synaptic transmission (21). This idea stems from the general concept that synapses, which do not have mechanisms for enzymatically degrading released neurotransmitters, possess presynaptic reuptake mechanisms for transmitter removal and for terminating their actions on the postsynaptic neurotransmitter receptors. At GABA-ergic and serotoninergic synapses, inhibitors of presynaptic neurotransmitter uptake were shown to prolong the postsynaptic currents, indicating that presynaptic reuptake carriers largely contribute to the termination of synaptic transmission (12,86). In glutamatergic synapses, however, the inhibition of glutamate transporters did not prolong the decay time-courses of fast excitatory postsynaptic potential (EPSC) in hippocampal CA1 pyramidal cells and cerebellar granule cells, when using brain slices or culture preparations (34,56,76,87). Based on studies using single neuron micro-islands prepared from hippocampus, Mennerick and Zorumski (56) explained why glutamatergic synapses are different from other synapses and why glutamate uptake inhibitors did dot affect the shape of the excitatory postsynaptic potential. In their preparation, they inhibited glutamate uptake by glial depolarization rather than with uptake inhibitors, which are known also to attenuate NMDA receptor-mediated responses. They found that inhibition of glutamate uptake prolongs autoptically induced NMDA responses, which are known to exhibit slow or little desensitization, but the inhibition did not affect the time-course of the EPSC mediated by non-NMDA receptors, which exhibit fast desensitization. In contrast, if desensitization of non-NMDA receptor-mediated responses was slowed down by cyclothiazide, the investigators were able to show that glutamate transporter inhibition significantly prolonged the time-course of non-NMDA receptor-mediated autoptic EPSC. Also consistent with these findings, the non-NMDA receptor-mediated EPSC recorded in cerebellar Purkinje cells after parallel fiber stimulation was prolonged by glutamate uptake inhibition, because the EPSC of Purkinje cells normally exhibits a slower decay time-course (6). Taken together, these data demonstrate that, because of the fast desensitization of non-NMDA receptor-mediated responses, glutamate transporters usually do not significantly affect the decay time-course of the fast EPSC. As is discussed in the following, however, glutamate transporters play important roles in removing released glutamate from the synaptic cleft.

Clements et al. (18) empirically estimated the decay time-course of the glutamate concentration in the synaptic cleft and concluded that it is slower than that derived from theoretical calculation based on simple diffusion out of the synaptic cleft. Consequently, these investigators proposed that diffusion of glutamate from the synaptic cleft is restricted by neighboring structures. This indicated that altering the location, density, and/or the function of glutamate transporters could influence the time-course of the transmitter clearance in the synaptic cleft. Wadiche et al. (97) recently determined the turnover rate of the human glutamate transporter GLT-1, based on the analysis of steady-state and presteady-state currents in response to voltage jumps. They found that the time constant for a complete cycle of transport at -80 mV and 22°C is approx 70 ms. This is significantly slower than the estimated glutamate decay time constant in hippocampal synapses, which is 1–2 ms (18). This difference was predicted to be true also at physiological temperatures (97). Consequently, it can be argued whether glutamate transporters really constitute a major mechanism for removing released glutamate (97). Binding of glutamate to glutamate transporters, however, exhibits fast kinetics. Tong and Jahr (87) demonstrated that glutamate binding to glutamate transporters, indeed, significantly contributes to the glutamate clearance in the synaptic cleft. This suggests that the density of glutamate transporters at the synaptic cleft is a factor that affects glutamate removal.

As Clements et al. (18) predicted, the geometry of the synapse is also an important determinant of the decay time-courses of the glutamate concentration at the synaptic cleft. For example, in cerebellar Purkinje cells, the non-NMDA receptor-mediated EPSC exhibits a slower decay time-course and this is thought to be the result of impaired transmitter diffusion, and, thereby, the continued presence of glutamate in the synaptic cleft (6). Based on our current knowledge, both diffusion of glutamate out of the synaptic cleft and binding of glutamate to glutamate transporters are the major factors affecting the decay time-course of the glutamate concentration in the synaptic cleft.

Role of Glutamate Transporters in Maintaining Extracellular Glutamate Concentration

Based on the stoichiometry of glutamate transporters and the prevailing ionic environment, it can be calculated that glutamate transporters concentrate glutamate more than 10,000-fold across cell membranes (40). Consistent with this, the glutamate concentration in the CSF is kept at ~1 μM, whereas the intracellular glutamate concentration in neurons is as high as 10 mM. Because of this high concentrating capacity of high-affinity glutamate transporters, these proteins are thought to play a major role in maintaining the extracellular glutamate concentration at low levels and in protecting neurons from the excitotoxic action of glutamate (40).

The importance of glutamate transporters in protecting neurons from glutamate excitotoxicity was experimentally demonstrated by Rothstein and coworkers, who treated organotypic rat spinal cord culture with the glutamate uptake inhibitors THA or PDC and observed a slight increase in glutamate concentration in the culture medium (70). Under this condition, motor neuron-specific degeneration was observed that was characterized by slow onset and gradual progression.

In order to determine which glutamate transporters are more important to protect neurons from glutamate excitotoxicity, Rothstein et al. (72) used organotypic culture preparation and incubated the spinal cord explant with antisense oligonucleotides, corresponding to the N-terminal part of the cloned glutamate transporters. They found that antisense oligonucleotides corresponding to the glial glutamate transporters GLT-1 and GLAST induced motor neuron-specific degeneration, similar to that observed when they used glutamate uptake inhibitors; antisense oligonucleotides, corresponding to the neuronal glutamate transporter EAAC1, did not induce neurodegeneration. The investigators also applied antisense oligonucleotides to the cerebroventricle of alert rats. Cerebroventricular administration of antisense GLT-1 or GLAST oligonucleotides also resulted in the degeneration of neurons, but EAAC1 antisense oligonucleotides did not induce neurodegeneration (72). Thus, primarily the glial, but not the neuronal, glutamate transporters protect neurons from glutamate excitotoxicity.

Antisense oligonucleotide inhibition was also used to determine the contribution of each glutamate transporter isoform to the total glutamate uptake in synaptosomes isolated from rat striatum. The contribution was 60% for GLT-1, 20% for GLAST, and 20% for EAAC1 (72). An important question arises as to why only antisense knockouts of glial, but not neuronal, glutamate transporters resulted in neurodegeneration. The answer to this question is related to the different functional roles glial and neuronal glutamate transporters play in the CNS. In neurons, the intracellular glutamate concentration is up to ~10 mM. Considering the low extracellular glutamate concentration of ~1 μM, this results in a steep glutamate concentration gradient across neuronal cell membranes that is essentially equal to the maximal concentration capacity of high-affinity glutamate transporters. Consequently, under normal conditions, neuronal glutamate transporters are almost at equilibrium and have little capacity to take up glutamate. It is therefore not too surprising that the antisense knockout of neuronal EAAC1 did not induce neurodegeneration. In glial cells, however, glutamate is taken up continuously and is then rapidly converted to glutamine by glutamine synthetase, an enzyme that is present in glial cells but not in neurons. The intracellular glutamate concentration in glia is therefore as low as ~50 μM. Consequently, glial glutamate transporters are not at equilibrium and keep pumping glutamate into glial cells; this generates a continuous flow of glutamate from glutamatergic synapses (source) to glial cells (sink) (*see also* ref. 38).

A recent study by Gundersen et al. (29) demonstrated that extracellularly applied D-aspartate was not taken up into glutamatergic terminals, but large amounts of D-aspartate were taken up in glial cells. This observation is consistent with the model that diffusion of glutamate out of the synaptic cleft determines the decay time-course of glutamate in the cleft. This result further raised the question of whether presynaptic glutamate transporters really exist. The existence of presynaptic glutamate uptake systems were originally postulated based on glutamate uptake studies of the synaptosomal fraction P_2. However, this fraction was subsequently found to contain large amounts of glial components (20,42). As discussed, the neuron-specific glutamate transporter EAAC1 was not detected at glutamatergic terminals (71). At present, there is no clear evidence for the existence of presynaptic glutamate transporters at glutamatergic terminals.

What are the major in vivo roles of the neuronal glutamate transporter EAAC1? This transporter probably functions to keep the intracellular neuronal glutamate concentration at high levels for use as a neurotransmitter and/or as a precursor for various metabolic reactions. Kanai et al. (36) also suggested the possibility that in GABAergic neurons, such as cerebellar Purkinje cells, EAAC1 provides glutamate as a precursor for GABA synthesis. Rothstein et al. (72) found that repeated administration of EAAC1 antisense oligonucleotide into the cerebroventricle caused rats to exhibit epileptic seizures within a week. Although the mechanism for induction of these seizures is not clear, it is reasonable to hypothesize that depletion of EAAC1 at GABA-ergic terminals results in a decrease in GABA synthesis, because of the decreased supply of glutamate to GABA-ergic terminals as the precursor of GABA synthesis.

Glutamate Transporters and Ischemia

Although the exact contribution of reversed glutamate transport to the increase in local glutamate concentration in brain ischemia after brain hemorrhage or thrombosis is still unclear, there is accumulating experimental evidence that alterations of the ionic environment and depletion of energy supply induces the efflux of glutamate through glutamate transporters (3,27,39,58,85). Since glutamate transport is driven by free energy stored in the form of electrochemical potential gradients across plasma membranes, the disturbance of the ionic gradients caused by insufficient energy supply, which occurs during brain ischemia, results in a decrease in the concentrating capacity of glutamate transporters. This favors the reversed operation of the glutamate transporter driven by the intracellular glutamate concentration (40). Since neurons have a much higher content of glutamate than glia, neuronal glutamate transporters are more likely to run in reverse in ischemia and to contribute to the extracellular rise in glutamate to excitotoxic levels. Selective inhibitors of neuronal glutamate transporters may therefore be of therapeutic interest for preventing reversed glutamate transport, without affecting the capability of glial glutamate transporters to keep the extracellular glutamate concentration at low levels. The availability of glutamate transporter subtype-specific inhibitors are required to test this hypothesis.

Because glial high-affinity glutamate transporters play a critical role in keeping the extracellular glutamate concentration below neurotoxic levels, alteration of their function or expression levels may affect the postischemic vulnerability of neurons. Torp et al. (89) recently showed that the GLT-1 message and protein content were decreased in the hippocampal CA1 region in rats following transient forebrain ischemia, while the expression of the other glial isoform GLAST and the neuronal isoform EAAC1 were not altered.

Consistent with this finding, glutamate uptake in synaptosomes (crude P_2 fraction) prepared from gerbils was shown to decrease after a transient ischemic treatment (*99*). It is therefore possible that the GLT-1 glutamate transporter decrease is one of several factors that contribute to the high sensitivity of neurons to the postischemic damage. In contrast, in the retina, it was shown that GLAST signals were markedly increased after transient occlusion of the central retinal artery (*61*). This increase, however, simply may have resulted from glial cell proliferation, which occurs after retinal ischemia, and may not necessarily represent a neuroprotective reaction.

Role of Glutamate Transporters in Amyotrophic Lateral Sclerosis

Amyotropic lateral sclerosis (ALS) typically affects individuals in mid-adult life, leading to degeneration of motor neurons and death by paralysis in 3–5 yr (*11*). Even though the disease is highly lethal, its cause is not completely known. About 10% of the cases are inherited as an autosomal dominant trait (familial ALS [FALS]). About 20% of these cases arise because of mutations in the gene for Cu/Zn superoxide dismutase (SOD1) (*11,69*) indicating that one element in the pathogenesis of ALS is a disturbance of free radical homeostasis, resulting in oxidative injury within the motor neurons (*see below*). A closely related hypothesis is that the disease results from excitotoxic stimulation by neurotransmitters, such as glutamate, and that the excitotoxicity is exacerbated when SOD1 function is altered. This hypothesis is supported by the observation that there are altered glutamate levels in ALS brain tissues (*64*) and reduced glutamate transport activity in synaptosomes prepared from affected regions of ALS brains (*73*). Excitotoxicity and abnormal glutamate transport are therefore widely investigated as the possible cause of motor neuron degeneration in ALS.

Recent studies, using specific antibodies against the recently cloned glutamate transporters EAAC1, GLT-1, and GLAST, revealed that the reduced glutamate uptake function that was observed in synaptosomes, prepared from the affected areas of postmortem sporadic ALS material, is associated with a major decrease of GLT-1 protein in the motor cortex (more than 70% reduction) and spinal cord (57% reduction) (*35,74*). The GLT-1 loss was not paralleled by changes in other glial protein markers, such as GFAP, indicating that loss of GLT-1 protein is not caused by general damage of astrocytes. A 20% defect was also seen for EAAC1 protein, which probably results from loss of neurons, but no defect was observed for GLAST. In spinal cord, GLT-1 is expressed in glial cells surrounding motor neurons that express EAAC1 mRNA and protein (*see* Figs. 7 and 8). Glutamate uptake inhibition, as well as GLT-1 antisense oligonucleotides, caused slow excitotoxic degeneration and death of motor neurons in organotypic spinal cord cultures (*72*). GLT-1 malfunction, may therefore be an important mechanism in the pathogenesis of ALS.

The studies by Rosen et al. (*69*) revealed that some forms of familial ALS arise from oxygen free radical toxicity and that missense mutations in the coding region of the SOD1 gene causes familial ALS in about 10% of all FALS patients studied. SOD1 is a metallo-enzyme that is ubiquitously expressed in eukaryotic cells. Its major function is believed to be the detoxification or dismutation of the superoxide anion to form hydrogen peroxide (*47*). This, in turn, is detoxified by either glutathione peroxidase or catalase to form water. Under normal circumstances, the superoxide anion (O_2^-) can also react with nitric oxide to form peroxynitrite ($ONOO^-$). Thus, defective SOD1 activity in familial ALS is predicted to result in disturbed free radical homeostasis and cytotoxicity by reactive oxygens. It was therefore postulated that a defect of the SOD1 enzyme causes neurodegeneration through stimulation, over a lifetime, of non-NMDA receptors and activation of voltage-dependent Ca^{2+} channels, leading to the production of oxygen free radicals through activation of xanthine oxidase and, because of the decreased SOD1 oxygen free radical scavenging capacity, to neuronal death (*55*) (*see* Fig. 1). Consistent with these hypotheses, studies by Rothstein et al. (*72*) using spinal cord organotypic cultures demonstrated that chronic inhibition of SOD1 activity, either by antisense oligonucleotides or diethyldithiocarbamate, resulted in the apoptotic degeneration of spinal neurons, including motor neurons, over several weeks. Moreover, motor neuron loss was significantly potentiated by the inhibition of glutamate transport. Troy et al. (*91*) showed that downregulation of SOD1 activity in PC12 cells by exposure to an appropriate antisense oligonucleotide also leads to apoptotic cell death, and that the nitric oxide–peroxynitrite pathway is a major contributor to the cell death. These data did not rule out another pathway as a possible contributor to cell death caused by SOD1 downregulation. According to this pathway, superoxide reduces Fe^{3+}, and the resulting Fe^{2+} reacts with hydrogen peroxide to form the highly reactive and destructive hydroxyl radical, which then leads to apoptotic cell death (*31*).

The etiology of sporadic ALS may involve a similar mechanism as the SOD1-dependent defects postulated to underlie familial ALS. It is conceivable that a small increase in local glutamate concentration caused by glutamate transport malfunction leads to sustained stimulation of nonNMDA receptors and an increase in the production of radicals, until it exceeds the capacity of SOD1 in motor neurons (Fig. 9). In Rothstein et al.'s (74) spinal cord organotypic cultures, motor neuron death by glutamate transporter inhibition was in fact mediated through nonNMDA receptors. Glutamate transporter malfunction, followed by accumulative injury of neurons by radicals over a long period of time, may therefore lead to the catastrophic death of neurons in sporadic ALS. Alternatively, the decrease in glutamate transport activity observed in sporadic ALS could be explained by a primary defect of the SOD1 enzyme, which causes inactivation of proteins, such as high-affinity glutamate transporters, through modification by reactive oxygen species. Future studies will be required to delineate the exact role of glutamate transporters in the pathophysiology of familial and sporadic ALS.

Glutamate Transporters, Oxidative Stress, and Arachidonic Acid

An event common to several neurodegenerative pathologies and pathologic conditions, such as ischemia after a stroke, is activation of phospholipases with release of free fatty acids, in particular polyunsaturated fatty acids, such as arachidonic acid, from membrane phospholipids (24). In most of these situations, fatty acids tend to accumulate in brain tissue, since reacylation in phospholipids, which is an ATP-dependent process, is compromised because of energy failure. Moreover, reactive oxygen species, including superoxide anion (O_2^-), hydrogen peroxide (H_2O_2), and hydroxyl radical (OH$^\bullet$), mostly formed as intermediates of mitochondrial respiration, may escape the impaired antioxidant defenses and target vital cell components (80) (see Fig. 9). Several lines of evidence suggest their participation in the mechanisms of neuronal damage (30). On the other hand, dysregulation of glutamatergic transmission is known to be one of the major components leading to neurotoxicity, and elevated extracellular levels of glutamate, which were observed both in in vitro and in vivo models of ischemia, trauma, and seizures were directly correlated with damage (16). Thus, excess stimulation of different types of glutamate receptors results in several forms of neuronal damage by both Ca^{2+}-dependent and Ca^{2+}-

independent mechanisms (broadly termed excitotoxicity), and often leads to irreversible degeneration of nerve cells (15). Arachidonic acid release, reactive oxygen species formation, and extracellular glutamate accumulation are interdependent phenomena, and not just parallel events. Arachidonic acid and reactive oxygen species are both liberated in response to glutamate receptor activation (21). As will be discussed in detail in the next section, arachidonic acid and reactive oxygen species oppose the removal of glutamate from the extracellular space by inhibiting certain high-affinity glutamate transporter isoforms (*see* Fig. 9). Accordingly, their feedback inhibition on glutamate uptake is predicted to trigger a vicious cycle that probably contributes to the elevation of extracellular glutamate to neurotoxic levels.

Inhibition of Glutamate Uptake by Arachidonic Acid

By using synaptosomes and cultured astrocytes from rat cerebral cortex, Volterra et al. (93) reported that arachidonic acid leads to a fast (within 30 sec) and largely reversible reduction in glutamate uptake activity. Inhibition of glutamate uptake could also be achieved through the modulation of the extracellular levels of endogenous arachidonic acid by using compounds that interfere with its deacylation-reacylation cycle into the membrane phospholipids, such as melittin (a phospholipase A_2 activator) and thimerosal (an inhibitor of the reacylation pathway). Inhibition of glutamate uptake into salamander retinal glial cells by arachidonic acid was shown by monitoring the inward current induced by the electrogenic glutamate transport (7). Moreover, arachidonic acid does not act through mechanisms mediated by eicosanoids formation or PKC activation (7,93).

The inhibitory effect of arachidonic acid on glutamate uptake was also demonstrated in a simple reconstituted system, consisting of purified glutamate transporter protein residing in liposomes (90). Therefore, it was possible to exclude indirect actions of arachidonic acid, such as changes in the ion gradients (inhibition of Na^+/K^+-ATPase, modification of ion channels, etc.), PKC activation, formation of downstream mediators (enzymatic derivatives of arachidonic acid, briefly eicosanoids), or changes in membrane lipid composition caused by active esterification of arachidonic acid in phospholipids by acetyl-transferase enzymes. Using this model, it was demonstrated that inhibition of glutamate uptake by arachidonic acid is caused by reversible binding of free aqueous arachidonic acid to either the transporter protein or the protein-lipid boundary. The binding, which requires both a hydrophobic *cis*-polyunsaturated carbon chain and a free carboxyl group, is probably of low affinity, since it was easily reversed by simple dilution. This procedure does not remove arachidonic acid bound to liposomal lipids (about 95% of the added arachidonic acid), suggesting that only the arachidonic acid partitioning to the aqueous phase affects transport by binding to the transporter protein, and that the binding to the phospholipid membranes does not seem to affect the function of the glutamate transporter. Arachidonic acid exerts an opposite effect on the uptake by two of four human glutamate transporters (*100*). Micromolar amounts of arachidonic acid inhibited glutamate uptake mediated by human GLAST (EAAT1) by reducing the maximal transport rate. In contrast, arachidonic acid increased transport mediated by human GLT-1 (EAAT2) by causing an increase in the apparent affinity for glutamate more than twofold. Human EAAC1 (EAAT3) activity was not affected, and the effect on EAAT4 has not yet been reported.

Inhibition of Glutamate Uptake by Oxygen Free Radicals

In pathological conditions such as ischemia after a stroke, oxygen radical production overcomes the endogenous protection system consisting of scavenger enzymes and antioxidant molecules. As a consequence, reactive species, including superoxide anion and, in particular, hydroxyl radicals, can attack cellular components. The high-affinity glutamate transporters are important targets of reactive oxygen species. Volterra et al. (*95*) have demonstrated that glutamate uptake in cortical glial cultures is persistently inhibited by brief exposures to reactive oxygen species, such as superoxide anion and H_2O_2. This effect is antagonized and partly reversed (>50%) by disulfide reducing agents (e.g., dithiothreitol), suggesting that cysteine residues of glutamate transporters are the target for inhibition. H_2O_2 attenuates the electrogenic glutamate uptake current in voltage-clamped astrocytes with minor or no effect on resting membrane conductance. Therefore, H_2O_2 probably directly reacts with glutamate transporters. Although both arachidonic acid and reactive oxygen species appear to directly modify glutamate transporters, their mechanism of action must be distinct and independent, since their effects were fully additive and different pharmacological agents selectively blocked their action (*96*).

Summary and Conclusions

Glutamate transporters have the capacity to take up the excitatory neurotransmitter glutamate from the extracellular space against its concentration gradient into neurons and glial cells. The major role of these transporters in the CNS is to keep the extracellular glutamate concentration at low levels and to protect neurons from glutamate toxicity. In contrast to other neurotransmitter transporters, glutamate transporters mostly do not contribute to the shape of the fast postsynaptic potential.

The recent isolation of cDNA clones encoding glutamate transporters and related proteins has revealed that these transporters belong to a large gene family that includes transporters for both acidic and neutral amino acids. The family is unique, in that transport is energized by coupling amino acid uptake to the cotransport of Na^+ and the countertransport of K^+ ions. Glutamate transporters are also coupled to pH-changing ions, either to the cotransport of H^+ or to the countertransport of OH^-. In addition, some of the glutamate transporter isoforms exhibit Cl^- permeability, which will be a new challenge for the study of channel/transporter correlation. The isolation of glutamate transporter cDNAs has not only provided valuable information on the transport processes through extensive functional analysis of the recombinant proteins, but has also facilitated the understanding of the mechanisms of disease in which transporter defects are involved. Some of the sporadic forms of ALS have been associated with the disturbance of glial glutamate transporters, leading to the manifestation of glutamate excitotoxicity through local rises in glutamate concentration. There are still many problems that need to be resolved. For example, are there specific glutamatergic presynaptic uptake carriers? What causes the defects of glial glutamate transporter observed in sporadic ALS? What structural attributes of glutamate transporters provide such a powerful concentrating ability necessary to satisfy their functional requirements? Given the rapid pace at which research is moving in this area of research, it can be expected that these questions will be resolved soon.

Acknowledgment

Work on the glutamate transporter EAACI was supported by NIH grants DK43171 and NS32001 to M. A. Hediger.

References

1. Arriza, J. L., Fairman, W. A., Wadiche, J. I., Murdoch, G. H., Kavanaugh, M. P., and Amara, S. G. Functional comparisons of three glutamate transporter subtypes cloned from human motor cortex. *J. Neurosci.* **14** (1994) 5559–5569.

2. Arriza, J. L., Kavanaugh, M. P., Fairman, W. A., Wu, Y.-N., Murdoch, G. H., North, R. A., and Amara, S. G. Cloning and expression of a human neutral amino acid transporter with structural similarity to the glutamate transporter gene family. *J. Biol. Chem.* **268** (1993) 15,329–15,332.

3. Attwell, D., Barbour, B., and Szatkowski, M. Nonvesicular release of neurotransmitter. *Neuron* **11** (1993) 401–407.

4. Barbour, B., Brew, H., and Attwell, D. Electrogenic glutamate uptake in glial cells is activated by intracellular potassium. *Nature* **335** (1988) 433–435.

5. Barbour, B., Brew, H., and Attwell, D. Electrogenic uptake of glutamate and aspartate into glial cells isolated from the salamander (Ambystoma) retina. *J. Physiol.* **436** (1991) 169–193.

6. Barbour, B., Keller, B. U., Llano, I., and Marty, A. Prolonged presence of glutamate during excitatory synaptic transmission to cerebellar Purkinje cells. *Neuron* **12** (1994) 1331–1343.

7. Barbour, B., Szakowski, M., Ingledew, N., and Attwell, D. Arachidonic acid induces a prolonged inhibition of glutamate uptake into glial cells. *Nature* **342** (1989) 918–920.

8. Bilups, B. and Attwell, D. Modulation of glutamate uptake by pH slows nonvesicular glutamate release in conditions mimicking stroke. *Nature* **379** (1996) 171–174.

9. Bouvier, M., Szatkowski, M., Amato, A., and Attwell, D. The glial cell glutamate uptake carrier countertransports pH-changing anions. *Nature* **360** (1992) 471–474.

10. Brew, H. and Attwell, D. Electrogenic glutamate uptake is a major current carrier in the membrane of axolotl retinal glial cells (erratum: *Nature* **328** [1987] 742). *Nature* **327** (1987) 707–709.

11. Brown, H. J. Amyotrophic lateral sclerosis: recent insights from genetics and transgenic mice. *Cell* **80** (1995) 687–692.

12. Bruns, D., Engert, F., and Lux, H. D. A fast activating presynaptic uptake current during serotonergic transmission in identified neurons of Hirudo. *Neuron* **10** (1993) 559–572.

13. Casado, M., Bendahan, A., Zafra, F., Danbolt, N. C., Aragon, C., Gimenez, C., and Kanner, B. I. Phosphorylation and modulation of brain glutamate transporters by protein kinase C. *J. Biol. Chem.* **268** (1993) 27,313–27,317.

14. Chaudhry, F., Lehre, K., van Lookeren-Campagne, M., Ottersen, O., Danbolt, N., and Storm-Mathisen, J. Glutamate transporters in glial plasma membranes: highly differentiated localizations revealed by quantitative ultrastructural immunocytochemistry. *Neuron* **15** (1995) 711–720.

15. Choi, D. Calcium-mediated neurotoxicity: relationship to specific channel types and role in ischemic damage. *TINS* **11** (1988) 465–469.

16. Choi, D. Glutamate neurotoxicity and diseases of nervous system. *Neuron* **1** (1988) 623–634.

17. Christensen, H. N. Role of amino acid transport and countertransport in nutrition and metabolism. *Physiol. Rev.* **70** (1990) 43–77.

18. Clements, J. D., Lester, R. A. J., Tong, G., Jahr, C. E., and Westbrook, G. L. The time course of glutamate in the synaptic cleft. *Science* **258** (1992) 1498–1501.

19. Cox, D. W., Headley, M. H., and Watkins, J. C. Actions of L- and D-homocysteate in rat CNS: a correlation between low-affinity uptake and the time

courses of excitation by microelectrophoretically applied L-glutamate analogues. *J. Neurochem.* **29** (1977) 579–588.

20. Danbolt, N. C., Storm-Mathisen, J., and Kanner, B. I. An [$Na^+ + K^+$]coupled L-glutamate transporter purified from rat brain is localized in glial cell processes. *Neuroscience* **51** (1992) 259–310.

21. Dumuis, A., Sebben, M., Haynes, L., Pin, J., and Bockaert, J. NMDA receptors activate the arachidonic acid cascade system in striatal neurons. *Nature* **336** (1988) 68–70.

22. Fairman, W. A., Vandenberg, R. J., Arriza, J. L., Kavanaugh, M. P., and Amara, S. G. An excitatory amino-acid transporter with properties of a ligand-gated chloride channel. *Nature* **375** (1995) 599–603.

23. Fairman, W. A., Vandenberg, R. J., Arriza, J. L., Shannon, E. M., Murdoch, G. H., Kavanaugh, M. P., and Amara, S. G. Functional characterization and localization of a human excitatory amino acid transporter with properties of a ligand-gated chloride channel. *Soc. Neurosci. Abstr.* **21** (1995) 1861.

24. Farooqui, A. and Horrocks, L. Excitatory amino acid receptors, neural membrane phospholipid metabolism and neurological disorders. *Brain Res. Rev.* **16** (1991) 171–191.

25. Fonnum, F. Glutamate: a neurotransmitter in mammalian bran. *J. Neurochem.* **42** (1984) 1–11.

26. Fukuhara, Y. and Turner, R. J. Cation dependence of renal outer cortical brush border membrane L-glutamate transport. *Am. J. Physiol.* **248** (1985) F869–F875.

27. Gemba, T., Oshima, T., and Ninomiya, M. Glutamate efflux via the reversal of the sodium-dependent glutamate transporter caused by glycolytic inhibition in rat cultured astrocytes. *Neuroscience* **63** (1994) 789–795.

28. Gerchman, Y., Olami, Y., Rimon, A., Taglicht, D., Schuldiner, S., and Padan, E. Histidine-226 is part of the pH sensor of NhaA, a Na^+/H^+ antiporter in *Escherichia coli. Proc. Natl. Acad. Sci. USA* **90** (1993) 1212–1216.

29. Gundersen, V., Shupliakov, O., Brodin, L., Ottersen, O., and Storm-Mathisen, J. Quantification of excitatory amino acid uptake at intact glutamatergic synapses by immunocytochemistry of exogenous D-aspartate. *J. Neurosci.* **15** (1995) 4417–4428.

30. Hall, E. and Braughler, J. Central nervous system trauma and stroke. Physiological and pharmacological evidence for involvement of oxygen radicals and lipid peroxidation. *Free Rad. Biol. Med* **6** (1989) 303–313.

31. Halliwell, B. and Gutteridge, J. C. M. Role of free radicals and catalytic metal ions in human disease: an overview. *Methods Enzymol.* **186** (1990) 1–88.

32. Hediger, M. A. and Rhoads, D. B. Molecular physiology of $Na^+/glucose$ cotransporters. *Physiol. Rev.* **74** (1994) 993–1026.

33. Heinz, E., Sommerfeld, D. L., and Kinne, R. K. H. Electrogenicity of sodium/L-glutamate cotransport in rabbit renal brush-border membranes. *Biochem. Biophys. Acta* **937** (1988) 300–308.

34. Isaacson, J. S. and Nicoll, R. A. The uptake inihibitor L-trans-PDC enhances responses to glutamate but fails to alter the kinetics of excitatory synaptic currents in the hippocampus. *J. Neurophysiol.* **70** (1993) 2187–2191.

35. Jin, L., Dykes, M. Hoberg, M., Kuncl, M., and Rothstein, J. D. Selective loss of glutamate transporter subtypes in amyotrophic lateral sclerosis. *Soc. Neurosci. Abstr.* **20** (1994) 927.

36. Kanai, Y., Bhide, P. G., DiFiglia, M., and Hediger, M. A. Neuronal high-affinity glutamate transport in the rat central nervous system. *Neuroreport* **6** (1995) 2357–2362.

37. Kanai, Y. and Hediger, M. A. High-affinity glutamate transporters: physiological and pathophysiological relevance in the central nervous system. In Brann, D. W. and Mahesh, V. B. (eds.), *Excitatory Amino Acids: Their Role in Neuroendocrine Function*, CRC, Boca Raton, FL, 1995, pp. 103–131.

38. Kanai, Y. and Hediger, M. A. Primary structure and functional characterization of a high-affinity glutamate transporter. *Nature* **360** (1992) 467–471.

39. Kanai, Y., Nussberger, S., Romero, M. F., Boron, W. F., Hebert, S. H., and Hediger, M. A. Electrogenic properties of the epithelial and neuronal high affinity glutamate transporter. *J. Biol. Chem.* **270** (1995) 16,561–16,568.

40. Kanai, Y., Smith, C. P., and Hediger, M. A. A new family of neurotransmitter transporters: the high affinity glutamate transporter. *FASEB. J.* **7** (1993) 1450–1459.

41. Kanai, Y. K., Stelzner, M., Nussberger, S., Khawaja, S., Hebert, S. C., Smith, C. P., and Hediger, M. A. The neuronal and epithelial human high affinity glutamate transporter: insights in structure and mechanism of transport. *J. Biol. Chem.* **269** (1994) 20,599–20,606.

42. Kanner, B. I. and Schuldiner, S. Mechanism of transport and storage of neurotransmitters. *CRC Crit. Rev. Biochem.* **22** (1987) 1–38.

43. Kimelberg, H. K., Pang, S., and Treble, D. H. Excitatory amino acid-stimulated uptake of $22Na^+$ in primary astrocyte cultures. *J. Neurosci.* **9** (1989) 1141–1149.

44. Kirschner, M., Arriza, J. L., Copeland, N. G., Gilbert D. J., Jenkins, N. A., Magenis, E., and Amara, S. G. The mouse and human excitatory amino acid transporter gene (EAAT1) maps to mouse chromosome 15 and a region of syntenic homology on human chromosome 5. *Genomics* **22** (1994) 631–633.

45. Klöckner, U., Storck, T., Conradt, M., and Stoffel, W. Electrogenic L-glutamate uptake in *Xenopus laevis* oocytes expressing a cloned rat brain L-glutamate/L-aspartate transporter (GLAST-1). *J. Biol. Chem.* **268** (1993) 14,594–14,596.

46. Koepsell, H., Korn, K., Ferguson, D., Menuhr, H., Ollig, D., and Haase, W. Reconstitution and partial purification of several Na^+ contransport systems from renal brush-border membranes. Properties of the L-glutamate transporter in proteoliposomes. *J. Biol. Chem.* **259** (1984) 6548–6558.

47. Koppenol, W. H., Moreno, J. J., Pryor, W. A., Ischiropoulos, H., and Beckman, J. S. Peroxynitrite, a cloaked oxidant formed by nitric oxide and superoxide. *Chem. Res. Toxicol.* **5** (1992) 834–842.

48. Krishnan, S. N., Desai, T., Wyman, R. J., and Haddad, G. G. Cloning of a glutamate transporter from human brain. *Soc. Neurosci. Abstr.* **19** (1993) 219.

49. Lehre, K., Levy, L., Ottersen, O., Strom-Mathisen, J., and Danbolt, N. Differential expression of the two glial glutamate transporters in the rat brain: quantitative and immunocytochemical observation. *J. Neurosci.* **15** (1995) 1835–1853.

50. Lerner, J. Acidic amino acid transport in animal cells and tissues. *Comp. Biochem. Physiol.* **87B** (1987) 443–457.

51. Levy, L., Lehre, K., Rolstad, B., and Danbolt, N. A monoclonal antibody raised against an $[Na^+/K^+]$coupled L-glutamate transporter purified from rat brain confirms glial cell localization. *FEBS Lett.* **317** (1993) 79–84.

52. Loo, D. D. F., Hazama, A., Supplisson, S., Turk, E., and Wright, E. M. Relaxation kinetics of the Na^+/glucose cotransporter. *Proc. Natl. Acad. Sci. USA* **90** (1993) 5767–5771.

53. Mager, S., Naeve, J., Quick, M., Labarca, C., Davidson, N., and Lester, H. A. Steady states, charge movements and rates for a cloned GABA transporter expressed in *Xenopus* oocytes. *Neuron* **10** (1993) 177–188.

54. Matteoli, M. and Volterra, A. Extrasynaptic localization of the glutamate transporter EAACI in cultured hippocampal neurons. Submitted (1996).

55. McNamara, J. O. and Fridovich, I. Did radicals strike Lou Gehrig? *Nature* **362** (1993) 59–62.

56. Mennerick, S. and Zorumski, C. F. Glial contributions to excitatory neurotransmission in cultured hippocampal cells. *Nature* **368** (1994) 59–62.

57. Nelson, P. J., Dean, G. E., Aronson, P. S., and Rudnick, G. Hydrogen ion cotransport by the renal brush border glutamate transporter. *Biochemistry* **22** (1983) 5459–5463.

58. Nicholls, D. and Attwell, D. The release and uptake of excitatory amino acids. *Trends Pharmacol Sci.* **11** (1990) 462–468.

59. Nussberger, S., Foret, F., Hebert, S. C., Karger, B. L., and Hediger, M. A. Non-radioactive monitoring of organic solute transport into single *Xenopus* oocytes by capillary zone electrophoresis. *Biophys. J.* **70** (1996) 998–1005.

60. O'Hara, P. J., Sheppard, P. O., Thogersen, H., Venezia, D., Haldeman, B. A., McGrane, V., Houamed, K. M., Thomsen, C., Gilbert, T. L., and Mulvihill, E. R. The ligand-binding domain in metabotropic glutamate receptors is related to bacterial periplasmic binding proteins. *Neuron* **11** (1993) 41–52.

61. Otori, Y., Shimada, S., Tanaka, K., Ishimoto, I., Tano, Y., and Tohyama, M. Marked increase in glutamate-aspartate transporter (GLAST/GluT-1) mRNA following transient retinal ischemia. *Mol. Brain Res.* **27** (1994) 310–314.

62. Pines, G., Danbolt, N. C., Bjoras, M., Zhang, Y., Bendahan, A., Eide, L., Koepsell, H., Storm-Mathisen, J., Seeberg, E., and Kanner, B. I. Cloning and expression of a rat brain L-glutamate transporter. *Nature* **360** (1992) 464–467.

63. Pines, G., Zhang, Y., and Kanner, B. I. Glutamate 404 is involved in the substrate discrimination of GLT-1, a $(Na^+ + K^+)$-coupled glutamate transporter from rat brain. *J. Biol. Chem.* **270** (1995) 17,093–17,097.

64. Plaitakis, A. P., Constantantakakis, E., and Smith, J. The neuroexcitotoxic amino acids glutamate and aspartate are altered in the spinal cord and brain in amyotrophic lateral sclerosis. *Ann. Neurol.* **24** (1988) 446–449.

65. Pourcher, T., Zani, M.-L., and Leblanc, G. Mutagenesis of acidic residues in putative membrane-spanning segments of the melibiose permease in *Escherichia coli*. Effect on Na^+-dependent transport and binding properties. *J. Biol. Chem.* **268** (1993) 3209–3215.

66. Puttner, I. B., Sarkar, H. K., Padan, E., Lolkema, J. S., and Kaback, H. R. Characterization of site-directed mutants in the *lac* permease of *Escherichia coli*. Replacement of histidine residues. *Biochemistry* **28** (1989) 2525–2533.

67. Puttner, I. B., Sarkar, H. K., Poonian, M. S., and Kaback, H. R. His-205 and His-322 play different roles in lactose/H^+ symport. *Biochemistry* **25** (1986) 4483–4485.

68. Romano, P. M., Ahearn, G. A., and Storelli, C. Na-dependent L-glutamate transport by eel intestinal BBMV: Role of K^+ and Cl^-. *Am. J. Physiol.* **257** (1989) R180–R188.

69. Rosen, D. R., Siddique, T., Patterson, D., Figlewicz, D. A., Sapp, P., Hentati, A., Donaldson, D., Goto, J., O'Regan, J. P., Deng, H. X., et al. Mutations in Cu/Zn

superoxide dismutase gene are associated with familial amyotrophic lateral sclerosis. *Nature* **362** (1993) 59–62.

70. Rothstein, J., Jin, L., Dykes-Hoberg, M., and Kuncl, R. W. Chronic inhibition of glutamate uptake produces a model of slow neurotoxicity. *Proc. Natl. Acad. Sci. USA* **90** (1993) 6591–6595.

71. Rothstein, J., Martin, L., Levey, A., Dykes-Hoberg, M., Jin, L., Wu, D., Nash, N., and Kunkl, R. Localization of neuronal and glial glutamate transporters. *Neuron* **13** (1994) 713–725.

72. Rothstein, J. D., Dykes-Hoberg, M., Pardo C. A., Bristol, L. A., Jin, L., Kuncl, R. W., Kanai, Y., Hediger, M. A., Wang, Y., Schielke, J., and Welty, D. F. Glial but not neuronal glutamate transporters are responsible for slow glutamate toxicity. *Neuron* **16** (1996) 675–686.

73. Rothstein, J. D., Martin, L. J., and Kuncl, R. W. Decreased glutamate transport by the brain and spinal cord in amyotrophic lateral sclerosis. *N. Engl. J. Med.* **326** (1992) 1464–1468.

74. Rothstein, J. D., Van Kammen, M., Levey, A. I., Martin, L., and Kuncl, R. W. Selective loss of glial glutamate transporter GLT-1 in amyotrophic lateral sclerosis. *Ann. Neurol.* **38** (1995) 73–84.

75. Sarantis, M. and Attwell, D. Glutamate uptake in mammalian retinal glia is voltage- and potassium-dependent. *Brain Res.* **516** (1990) 322–325.

76. Sarantis, M., Ballerini, L., Miller, B., Silver, R. A., Edwards, M., and Attwell, D. Glutamate uptake from the synaptic cleft does not shape the decay of the non-NMDA component of the synaptic current. *Neuron* **11** (1993) 541–549.

77. Schousboe, A. Transport and metabolism of glutamate and GABA in neurons are glial cells. *Int. Rev. Neurobiol.* **22** (1981) 1–45.

78. Shafqat, S., Tamarappoo, B. K., Kilberg, M. S., Puranam, R. S., McNamara, J. O., Guadano-Ferraz, A., and Fremeau, J., R. T. Cloning and expression of a novel Na$^+$-dependent neutral amino acid transporter structurally related to mammalian Na$^+$/glutamate cotransporters. *J. Biol. Chem.* **268** (1993) 15,351–15,355.

79. Shibata, T., Watanabe, M., Tanaka, K., Wada, K., and Inoue, Y. Dynamic changes in expression of glutamate transporter mRNAs in developing brain. *NeuroReport* **7** (1996) 705–709.

80. Siesjo, B., Argardh, C., and Bengtsson, F. Free radicals and brain damage. *Cerebrosvasc. Brain Metab. Rev.* **1** (1989) 165–211.

81. Smith, C. P., Weremowicz, S., Kanai, Y., Stelzner, M., Morton, C., and Hediger, M. A. Assignment of the gene coding for the human high affinity glutamate transporter EAAC1 to 9p24: implications for neurodegenerative disorders and dicarboxylic aminoaciduria. *Genomics* **20** (1994) 335,336.

82. Somohano, F. and Lopez-Colome, A. M. Characteristics of excitatory amino acid uptake in cultures from neurons and glia from the retina. *J. Neurosci. Res.* **28** (1995) 556–562.

83. Stallcup, W. B., Bulloch, K., and Baetge, E. E. Coupled transport of glutamate and sodium in a cerebellar nerve cell line. *J. Neurochem.* **32** (1979) 57–65.

84. Storck, T., Schulte, S., Hofmann, K., and Stoffel, W. Structure, expression and functional analysis of a Na$^+$-dependent glutamate/aspartate transporter from rat brain. *Proc. Natl. Acad. Sci. USA* **89** (1992) 10,955–10,959.

85. Szatkowski, M. and Attwell, D. Triggering and execution of neuronal death in brain ischaemia: Two phases of glutamate release by different mechanisms. *Trends Neurosci.* **17** (1994) 359–365.

86. Thompson, S. M., and Gahwiler, B. H. Effects of the GABA uptake inhibitor tiagabine on inhibitory synaptic potentials in rat hippocampal slice cultures. *J. Neurophysiol.* **67** (1992) 1698–1701.

87. Tong, G. and Jahr, C. E. Block of glutamate transporters potentiates postsynaptic excitation. *Neuron* **13** (1994) 1195–1203.

88. Torp, R., Danbolt, N., Babaie, E., Bjoras, M., Seeberg, E., Storm-Mathisen, J., and Otterson, O. P. Differential expression of two glial glutamate transporters in the rat brain: an *in situ* hybridization study. *Eur. J. Neurosci.* **6** (1994) 936–942.

89. Torp, R. Lekieffre, D., Levy, L. M., Haug, F. M., Danbolt, N. C., Meldrum, B. S., and Ottersen, O. P. Reduced postischemic expression of a glial glutamate transporter, GLT1, in the rat hippocampus. *Exp. Brain Res.* **103** (1995) 51–58.

90. Trotti, D., Volterra, A., Lehre, K. P., Rossi, D., Gjesdal, O., Racagni, G., and Danbolt, N. Arachidonic acid inhibits a purified and reconstituted glutamate transporter directly from the water phase and not via the phospholipid membrane. *J. Biol. Chem.* **270** (1995) 9890–9895.

91. Troy, C. M., Derossi, D., Prochiantz, A., Greene, L. A., and Shelanski, M. Downregulation of Cu/Zn superoxide dismutase leads to cell death via the nitric oxide-peroxynitrite pathway. *J. Neurosci.* **16** (1996) 253–261.

92. Utsunomiya-Tate, N., Endou, H., and Kanai, Y. Cloning and functional characterization of a system ASC-like Na$^+$-dependent neutral amino acid transporter. *J. Biol. Chem.* **271** (1996) 14,883–14,890.

93. Volterra, A., Trotti, D., Cassutti, P., Salvaggio, A., Melcangi, R., and Racagni, G. High sensitivity of glutamate uptake to extracellular free arachidonic acid levels in rat cortical synaptosomes and astrocytes. *J. Neurochem.* **59** (1992) 600–606.

94. Volterra, A., Trotti, D., and Racagni, G. Glutamate uptake is inhibited by arachidonic acid and oxygen free radicals via two distinct and additive mechanisms. *Mol. Pharmacol.* **46** (1994) 986–992.

95. Volterra, A., Trotti, D., Tromba, C., Floridi, S., and Racagni, G. Glutamate uptake inhibition by oxygen free radicals in rat cortical astrocytes. *J. Neurosci.* **14** (1994) 2924–2932.

96. Wadiche, J. I., Amara, S. G., and Kavanaugh, M. P. Ion fluxes associated with excitatory amino acid transport. *Neuron* **75** (1995) 721–728.

97. Wadiche, J. I., Arriza, J. L., Amara, S. G., and Kavanaugh, M. P. Kinetics of a human glutamate transporter. *Neuron* **14** (1995) 1019–1027.

98. Wingrove, T. G. and Kimmich, G. A. Low-affinity intestinal L-aspartate transport with 2:1 coupling stoichiometry for Na$^+$/Asp. *Am. J. Physiol.* **255** (1988) C737–C744.

99. Zanchin, G., De Boni, A., Lauria, G., Maggioni, F., Rossi, P., and Villacara, A. Synaptosomal glutamate uptake in a model of experimental cerebral ischemia. *Neurochem. Res.* **20** (1995) 195–199.

100. Zerague, N., Arriza, J., Amara, S., and Kavanaugh, M. Differential modulation of human glutamate transporter subtypes by arachidonic acid. *J. Biol. Chem.* **270** (1995) 6433–6435.

101. Zhang, Y., Pines, G., and Kanner, B. I. Histidine 326 is critical for the function of GLT-1, a (Na$^+$+K$^+$)-coupled glutamate transporter from rat brain *J. Biol. Chem.* **269** (1994) 19,573–19,577.

CHAPTER 7

Vesicular Neurotransmitter Transporters

Pharmacology, Biochemistry, and Molecular Analysis

Shimon Schuldiner

Transporters and Neurotransmission

Synaptic transmission involves the regulated release of transmitter molecules to the synaptic cleft, where they interact with postsynaptic receptors that subsequently transduce the information. Removal of the transmitter from the cleft enables termination of the signal and usually occurs by its reuptake back into the presynaptic terminal or into glial elements by a sodium-dependent process. This process assures constant and high levels of neurotransmitters in the neuron and low concentrations in the cleft.

Storage of neurotransmitters in subcellular organelles is also crucial for protecting the accumulated molecules from leakage or intraneuronal metabolism and the neuron from possible toxic effects of the transmitters. In addition, the removal of intraneuronal molecules into the storage system effectively lowers the concentration gradient across the neuronal membrane and thus acts as an amplification stage for the overall process of uptake. Drugs that interact with either transport system have profound pharmacological effects as they modify the levels of neurotransmitter in the cleft.

Vesicular transport has been observed for several classical transmitters, including acetylcholine (ACh), the monoamines, glutamate, γ-amino butyric acid, and glycine (reviewed in ref. 73). All the transporters are driven by the proton electrochemical gradient ($\Delta\mu_{H^+}$),

Neurotransmitter Transporters: Structure, Function, and Regulation
Ed.: M.E.A. Reith Humana Press Inc, Totowa, NJ

generated by the vacuolar type adenosine triphosphatase (V-ATPase). This ubiquitous enzyme utilizes the energy of cytoplasmic ATP to translocate H^+ ions into the vesicle and generates a $\Delta\mu_{H^+}$ (acid and positive inside). The vesicular neurotransmitter transporters (VNTs) utilize this energy by exchanging one or more protons with a neurotransmitter molecule (for extensive reviews on the bioenergetics of the transport system, *see* refs. *32,48,49,73*). The vesicular monoamine (VMAT) and ACh (VAChT) transporters have been the most intensively studied and are the ones for which most molecular information has been obtained; we will review the most salient features of both, (for recent reviews on the topic, *see also* refs. *17,70,73,81*). In both cases, the key for this knowledge resides in the availability of potent and specific inhibitors and excellent experimental paradigms.

Pharmacology of VNTs

The best-characterized inhibitors of VNTs are reserpine and tetrabenazine, the two principal agents that inhibit vesicular monoamine transport (*35,56*). In recent years, vesamicol, a novel inhibitor of VAChT, has been introduced and studied in detail (*42,43,52*).

Molecular Mechanism of Reserpine Action

Reserpine presumably binds at the site of amine recognition, based on the fact that it inhibits transport in an apparent competitive way. With a K_i in the subnanomolar range (*13,68*), it binds to the transporter with a K_d similar to its K_i (*13,68*), and transport substrates prevent its association in a concentration range similar to the range of their apparent K_ms (*68*). Its effect in vitro is practically irreversible (*64*), in line with the in vitro effect of the drug, which is extremely long lasting and is relieved only when new vesicles replace the ones that were hit (*78*). As a result of this action, it depletes monoamine stores, providing considerable information on the physiological role of biogenic amines in the nervous system (*10*). Reserpine has been in clinical use because it potently reduces blood pressure; however, it frequently produces a disabling effect of lethargy that resembles depression and this has limited its clinical utility (*21*). This observation has given rise to the amine hypothesis of affective disorders, which, in modified form, still produces a useful framework for considering this group of major psychiatric disorders.

The time-course of reserpine binding is relatively slow. This low rate of association is consistent with a similar time-course for inhibition of monoamine transport (*64*). Reserpine binding is accelerated by $\Delta\mu_{H^+}$, whether generated by the H^+-ATPase (*68,84*) or artificially imposed (*64*). This acceleration is observed also in proteoliposomes reconstituted with the purified protein (*75*).

In all cases, in the presence or absence of $\Delta\mu_{H^+}$ and in the native as well as in the purified protein, two distinct populations of sites have been detected (*68,75*): a high-affinity site, $K_d = 0.5$ nM, $B_{max} = 7$–10 pmol/mg protein in the native chromaffin granule membrane vesicle preparation (0.3 and 310, respectively, for the purified protein), and a low-affinity site, $K_d = 20$ nM, $B_{max} = 60$ pmol/mg protein in the native system (30 and 4200, respectively, for the purified preparation). Surprisingly, the apparent K_d does not change with an imposition of a $\Delta\mu_{H^+}$, even though the on rate increases several-fold (*68*). It has to be assumed that the off rate changes accordingly also, although it is so slow that it has not been possible to measure. When the K_d is measured under conditions in which the concentration of ligand binding sites does not exceed the value of the dissociation constant, it is 30 pM, i.e., about 10 times higher affinity than previously estimated (*13*).

The reserpine binding rate is less sensitive than transport to changes in the ΔpH, and is stimulated equally efficiently by ΔpH and $\Delta\psi$ (*64*). These findings suggest that fewer protons are translocated in the step that generates the high-affinity binding site than in the overall transport cycle. Changes in binding rate probably reflect changes in the availability of reserpine binding sites and translocation of a single H^+ generates the binding form of the transporter. The high-affinity form of the transporter is apparently achieved by either protonation of VMAT or by H^+ translocation. The energy invested in the transporter may be released by ligand binding and converted into vectorial movement of a substrate molecule across the membrane, or directly into binding energy, in the case of reserpine. In the case of a substrate, a second conformational change results in the ligand binding site being exposed to the vesicle interior, where the substrate can dissociate. The second H^+ in the cycle may be required to facilitate the conformational change or to allow for release of the positively charged substrate from the protein. In the model, this second H^+ binding and release is arbitrarily located, since there is no information about the order of the reactions. Interesting, in this respect, are the observations that the apparent affinity of the transporter for substrates drops when the pH decreases (*12,67*). This could reflect a mechanism for releasing the substrate in the acidic lumenal milieu. Substrate and H^+ release regenerates the transporter, which can now start a new cycle. In the case of reserpine, however, its structure (bulk of its side chain?) restricts the conformational change, so that, instead of releasing the ligand into the interior, the complex becomes trapped in a state from which reserpine cannot readily dissociate and which cannot translocate another H^+ to regenerate the high-affinity form. It is not known whether the slow binding of reserpine also requires protonation of VMAT. If this is the case, protonation in the absence of $\Delta\mu_{H^+}$ would be the rate-limiting step.

A Second Site for Inhibitor Action on VMAT

Tetrabenazine (TBZ) is another potent inhibitor of the transporter. Radiolabeled dihydrotetrabenazine (TBZOH) has been used in binding studies to characterize the protein (28,68), to study the regulation of its synthesis (14,15,77), and its distribution in various tissues (65). Binding of TBZOH to the transporter is not modified by the imposition of a $\Delta\mu_{H^+}$, as shown for reserpine. In addition, binding is not inhibited by reserpine at concentrations that fully inhibit transport. Moreover, transport substrates block binding only at concentrations 100-fold higher than their apparent K_m values. These findings have led Henry and collaborators (13,28,69) to suggest that TBZOH binds to a site on the protein that is different from the reserpine and substrate binding site. It has been suggested that both sites are mutually exclusive, i.e., VMAT exists in two different conformations, each conformation binding only one type of ligand, TBZ or reserpine. According to this interpretation, addition of TBZ would pull the conformational equilibrium toward the TBZ binding conformation, which is unable to bind reserpine. Indeed, under proper conditions (low protein concentration and short incubation times), 50 nM TBZOH inhibits reserpine binding by 70%. ATP, through the generation of $\Delta\mu_{H^+}$, would pull the conformational equilibrium towards the reserpine binding site (13). Although elegant and attractive, this model has yet to explain the lack of effect of $\Delta\mu_{H^+}$ on TBZ binding, which should be inhibited, were the two forms mutually exclusive. Also, the concentrations of reserpine required to inhibit TBZ binding are higher than those required for site occupancy (binding and inhibition of transport).

ACh Transporter

An important development in the study of VAChT was the discovery of a specific inhibitor, *trans*-2-(4-phenylpiperidino)cyclohexanol, code named AH5183 and now called vesamicol, which blocks neuromuscular transmission and shows unusual character-istics of action. Marshall (*42*) hypothesized that AH5183 blocks storage by synaptic vesicles and, indeed, it inhibits ACh storage by purified *Torpedo* synaptic vesicles with an IC_{50} of 40 nM. The drug was the most potent inhibitor found among at least 80 compounds initially screened (*59,62*) and *see* ref. *52* for review). [^{3}H]Vesamicol binding showed an apparent K_d of 34 nM (*3–6,34*). ACh inhibits vesamicol binding only at very high concentrations (20–50 mM) and other high-affinity analogs were shown to competitively inhibit binding. However, in all cases where the analogs are trans-ported, the inhibition constants are about 20-fold higher than the apparent constants for transport. Nontransported analogs show the same efficiency for inhibition of both ACh transport and [^{3}H]vesamicol binding (*11*). A kinetic model has been suggested in which it is assumed that vesamicol binds to an allosteric site to form a dead-end complex when ACh is not bound. As described in the previous section, the existence of two sites with similar proper-ties has been observed also for VMAT. In the latter, TBZ is a potent inhibitor of monoamine accumulation, but its binding is inhibited by monoamines only at very high concentrations (*see* A Second Site for Inhibitor Action on VMAT for detailed discussion and refer-ences). In the case of VMAT, both binding sites are present in one protein, since the purified and the recombinant proteins show high sensitivity to TBZ. In the case of VAChT, the existence of a receptor has been postulated that could lie on the same protein or on a sep-arate one. The vesamicol receptor has been extensively studied by Parsons and collaborators; it has been purified (*5*) and labeled with photoaffinity labels (*52,60,61*). The receptor solubilized in cholate and stabilized with glycerol and a phospholipid mixture was puri-fied to yield a specific binding of 4400 pmol/mg protein, a purifi-cation factor of about 15. Unfortunately, the purified receptor exhibits very heterogeneous electrophoretic mobility in sodium dodecyl sulfate-polyacrylamide gel electrophoresis (SDS-PAGE) with very diffuse staining at about 240 kDa. This is the typical behavior of membrane glycoproteins that are not fully monodis-persed because of boiling and because of the nature of the deter-gent used.

Recently, glycoproteins from various species that bind vesamicol with high affinity have been expressed in CV1-fibroblasts (*19,63,82*) (*see also* section on Cloning and Functional Expression of VMATs). In addition, the rat VAChT expressed in CV1-fibroblasts catalyzes vesamicol-sensitive ACh accumulation (*19*). As will be seen, the evidence available now clearly demonstrates that vesamicol binds to the vesicular ACh transporter itself.

Identification of Functional Transporters

The only VNT purified in a functional form is the bovine VMAT. The high stability of the complex [^{3}H]reserpine-transporter has been used to label the transporter and follow its separation through a variety of procedures. In these experiments, a small amount of Triton X100-extracts from prelabeled membranes were mixed with a four- to five fold higher amount of extract from unlabeled membranes (Fig. 1). Purification of the material labeled in this way has revealed the presence of two proteins that differ in pI, a very acidic one (pI 3.5) and a moderately acidic one (pI 5.0) (*75*). Reconstitution in proteoliposomes has shown both to catalyze monoamine transport with the expected properties. The more acidic isoform is a glycoprotein of 80 kDa, which has been purified and reconstituted in proteoliposomes. It catalyzes transport of serotonin with an apparent K_m of 2 μM and a V_{max} of 140 nmol/mg/min, about 200-fold higher than the one determined in the native system. Transport is inhibited by reserpine and tetrabenazine, ligands that bind to two distinct sites on the transporter. In addition, the reconstituted purified transporter binds reserpine with a biphasic kinetic behavior, typical of the native system. The results demonstrate that a single polypeptide is required for all the activities displayed by the transporter, i.e., reserpine- and tetrabenazine-sensitive, ΔpH-driven serotonin accumulation, and binding of reserpine in an energy-dependent and -independent way. Based on these and additional findings, it is estimated that the transporter represents about 0.2–0.5% of the chromaffin granule membrane vesicle and has a turnover of about 30 min^{-1}.

The assignment of the activity to the 80-kDa polypeptide and the localization of the tetrabenazine and reserpine binding sites in the same polypeptide is confirmed by several independent approaches, including direct sequencing of the purified protein (*37,76*) and cloning and analysis of the recombinant protein (*18,39,72*). Vincent and Near (*83*) purified a TBZOH-binding glycoprotein from bovine adrenal medulla using a protocol identical to the one used to purify the functional transporter. The TBZOH-binding protein displays an apparent M_r of 85 kDa. In addition, Isambert and Henry (*31*) labeled bovine VMAT with 7-azido-8-[^{125}I] iodoketanserin, a photoactive derivative of ketanserin, that is thought to interact with the TBZ bind-

Purification of VMAT

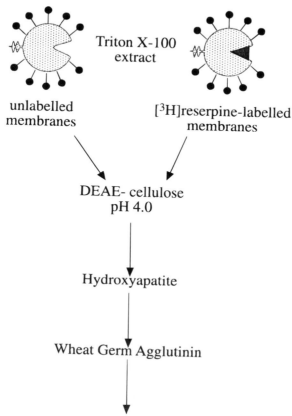

Triton X-100
extract

unlabelled
membranes

[³H]reserpine-labelled
membranes

DEAE- cellulose
pH 4.0

Hydroxyapatite

Wheat Germ Agglutinin

"80 kDa glycoprotein"; upon reconstitution
transports serotonin in a reserpine and
tetrabenazine sensitive mode

Fig. 1. Purification of bovine VMAT from bovine chromaffin granules. The only VNT purified in a functional form is the bovine VMAT. The high stability of the complex [³H]reserpine-transporter has been used to label the transporter and follow its separation through a variety of procedures. In these experiments, a small amount of Triton X-100-extracts from membranes prelabeled with [³H]reserpine were mixed with a 4- to 5-fold higher amount of extract from unlabeled membranes. The major isoform, which accounts for most of the activity in the membranes, displays an extremely acidic pI, which allowed for an efficient purification on an ion exchange column at low pH. Bovine VMAT is a glycoprotein with an apparent molecular mass of 80 kDa, which on reconstitution is fully functional and is inhibited by reserpine and tetrabenazine, (for experimental details, *see* ref. 75).

ing site. The labeled polypeptide displayed an apparent M_r of 70 kDa and a pI ranging from 3.8–4.6. In all cases, broad diffuse bands, characteristic of membrane proteins, were detected, so that the differences in the M_rs reported (70, 80, and 85 kDa) are probably caused by a different analysis of the results and not by innate variations. Sequencing of the azidolodoketanserine-labeled protein confirmed that it is identical with the functional transporter (37).

The basis of the difference between the two isoforms has not yet been studied and could be caused by either covalent modification (i.e., phosphorylation or different glycosylation levels) of the same polypeptide backbone, by limited proteolysis during preparation, or by a different polypeptide backbone. Since we know now that there are two types of VMATs—VMAT2, which is sensitive to TBZ, and VMAT1, which is less sensitive—it should be determined whether the activity of the high pI form is less sensitive to TBZ. The sequence of 26 N-terminal amino acids of the purified protein (low pI, high TBZ sensitivity) is practically identical to the predicted sequence of the bovine adrenal VMAT2 (29,37,76). Antibodies raised against a synthetic peptide, based on the described sequences, specifically recognize the pure protein on Western blots and immunoprecipitate reserpine binding activity under conditions in which the 80-kDa protein alone is precipitated (76).

Cloning and Functional Expression of VMATs

Several sequences of VMAT and VAChT from various species are now available. Rat VMAT was cloned by Edwards et al. (39) and Erickson et al. (18) practically at the same time, using different strategies reviewed elsewhere (17,73). Erickson et al. (18) used expression cloning in CV-1 cells transfected with c-DNA prepared from rat basophilic leukemia (RBL) cells mRNA. Edwards et al. took advantage of the ability of VMAT1 to render CHO cells resistant to MPP^+ by means of its ability to transport the neurotoxin into intracellular acidic compartments, thereby lowering its effective concentration in the cytoplasm (Fig. 2) (39).

Sequence analysis of the cDNA conferring MPP^+ resistance (VMAT1) shows a single large open reading frame that predicts a 521 amino acid protein. Analysis by the method of hydrophobic moments predicts 12 putative transmembrane segments (TMS). A large hydrophilic loop occurs between membrane domains 1 and 2 and contains three potential sites for N-linked glycosylation. According to the 12 TMS model (39), this loop faces the lumen of the vesicle, and both termini face the cytoplasm.

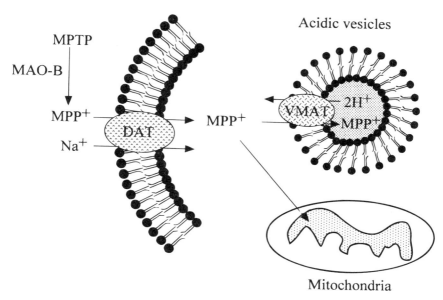

Fig. 2. VMAT renders cells resistant to the neurotoxin MPP$^+$ because it removes the neurotoxin away from its presumed target. The ability of the neurotoxin MPTP to induce Parkinsonism has been explained by its ability to cross the blood–brain barrier and its oxidation in astrocytes to MPP$^+$ by monoamine oxidase B (MAO-B). The higher sensitivity of dopaminergic cells to MPP$^+$ is probably caused by its accumulation into these cells by DAT, the Na$^+$-coupled plasma membrane dopamine transporter. VMAT renders CHO cells resistant to MPP$^+$ by means of its ability to transport the neurotoxin into intracellular acidic compartments, thereby lowering its effective concentration in the cytoplasm and in its presumed target, the respiratory chain of the mitochondria (*17,39*). These findings have suggested a novel type of drug resistance in eukaryotic cells: protection of the devices essential for life by compartmentalization.

Biochemical and quantitative evidence for the identity of the cloned cDNA was provided by developing a cell-free system in which membranes were assayed for dopamine transport and reserpine binding (*39,72*).

VMAT1 expressed in MPP$^+$-resistant Chinese hamster ovary (CHO) cells accounts for about 0.1% of the total cell membrane protein (*72*), and the bovine vesicular transporter accounts for 0.2–0.5% of the chromaffin granule membrane protein (*75*).

A transporter distinct from VMAT1 has been identified in rat brain (VMAT2) (*39*) and in RBL cells (*18*). The predicted protein shows an overall identity of 62% and a similarity of 78% to VMAT1. The major sequence divergences occur at the large lumenal loop located between the first and the second transmembrane domains and at the N- and C-termini.

The Two VMAT Subtypes Differ Also in Some Functional Properties

A comprehensive comparison between the functions of rat VMAT1 and VMAT2 has been performed by Peter et al. (*54*) in membrane vesicles prepared from CHO stable transformed cells lines in which the respective proteins are expressed. According to these studies, VMAT2 has a consistently higher affinity for all the monoamine substrates tested. In the cases of serotonin, dopamine, and epinephrine, the apparent K_m of VMAT1 for ATP-dependent transport is 0.85, 1.56, and 1.86 μM, respectively; the corresponding $K_m s$ measured for VMAT2 are four- to fivefold lower, 0.19, 0.32, and 0.47 μM, correspondingly. Although the affinities are slightly different, the rank order for the various monoamines is similar. Also, other substrates, such as MPP$^+$ (1.6 vs 2.8 μM, respectively) and methamphetamine (2.7 vs 5.5 μM respectively, as estimated from measurements of the ability to inhibit reserpine binding) display a similar pattern. A most striking difference is detected for histamine: 3 μM for VMAT2 and 436 μM for VMAT1. Also, VMAT1 is significantly less sensitive to tetrabenazine, IC$_{50}$ = 3–4 μM (*39,54*), than either VMAT2 (IC$_{50}$ = 0.3–0.6 μM) (*18,54*) or the native (*13,56*) and the purified transporter (IC$_{50}$ = 25 nM) (*75*) from bovine adrenal medulla. The apparent affinities, determined in heterologous expression systems or in proteoliposomes reconstituted with the purified transporter, are higher than those determined in chromaffin granules membrane vesicles (*see* ref. *32* for references). The turnover number (TO) of the recombinant protein has been calculated based on the V_{max} for serotonin transport and the number of reserpine binding sites. The TO for VMAT1 is 10/min and that for VMAT2 is 40/min (*54*). A similar analysis of the purified bovine transporter (VMAT2 type) showed a TO of 30/min (*75*). These values are lower than the 135/min estimated for intact bovine chromaffin granules (*66*), but coincide well with the values obtained from brain regions (10–35/min) (*65*) and other estimates (15 and 35/min) in chromaffin granules (*69*).

Tissue Distribution

Tissue distribution of rat VMAT subtypes has been studied very intensively using a variety of techniques, including Northern analysis

(18,39), *in situ* hybridization (39), and immunohistochemistry (55,85). From these studies it is concluded that expression of VMAT1 and VMAT2 is mutually exclusive: VMAT1 is restricted to nonneuronal cells and VMAT2 to neuronal cells. VMAT1 is expressed in endocrine/paracrine cells: in the adrenal medulla chromaffin cells, in the intestine and gastric mucose in serotonin and histamine-containing endocrine and paracrine cells, and in dopamine-containing SIF cells of sympathetic ganglia. VMAT2 is expressed in neuronal cells throughout, including in the intestine and stomach. There are two exceptions for this restriction: a subpopulation of VMAT2-expressing chromaffin cells in the adrenal medulla, and a population of VMAT2, chromogranin A-positive endocrine cells of the oxyntic mucose of the rat stomach (85).

Although the studies in rat are very definitive, the situation is very different in other species. In human pheochromocytoma, mRNA for both subtypes is found (85). The bovine adrenal medulla expresses a VMAT2 type transporter whose message also has been detected in brain (29,37). VMAT2 is the main adrenal medulla transporter, as was found in direct protein purification studies (29,37,75,76). The purified transporter from bovine adrenal is VMAT2 and accounts for at least 60% of the activity in the gland.

Subcellular Targeting of VMAT

Storage of monoamines differs from that of other classical neurotransmitters. Thus, the latter are stored in small synaptic vesicles, but monoamines in the adrenal medulla are stored with neural peptides in large dense core chromaffin granules. In the central nervous system, neurons store monoamines in vesicles that may contain a dense core. The difference in the storage of the monoamines, compared to that of classical transmitters, may reflect differential sorting of the VNTs. Sorting of VMAT was studied with immunohystochemical and biochemical tools (38,47).

In heterologous expression of VMAT1 in CHO cells, the transporter is targeted to a population of recycling vesicles and co-localizes with the transferrin receptor. Thus, localization in CHO cells is similar to that of other neuronal vesicle proteins, such as synaptophysin and SV2 (38).

In PC12 cells, endogenous VMAT1 occurs principally in large dense core vesicles (LDCVs) (38). Only small amounts are found in synaptic-like microvesicles (SLMVs) and in endosomes (38). In the rat adrenal medulla, immunoreactivity for VMAT1 occurs at several sites in the secretory pathway, but most prominently in the chromaf-

fin granules, supporting the results in PC12 cells (*39*). In central neurons, localization of r-VMAT2's was studied in the nuclei of solitary
tract, a region known to contain a dense and heterogenous population of monoaminergic neurons (*47*). VMAT2 localizes primarily to
LDCVs in axon terminals, but it is also detected in less prominent
amounts in small synaptic vesicles, the trans-Golgi network, and
other sites of vesicle transport and recycling. Thus, both VMAT1 and
VMAT2 are primarily sorted to LDCVs in all the cell types studied.

Regulation of Expression of VMAT

Evidence for regulation of expression of VMAT was first obtained
in insulin-shocked rats in which an increase in the number of
[^{3}H]TBZOH binding sites in the adrenal medulla was detected. The
increase was maximal after 4–6 d (*77*). A similar increase was
observed in vitro in bovine chromaffin cells in culture in the presence
of carbamylcholine or depolarizing concentrations of potassium ions
(*14*). The response was mimicked by forskolin and by phorbol esters
and was blocked by actinomycin and cycloheximide, suggesting
involvement of transcriptional activation.

This suggestion was supported by the detection of an increase in
message for VMAT2 after a 6 h depolarization (*37*). After 5 d, the cells
contained less secretory granules and those left had a higher density,
suggesting that they were newly synthesized and immature. Although
the catecholamine, chromogranin A, and cytochrome b561 content
decreased, [^{3}H]TBZOH binding sites increased about 1.5 fold. The
physiological significance of these findings is not obvious. It has been
speculated that this phenomenon may reflect the fact that vesicular
uptake might be rate-limiting and, thereby, to accelerate refilling, an
increase in VMAT is needed. Mahata et al. (*40,41*) suggested, however,
that there is no increase in other membrane proteins in the rat granule.
They have reported no changes in the level of VMAT1 message (the
main subtype in rat adrenal) under conditions at which mRNA for the
matrix peptide NPY increased (*40,41*). Since the [^{3}H] TBZOH binding
sites increased in the same system, the latter findings may suggest a
novel mode of regulation of activity of preexisting protein.

Cloning and Functional Expression
of VAChT Transporters

The powerful genetics of the nematode *Caenorhabditis elegans* has
provided important information regarding VAChT. The elegant

approach used by Alfonso et al. (2) was based on the analysis of one of the mutants described by Brenner (9) 20 yr ago. Mutations in the *unc-17* gene of the nematode result in impaired neuromuscular function, which suggests that cholinergic processes might be defective in the mutant. In addition, *unc-17* mutants were resistant to cholinesterase inhibitors (9), a resistance that may result from decreased synthesis or release of the transmitter. Moreover, *unc-17* was found closely linked to *cha-1* gene, which encodes choline acetyltransferase (58). The genomic region of *unc-17* was cloned by walking from the *cha-1* gene and thereafter cDNA was isolated from a library (2). Injection of a cosmid containing the complete coding sequence of the isolated cDNA rescues the mutant phenotypes of *unc-17* animals. A protein with 532 amino acids is predicted from the isolated DNA sequences. This protein (UNC-17 = VAChT) is 37% identical to VMAT1 and 39% identical to VMAT2. The findings strongly suggested that UNC-17 is VAChT. This was supported by the fact that antibodies against specific peptides stain most regions of the nervous system. Within individual cells, staining was punctate and concentrated near synaptic regions. Double labeling with anti-synaptotagmin showed colocalization of the two antigens. In addition, in *unc-104* mutants, a mutation in a kinesin-related protein required for the axonal transport of synaptic vesicles, synaptic vesicles accumulate in cell bodies. In these animals, anti-UNC-17 staining was restricted to neuronal cell bodies. More than 20 alleles, viable as homozygotes, have now been identified. Their phenotypes vary from mild to severe. In two of these mutants, staining was dramatically decreased throughout the nervous system. Two other alleles were isolated that are lethal as homozygotes and they seem to represent the null *unc-17* phenotype. This is the first demonstration that the function encoded by a VNT is essential for survival.

Homology screening with a probe from *unc-17* allowed for the isolation of DNA clones from *Torpedo marmorata* and *Torpedo ocellata* (82). The *Torpedo* proteins display approximately 50% identity to UNC-17 and 43% identity to VMAT1 and VMAT2. Message is specifically expressed in the brain and the electric lobe. The *Torpedo* protein, expressed in CV-1 fibroblast cells, binds vesamicol with high affinity (K_d = 6 nM). The UNC-17 protein expressed in the same cells binds also vesamicol, albeit with a lower affinity (124 nM) (82). Mammalian VAChTs (human and rat) have been identified (19,63). The predicted sequences of both proteins are highly similar to those of the *Torpedo* and *C. elegans* counterparts. The rat VAChT has been shown to bind vesamicol with high affinity (K_d = 6 nM). It also catalyzes proton-dependent, vesamicol-sensitive ACh accumulation in transfected CV1 cells (19). The distribution of rat VAChT mRNA coincides with that reported for choline acetyltransferase (ChAT), the enzyme required for ACh biosynthesis, in the peripheral and central cholinergic nervous systems. The human VAChT gene localizes to chromosome 10q11.2, which is also the location of the ChAT gene. The entire sequence of the human VAChT coding area is contained uninterrupted within the first intron of the ChAT gene locus (19). Transcription of both genes from the same or contiguous promoters provides a novel mechanism for coordinate regulation of two proteins whose expression is required to establish a phenotype.

Structure–Function Studies: Identification of Residues/Domains with Putative Roles in Structure and Function

Hydropathic analysis of the VNT's protein sequence predict 12 putative transmembrane segments and a large hydrophilic loop between transmembrane domains 1 and 2 (Fig. 3). The loop contains potential sites for N-linked glycosylation. Previous studies have demonstrated that all the glycan moieties in glycoproteins of chromaffin granules and ACh storage vesicles face the lumen. Therefore, according to the latter finding and the model, the loop faces the lumen and both termini face the cytoplasm.

Identification of functional residues in VNTs is based on studies using site-directed mutagenesis and relatively specific chemical modifiers. These studies are facilitated by the availability of sequences from different species and subtypes. It is usually assumed that residues that play central roles in catalysis are conserved throughout species. The degree of conservation in the group of VNTs is rather high. The members that are farther away in the group (human VMAT2 and the *C. elegans* VAChT) are still 38% identical and 63% similar (73). The highest divergence is detected in the N- and C-termini and in the glycosylation loop between putative TMS1 and 2. The highest identity is observed in TM 1, 2, and 11, where at least 11 amino acids are fully conserved. In TMS 11 the conservation is particularly striking, since practically all the amino acids conserved are in a contiguous stretch SVYGSVYAIAD.

Carboxyl Residues

Particularly striking are four conserved Asp residues—D34, D267, D404, and D431 (numbers of rVMAT1)—in the middle of TMS 1, 6,

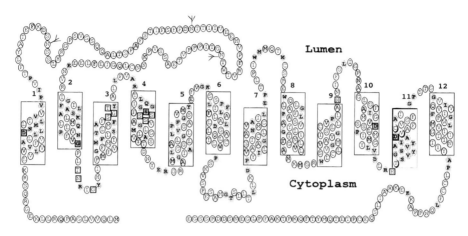

Fig. 3. Model of rVMAT1. Analysis by the method of hydrophobic moments predicts 12 putative transmembrane segments (TMS). A large hydrophilic loop occurs between membrane domains 1 and 2 and contains three potential sites for N-linked glycosylation. According to the 12 TMS model (*39*), this loop faces the lumen of the vesicle, and both termini face the cytoplasm. In this model, the residues conserved in all VNTs are highlighted. The residues that have been mutagenized are shown in squares. Details of the effect of the mutations are given in the text.

10, and 11, respectively (Fig. 3). In addition to these conserved charged residues in the membrane, biochemical evidence is available that N,N'-dicyclohexylcarbodiimide (DCC) inhibits VMAT-mediated transport (*22,71,80*). DCC reacts with a carboxyl residue whose availability is influenced by the occupancy of the tetrabenazine binding site (*80*). Reaction with the above carboxyl residue inhibits not only overall transport activity but also TBZ and reserpine binding, suggesting that the residue plays a role in one of the first steps of the transport cycle. As with all chemical modifiers, indirect effects, such as steric hindrance by the DCC moiety or indirect effect on the structure of the protein, cannot be ruled out at present. Therefore, mutagenesis studies of the roles of these four Asp residues on VMAT should be instructive.

Conservative replacement of Asp33 with Glu in rVMAT2 (equivalent to Asp34 in rVMAT1) reduced activity but did not abolish it (*44*). Replacement with Asn abolished transport, indicating the crucial role of a negative charge at this position. However, D33Q rVMAT2 could still bind [^{3}H]reserpine, and binding was accelerated by $\Delta\mu_{H^+}$ (*44*).

Inhibition of reserpine binding in D33N by serotonin differs dramatically from the wild type, suggesting interference with substrate recognition. Similarly, replacements in positions 404 and 431 in rVMAT1, located in TMS 10 and 11, had dramatic effects on activity (74a). In the case of 431, even a conservative replacement with Glu led to transport inhibition. Replacement of Asp404 with Glu generated a very interesting protein; the pH optimum of transport was shifted by about 1 pH unit to the acid side. In addition, the affinity of the mutant protein to TBZ dramatically increased to levels comparable to those observed in the VMAT2 subtype. It is concluded that the environment around the carboxyl moiety at position 404 is critical for the recognition of TBZ and influences the pK of one or more groups in the protein involved in the last steps of the catalytic cycle. Replacement with either Cys or Ser on both positions yielded proteins that displayed no transport at all. The Asp431 replacements, D431E and D431S, but not D431C, which was not expressed at detectable levels, bound [³H] reserpine normally and binding was accelerated by $\Delta\mu_{H^+}$. The Asp404 replacements D404S and D404C showed no binding at all (74a).

An important conclusion from these studies is that replacements of negative charges in the middle of putative transmembrane segments have dramatic effects on transport, but do not necessarily induce major changes in the protein structure, since some of the mutants still bind a high-affinity ligand and respond to $\Delta\mu_{H^+}$. The ability to measure partial reactions in VMAT allows for a more sophisticated analysis of mutagenized proteins than was previously possible. Thus, although it does not transport, it was shown that the D33N mutant protein has a lower affinity to serotonin than the wild type. Also, the mutant D404E shows an acid shift on the overall cycle but not on partial reactions, suggesting an effect on a pK_a important for the final steps of transport. It is tempting to speculate a direct role of D404 in the translocation of the second H^+ needed for the overall cycle. Direct proof of this contention will need further experimentation. In this context, it is interesting to point out that only two of the 19 mutants described thus far are completely inactive. In addition, one of them is not expressed to detectable levels.

His and Arg Residues

Also it has been suggested that His residues play a role in H^+ translocation and sensing in other H^+-coupled transporters (23,57). In VMATs, there is only one His conserved (His419) in loop 10, between

TMS 9 and 10. This His is immediately behind an Arg residue conserved throughout the whole VNT family and is very close to the longest conserved sequence stretch. Although also present in the rat, human, and *C. elegans* VAChT, it is replaced by a Phe in the *Torpedo* VAChT. Biochemical evidence also suggested a role for His in VMAT. Phenylglyoxal (PG) and diethyl pyrocarbonate (DEPC) are reagents relatively specific for Arg and His residues, respectively. They both inhibit serotonin accumulation in chromaffin granule membrane vesicles in a dose-dependent manner (IC_{50} of 8 and 1 mM, respectively) (*30,79*). The inhibition by DEPC was specific for His groups, since transport could be restored by hydroxylamine (*79*). Neither PG nor DEPC inhibited binding of either reserpine or tetrabenazine, indicating that the inhibition of transport is not caused by a direct interaction with either of the known binding sites. However, the acceleration of reserpine binding by a transmembrane H^+ gradient was inhibited by both reagents (*79*). The results suggest either proton transport or a conformational change induced by proton transport is inhibited by both types of reagents. Several other transport systems are sensitive to DEPC and phenylglyoxal (reviewed in refs. *33,51,79*).

A more direct analysis of the role of histidines in VMAT has been carried out by site-directed mutagenesis of rVMAT1 (*74*). Replacement of His419, the only His conserved in VMAT1, with either Cys (H419C) or Arg (H419R), completely abolishes transport as measured in permeabilized CV1 cells transiently transformed with the mutants DNA. In the absence of $\Delta\mu_{H^+}$ reserpine binding to the mutant proteins is at levels comparable to those detected in the wild type. However, acceleration of binding in the presence of $\Delta\mu_{H^+}$ is not observed in either H419C or H419R. These results suggest that His419 plays a role in a step other than binding and may be associated directly with H^+ translocation or in conformational changes occurring after substrate binding.

Serine Residues

It has been suggested that serines play a role in ligand recognition in the β-adrenergic receptor and in the dopamine plasma membrane transporter (*36*). Two groups of serine residues occur in VMAT2, in TM 3 and TM 4. Simultaneous replacement of 4 serines in TM 4 (S197, 198, 200, and 201) with alanine does not affect transport activity. On the other hand, mutant VMAT2, in which serines 180, 181, and 182 (in

TM 3) were replaced with alanine, showed no transport activity. Moreover, binding of [^{3}H] reserpine was at normal levels and it was accelerated by $\Delta\mu_{H^+}$. However, in contrast to wild type, and similar to D33N, binding was not inhibited by serotonin, even at concentrations of 500 μM. The results suggest a possible role of Ser 180–182 in substrate recognition (44).

Mutations in TetA and BMR Proteins

Interesting information can also be inferred from studies in homologous proteins performing similar or identical functions. Toxin extruding antiporters (TEXANs) have evolved in many living organisms as transport proteins that play central roles in survival. Because of the overall similarities in mechanism (H$^+$/substrate antiporters), secondary structure, and sharing of some of the substrates, the information obtained in studies with other TEXANs deserves some attention. Two proteins, TetA and Bmr, have been studied in detail and a large number of mutants were characterized (1,87–89).

Comparison to VMAT has suggested a number of residues that may be involved in catalysis. Replacement of N155 in VMAT2 with the Asp found in related bacterial protein does not affect transport activity. Also, replacement of the adjacent potential phosphorylation site (T154) with alanine does not impair function, indicating that phosphorylation at this site is not required for activity. Replacement of Gly151 and 158 in the conserved motif GXXXXRXG in loop 3 has no effect on transport.

Random mutagenesis of *B. subtilis* multidrug transporter (Bmr) gave rise to several independent mutants exhibiting altered spectra of cross-resistance to various drugs (Neyfakh, A., personal communication). All these mutants were located within the region of transmembrane domains 9–11. In addition, a reserpine-insensitive mutant located in the same region was identified (1). Four more site-directed mutations in this region were engineered and all of them changed quantitatively the cross-resistance profile of bacteria expressing Bmr (Neyfakh, A., personal communication). These site-directed mutations were designed based on the following principle. Amino acids conserved between Bmr and its *S. aureus* homolog NorA, which is very similar to Bmr in the cross-resistance profile it confers to *B. subtilis* (46), but different from their homologous Tet transporters, were converted into the Tet-specific amino acids. For example, if a certain residue in Bmr and NorA is Met, but in the Tet proteins the corresponding residue is Gly, Met was converted in Bmr into Gly. Using the latter principle, control mutations in some other regions of the transporter were made, one in the seventh TM domain, another in the fourth TM domain. Both these control mutations gave changes in the resistance profile as large as the ones observed with the mutations in the 9–11 region, indicating that other residues in different areas of the protein are needed for substrate specificity. It is not clear, therefore, why all the random mutations showing altered cross-resistance profile were clustered in the 9–11 region (the probability of such a clustering by pure chance is just 1.2%).

An extensive mutagenesis study has been performed, also, in the *Escherichia coli* TetA protein (*87–89*). These studies highlight residues with putative roles in catalysis in TM domains 8–9, as well as in 1–3. Other transport proteins, like the *lac* permease from *E. coli*, a 12 TM protein that catalyzes symport of H^+ and β-galactosides, but does not belong to the TEXAN superfamily, imply a similar conclusion. In addition to important residues in TM 9 and 10, it was found by Kaback (*33*) that very few of the residues in the other TM areas are essential. In fact, TM 2–7 can be completely deleted and the protein still catalyzes facilitated diffusion of lactose (*8*). Studies by Hama and Wilson (*27*) on the melibiose symporter suggest that the above suggestions may be an oversimplification, since more than one domain is involved in substrate recognition (*27*).

TEXANs

The VNTs are part of a family that includes at least 40 proteins from prokaryotes and eukaryotes and has been surveyed in several monographs (*26,53,70,73*). Based on an analysis of the evolutionary relationships, four subgroups have been identified. All the proteins present in microorganisms are presumed to be exporters located in the cytoplasmic membrane of these cells, which confer resistance to a large list of compounds because of their ability to actively remove them from the cell. The VNTs, on the other hand, are located in intracellular vesicles. Though the bacterial transporters extrude the toxic compounds to the medium, those presently known in mammals remove neurotransmitters from the cytoplasm into intracellular storage compartments. In both cases, as a result of their functioning, the concentration of the substrates in the cytoplasm is reduced. When the substrate of the VNTs is cytotoxic, such as MPP^+, a substrate of the VMAT, the removal of the toxic compound from the cytoplasm, away from its presumed target, will ameliorate the toxicity of the compound. Indeed, CHO cells expressing VMAT are more resistant to MPP$^+$ (38). These findings suggest a novel type of drug resistance in eukaryotic cells: protection of the devices essential for life by compartmentalization. Similar strategies have previously been suggested to explain tolerance to high salt and toxic compounds in plants and yeasts (20,50,86) however, no molecular description of these phenomena has yet been proposed. One orphan mammalian protein, more similar in sequence to the bacterial Tet A-Bmr cluster than to the VNTs, has been described thus far (16).

Most transporters of the family have a very broad specificity for substrates. All of the substrates are aromatic compounds, usually bearing an ionizable or permanently charged nitrogen moiety. In some substrates, however, carboxylic groups are also present (i.e., norfloxacin); in others, a phosphonium moiety is present (i.e., TPP$^+$), and yet in others, no positive charge is present at all (i.e., actinorhodin, uncouplers). Many of the substrates are common to many multidrug transporters and this large overlap in substrate recognition may hint at common solutions to the problem of recognition of multiple substrates with high affinity.

All the transporters of the TEXAN family are located in membranes across which H$^+$ electrochemical gradients exist. The gradients are generated by primary pumps, such as the bacterial respiratory chain or the H$^+$-translocating ATPases of both bacteria and intracellular storage organelles. The gradient is utilized by the protein through the exchange of a substrate molecule with one or more hydrogen ions. All the neurotransmitter storage vesicles studied thus far, in brain, platelets, mast cells, and adrenal medulla, contain a vacuolar type H$^+$ pumping ATPase, similar in composition to the ATPase of lysosomes, endosomes, Golgi membranes, and clathrin-coated vesicles (24,25,45). In all these organelles, the activity of this proton pump generates an H$^+$ electrochemical gradient ($\Delta\mu_{H^+}$ acid and positive inside). In synaptic vesicles and neurotransmitter storage organelles, the proton electrochemical gradient is utilized by the VNTs, which couple efflux of H$^+$ ions to the uptake of a neurotransmitter molecule (for review, *see* ref. 73). In the case of Tet proteins, it has been suggested that the exchange is between a Metal–Tetracycline complex and one proton in an electroneutral process. Also BMR-mediated drug efflux is apparently driven by a transmembrane pH gradient. Although very little is known about the other transporters, the fact that they all display sequence similarities, and none of them show any ATP binding domains, in addition to the fact that they are all found in membranes with H⁺ gradients, suggests that they all are antiporters that exchange one or more H⁺ ions with a substrate molecule.

Acknowledgments

This work was supported by grants from the National Institute of Health (NH16708), the United States–Israel Binational Science Foundation (93-00051), and the National Institute of Psychobiology in Israel.

References

1. Ahmed, M., Borsch, C., Neyfakh, A., and Schuldiner, S. Mutants of the *Bacillus-subtilis* multidrug transporter Bmr with altered sensitivity to the antihypertensive alkaloid reserpine. *J. Biol. Chem.* **268** (1993) 11,086–11,089.

2. Alfonso, A., Grundahl, K., Duerr, J. S., Han, H. P., and Rand, J. B. The *Caenorhabditis elegans* Unc-17 Gene—A putative vesicular acetylcholine transporter. *Science* **261** (1993) 617–619.

3. Bahr, B. and Parsons, S. Acetylcholine transport and drug inhibition kinetics in *Torpedo* synaptic vesicles. *J Neurochem.* **46** (1986) 1214–1218.

4. Bahr, B. and Parsons, S. Demonstration of a receptor in *Torpedo* synaptic vesicles for the acetylcholine storage blocker L-trans-2-(4-phenyl[3,4-3H]piperidino) cyclohexanol. *Proc. Natl. Acad. Sci. USA* **83** (1986) 2267–2270.

5. Bahr, B. and Parsons, S. Purification of the vesamicol receptor. *Biochemistry* **31** (1992) 5763–5769.

6. Bahr, B., Clarkson, E., Rogers, G., Noremberg, K., and Parsons, S. A kinetic and allosteric model for the acetylcholine transporter-vesamicol receptor in synaptic vesicles. *Biochemistry* **31** (1992) 5752–5762.

7. Bahr, B., Noremberg, K., Rogers, G., Hicks, B., and Parsons, S. Linkage of the acetylcholine transporter–vesamicol receptor to proteoglycan in synaptic vesicles. *Biochemistry* **31** (1992) 5778–5784.

8. Bibi, E., Verner, G., Chang, C., and Kaback, H. Organization and stability of a polytopic membrane protein: deletion analysis of the lactose permease of *Escherichia coli. Proc. Natl. Acad. Sci. USA* **88** (1991) 7271–7275.

9. Brenner, S. The genetics of *Caenorhabditis elegans. Genetics* **77** (1974) 71–94.

10. Carlsson, A. Drugs which block the storage of 5-hydroxytryptamine and related amines. *Hand. Exp. Pharmacol.* **19** (1965) 529–592.

11. Clarkson, E., Rogers, G., and Parsons, S. Binding and active transport of large analogues of acetylcholine by cholinergic synaptic vesicles *in vivo. J. Neurochem.* **59** (1992) 695–700.

12. Darchen, F., Scherman, D., Desnos, C., and Henry, J.-P. Characteristics of the transport of the quaternary ammonium 1-methyl-4-phenylpyridinium by chromaffin granules. *Biochem. Pharmacol.* **37** (1988) 4381–4387.

13. Darchen, F., Scherman, D., and Henry, J.-P. Reserpine binding to chromaffin granules suggests the existence of two conformations of the monoamine transporter. *Biochemistry* **28** (1989) 1692–1697.

14. Desnos, C., Laran, M., and Scherman, D. Regulation of the chromaffin granule catecholamine transporter in cultured bovine adrenal medullary cells—stimulus biosynthesis coupling. *J Neurochem.* **59** (1992) 2105–2112.

15. Desnos, C., Raynaud, B., Vidal, S., Weber, M., and Scherman, D. Induction of the vesicular monoamine transporter by elevated potassium concentration in cultures of rat sympathetic neurons. *Dev. Brain Res.* **52** (1990) 161–166.

16. Duyao, M., Taylor, S., Buckler, A., Ambrose, C., Lin, C., Groot, N., Church, D., Barnes, G., Wasmuth, J., Housman, D., MacDonald, M., and Gusella, J. A gene from chromosome 4p16.3 with similarity to a superfamily of transporter proteins. *Hum. Mol. Genet.* **2** (1993) 673–676.

17. Edwards, R. The transport of neurotransmitters into synaptic vesicles. *Curr. Opin. Neurobiol.* **2** (1992) 586–594.

18. Erickson, J., Eiden, L., and Hoffman, B. Expression cloning of a reserpine-sensitive vesicular monoamine transporter. *Proc. Natl. Acad. Sci. USA* **89** (1992) 10,993–10,997.

19. Erickson, J. D., Varoqui, H., Schafer, M. K. H., Modi, W., Diebler, M. F., Weihe, E., Rand, J., Eiden, L., Bonner, T. I., and Usdin, T. B. Functional identification of a vesicular acetylcholine transporter and its expression from a 'cholinergic' gene locus. *J. Biol. Chem.* **269** (1994) 21,929–21,932.

20. Flowers, T. J., Troke, P. F., and Yeo, A. R. The mechanism of salt tolerance in halophytes. *Ann. Rev. Plant. Physiol.* **28** (1977) 89–121.

21. Frize, E. Mental depression in hypertensive patients treated for long periods with high doses of reserpine. *N. Engl. J. Med.* **251** (1954) 1006–1008.

22. Gasnier, B., Scherman, D., and Henry, J. Dicyclohexylcarbodiimide inhibits the monoamine carrier of bovine chromaffin granule membrane. *Biochemistry* **24** (1985) 1239–1244.

23. Gerchman, Y., Olami, Y., Rimon, A., Taglicht, D., Schuldiner, S., and Padan, E. Histidine 226 is part of the pH sensor of NhaA, a Na^+/H^+ antiporter in *Escherichia coli. Proc. Natl. Acad. Sci. USA* **90** (1993) 1212–1216.

24. Gluck, S. The structure and biochemistry of the vacuolar H^+ ATPase in proximal and distal urinary acidification. *J Bioenerg. Biomembr.* **24** (1992) 351–359.

25. Gogarten, J. P., Kibak, H., Dittrich, P., Taiz, L., Bowman, E. J., Bowman, B. J., Manolson, M. F., Poole, R. J., Date, T., Oshima, T., Konishi, J., Denda, K., and Yoshida, M. Evolution of the vacuolar H^+-ATPase: implications for the origin of eukaryotes. *Proc. Natl. Acad. Sci. USA* **86** (1989) 6661–6665.

26. Griffith, J., Baker, M., Rouch, D., Page, M., Skurray, R., Paulsen, I., Chater, K., Baldwin, S., and Henderson, P. Evolution of transmembrane transport: relationships between transport proteins for sugars, carboxylate compounds, antibiotics and antiseptics. *Curr. Opinions Cell Biol.* **4** (1992) 684–695.

27. Hama, H. and Wilson, T. Cation-coupling in chimeric melibiose carriers derived from *E. coli* and *Klebsiella pneumonia. J. Biol. Chem.* **268** (1993) 10,060–10,065.

28. Henry, J.-P. and Scherman, D. Radioligands of the vesicular monoamine transporter and their use as markers of monoamine storage vesicles. *Biochem. Pharmacol.* **38** (1989) 2395–2404.

29. Howell, M., Shirvan, A., Sternbach, Y., Steinermordoch, S., Strasser, J. E., Dean, G. E., and Schuldiner, S. Cloning and functional expression of a tetrabenazine sensitive vesicular monoamine transporter from bovine chromaffin granules. *FEBS Lett.* **338** (1994) 16–22.

30. Isambert, M. and Henry, J. Effect of diethylpyrocarbonate on pH-driven monoamine uptake by chromaffin granule ghosts. *FEBS Lett.* **136** (1981) 13–18.

31. Isambert, M., Gasnier, B., Botton, D., and Henry, J. Characterization and purification of the monoamine transporter of bovine chromaffin granules. *Biochemistry* **31** (1992) 1980–1986.

32. Johnson, R. Accumulation of biological amines in chromaffin granules: a model for hormone and neurotransmitter transport. *Physiol. Rev.* **68** (1988) 232–307.

33. Kaback, H. The lactose permease of *Escherichia-coli*—a paradigm for membrane transport proteins. *Biochim. Biophys. Acta* **1101** (1992) 210–213.

34. Kaufman, R., Rogers, G. A., Fehlmann, C., and Parsons, S. M. Fractional vesamicol receptor occupancy and acetylcholine active transport inhibition in synaptic vesicles. *Mol. Pharmacol.* **36** (1989) 452–456.

35. Kirshner, N. Uptake of catecholamines by a particulate fraction of the adrenal medulla. *J. Biol. Chem.* **237** (1962) 2311–2317.

36. Kitayama, S., Shimada, S., Xu, H., Markham, L., Donovan, D., and Uhl, G. Dopamine transporter site-directed mutations differentially alter substrate transport and cocaine binding. *Proc. Natl. Acad. Sci. USA* **89** (1992) 7782–7785.

37. Krejci, E., Gasnier, B., Botton, D., Isambert, M. F., Sagne, C., Gagnon, J., Massoulie, J., and Henry, J. P. Expression and regulation of the bovine vesicular monoamine transporter gene. *FEBS Lett.* **335** (1993) 27–32.

38. Liu, Y., Schweitzer, E., Nirenberg, M., Pickel, V., Evans, C., and Edwards, R. Preferential localization of a vesicular monoamine transporter to dense core vesicles in PC12 cells. *J. Cell Biol.* **127** (1994) 1419–1433.

39. Liu, Y., Peter, D., Roghani, A., Schuldiner, S., Prive, G., Eisenberg, D., Brecha, N., and Edwards, R. A CDNA that suppresses MPP⁺ toxicity encodes a vesicular amine transporter. *Cell* **70** (1992) 539–551.

40. Mahata, S. K., Mahata, M., Fischercolbrie, R., and Winkler, H. Reserpine causes differential changes in the messenger RNA levels of chromogranin-B, secretogranin-II, carboxypeptidase-H, alpha-amidating monooxygenase, the vesicular amine transporter and of synaptin/synaptophysin in rat brain. *Mol. Brain Res.* **19** (1993) 83–92.

41. Mahata, S. K., Mahata, M., Fischercolbrie, R., and Winkler, H. Vesicle monoamine transporter-1 and transporter-2—Differential distribution and regulation of their messenger RNAs in chromaffin and ganglion cells of rat adrenal medulla. *Neurosci. Lett.* **156** (1993) 70–72.

42. Marshall, I. Studies on the blocking action of 2-(4-phenyl piperidino) cyclohexanol (AH5183). *Br. J. Pharmacol.* **38** (1970) 503–516.

43. Marshall, I. and Parsons, S. The vesicular acetylcholine transport system. *Trends Neurosci.* **10** (1987) 174–177.

44. Merickel, A., Rosandich, P., Peter, D., and Edwards, R. Identification of residues involved in substrate recognition by a vesicular monoamine transporter. *J. Biol. Chem.* **270** (1995) 25,798–25,804.

45. Nelson, N. Structural conservation and functional diversity of V-ATPases, *J. Bioenerg. Biomembr.* **24** (1992) 407–414.

46. Neyfakh, A. The multidrug efflux transporter of *Bacillus subtilis* is a structural and functional homolog of the *Staphylococcus* NorA protein. *Antimicrob. Agents Chemother.* **36** (1992) 484, 485.

47. Nirenberg, M., Liu, Y., Peter, D., Edwards, R., and Pickel, V. The vesicular monoamine transporter-2 is preferentially localized to large dense core vesicles in the rat solitary tract nuclei. *Proc. Natl. Acad. Sci. USA* **92** (1995) 8773–8777.

48. Njus, D., Kelley, P. M., and Harnadek, G. J. Bioenergetics of secretory vesicles. *Biochim. Biophys. Acta* **853** (1986) 237–265.

49. Njus, D., Knoth, J., and Zallakian, M. Proton-linked transport in chromaffin granules, *Curr. Top. Bioenerg.* **11** (1981) 107–147.

50. Ohya, Y., Umemoto, N., Tanida, I., Ohta, A., Iida, H., and Anraku, Y. Calcium sensitive *cls* mutants of *Saccharomyces cerevisiae* showing a Pet-phenotype are ascribable to defects of vacuolar membrane H⁺-ATPase activity. *J. Biol. Chem.* **266** (1991) 13,971–13,977.

51. Padan, E., Sarkar, H., K, Vitanen, P. V., Poonian, M. S., and Kaback, H. R. Site-specific mutagenesis of histidine residues in the *lac* permease of *Escherichia coli*. *Proc. Natl. Acad. Sci. USA* **82** (1985) 6765–6768.

52. Parsons, S. M., Bahr, B. A., Rogers, G. A., Clarkson, E. D., Noremberg, K., and Hicks, B. W. Acetylcholine transporter vesamicol receptor pharmacology and structure. *Prog. Brain Res.* **98** (1993) 175–181.

53. Paulsen, I. and Skurray, R. Topology, structure and evolution of two families of proteins involved in antibiotic and antiseptic resistance in eukaryotes and prokaryotes—an analysis. *Gene* **124** (1993) 1–11.

54. Peter, D., Jimenez, J., Liu, Y. J., Kim, J., and Edwards, R. H. The chromaffin granule and synaptic vesicle amine transporters differ in substrate recognition and sensitivity to inhibitors. *J Biol. Chem.* **269** (1994) 7231–7237.

55. Peter, D., Liu, Y., Sternini, C., de Giorgio, R., Brecha, N., and Edwards, R. Differential expression of two vesicular monoamine transporters. *J Neurosci.* **15** (1995) 6179–6188.

56. Pletscher, A. Effect of neuroleptics and other drugs on monoamine uptake by membrane of adrenal chromaffin granules. *Br. J. Pharmacol.* **59** (1977) 419–424.

57. Puettner, I. B., Sarkar, H. K., Padan, E., Lolkema, J. S., and Kaback, H. R. Characterization of site-directed mutants in the *lac* permease of *Escherichia coli* Replacement of histidine residues. *Biochemistry* **28** (1989) 2525–2533.

58. Rand, J. Genetic analysis of the *cha1-unc17* gene complex in *Caenorhabditis*. *Genetics* **122** (1989) 73–80.

59. Rogers, G. and Parsons, S. Inhibition of acetylcholine storage by acetylcholine analogs in vitro. *Mol. Pharmacol.* **36** (1989) 333–341.

60. Rogers, G. and Parsons, S. Photoaffinity labeling of the acetylcholine transporter. *Biochemistry* **31** (1992) 5770–5777.

61. Rogers, G. A. and Parsons, S. M. Photoaffinity labeling of the vesamicol receptor of cholinergic synaptic vesicles. *Biochemistry* **32** (1993) 8596–8601.

62. Rogers, G., Parsons, S., Anderson, D., Nilsson, L., Bahr, B., Kornreich, W., Kaufman, R., Jacobs, R., and Kirtman, B. Synthesis, in vitro acetylcholine-storage-blocking activities, and biological properties of derivatives and analogues of *trans*-2-(4-phenylpiperidino) cyclohexanol (vesamicol). *J. Med. Chem.* **32** (1989) 1217–1230.

63. Roghani, A., Feldman, J., Kohan, S. A., Shirzadi, A., Gundersen, C. B., Brecha, N., and Edwards, R. H. Molecular cloning of a putative vesicular transporter for acetylcholine. *Proc. Natl. Acad. Sci. USA* **91** (1994) 10,620–10,624.

64. Rudnick, G., Steiner-Mordoch, S. S., Fishkes, H., Stern-Bach, Y., and Schuldiner, S. Energetics of reserpine binding and occlusion by the chromaffin granule transporter. *Biochemistry* **29** (1990) 603–608.

65. Scherman, D. Dihydrotetrabenazine binding and monoamine uptake in mouse brain regions. *J. Neurochem.* **47** (1986) 331–339.

66. Scherman, D. and Boschi, G. Time required for transmitter accumulation inside monoaminergic storage vesicles differs in peripheral and in central systems. *Neuroscience* **27** (1988) 1029–1035.

67. Scherman, D. and Henry, J. pH-dependence of the ATP-driven uptake of noradrenaline by bovine chromaffin-granule ghosts. *Eur. J. Biochem.* **116** (1981) 535–539.

68. Scherman, D. and Henry, J.-P. Reserpine binding to bovine chromaffin granule membranes. *Mol. Pharm.* **25** (1984) 113–22.

69. Scherman, D., Jaudon, P., and Henry, J. Characterization of the monoamine transporter of chromaffin granules by binding of [^{3}H]dihydrotetrabenazine. *Proc. Natl. Acad. Sci. USA* **80** (1983) 584–588.

70. Schuldiner, S. A molecular glimpse of vesicular monoamine transporters. *J. Neurochem.* **62** (1994) 2067–2078.

71. Schuldiner, S., Fishkes, H., and Kanner, B. I. Role of a transmembrane pH Gradient in epinephrine transport by chromaffin granule membrane vesicles. *Proc. Natl. Acad. Sci. USA.* **75** (1978) 3713–3716.

72. Schuldiner, S., Liu, Y., and Edwards, R. Reserpine binding to a vesicular amine transporter expressed in chinese hamster ovary fibroblasts. *J. Biol. Chem.* **268** (1993) 29–34.

73. Schuldiner, S., Shirvan, A., and Linial, M. Vesicular neurotransmitter transporters: from bacteria to human. *Physiol. Rev.* **75** (1995) 369–392.

74. Shirvan, A., Laskar, O., Steiner-Mordoch, S., and Schuldiner, S. Histidine-419 plays a role in energy coupling in the vesicular monoamine transporter from rat. *FEBS Lett.* **356** (1994) 145–150.

74a. Steiner-Mordoch, S., Shirvan, A., and Schuldiner, S. Modification of the pH profile and tetrabenazine sensitivity of rat VMAT1 by replacement of aspartate 404 with glutamate. *J. Biol. Chem.* **271** (1996) 13,048–13,054.

75. Stern-Bach, Y., Greenberg-Ofrath, N., Flechner, I., and Schuldiner, S. Identification and purification of a functional amine transporter from bovine chromaffin granules. *J. Biol. Chem.* **265** (1990) 3961–3966.

76. Stern-Bach, Y., Keen, J., Bejerano, M., Steiner-Mordoch, S., Wallach, M., Findlay, J., and Schuldiner, S. Homology of a vesicular amine transporter to a gene conferring resistance to 1-methyl-4-phenylpyridinium. *Proc. Natl. Acad. Sci. USA.* **89** (1992) 9730–9733.

77. Stietzen, M., Schober, M., Fischer-Colbrie, R., Scherman, D., Sperk, G., and Winkler, H. Rat adrenal medulla: levels of chromogranins, enkephalins, dopamine b-hydroxylase and of the amine transporter are changed by nervous activity and by hypophysectomy. *Neuroscience* **22** (1987) 131–139.

78. Stitzel, R. E. The biological fate of reserpine. *Pharm. Rev.* **28** (1977) 179–205.

79. Suchi, R., Stern-Bach, Y., and Schuldiner, S. Modification of arginyl or histidyl groups affects the energy coupling of the amine transporter. *Biochemistry* **31** (1992) 12,500–12,503.

80. Suchi, R., Stern-Bach, Y., Gabay, T., and Schuldiner, S. Covalent modification of the amine transporter with N, N'-dicyclohexylcarbodiimide. *Biochemistry* **30** (1991) 6490–6494.

81. Usdin, T., Eiden, L., Bonner, T., and Erickson, J. Molecular biology of the vesicular ACh transporter. *TINS* **18** (1995) 218–224.

82. Varoqui, H., Diebler, M., Meunier, F., Rand, J., Usdin, T., Bonner, T., Eiden, L., and Erickson, J. Cloning and expression of the vesamicol binding protein from the marine ray *Torpedo*: homology with the putative vesicular acetylcholine transporter *unc-17* from *Caenorhabditis elegans*, *FEBS Lett.* **342** (1994) 97–102.

83. Vincent, M. and Near, J. Purification of a [H-3]dihydrotetrabenazine-binding protein from bovine adrenal medulla. *Mol. Pharmacol.* **40** (1991) 889–894.

84. Weaver, J. A. and Deupree, J. D. Conditions required for reserpine binding to the catecholamine transporter on chromaffin granule ghosts. *Eur. J. Pharm.* **80** (1982) 437–438.

85. Weihe, E., Schafer, M.-H., Erickson, J., and Eiden, L. Localization of vesicular monoamine transporter isoforms (VMAT1 and VMAT2) to endocrine cells and neurons in rat. *J Mol. Neurosci.* **5** (1995) 149–164.

86. Wink, M. The plant vacuole: a multifunctional ccompartment. *J. Exp. Botany*, **44** (1993) 231–246.

87. Yamaguchi, A., Kimura, T., Someya, Y., and Sawai, T. Metal-tetracycline/H$^+$ antiporter of *Escherichia-coli* encoded by transposon Tn10—The structural resemblance and functional difference in the role of the duplicated sequence motif between hydrophobic segment-2 and segment-3 and segment-8 and segment-9. *J. Biol. Chem.* **268** (1993) 6496–6504.

88. Yamaguchi, A., Oyauchi, R., Someya, Y., Akasaka, T., and Sawai, T. Second-site mutation of Ala-220 to Glu or Asp suppresses the mutation of Asp-285 to Asn in the transposon Tn10-encoded metal-tetracycline/H($^+$) antiporter of *Escherichia-coli*. *J. Biol. Chem.* **268** (1993) 26,990–26,995.

89. Yamaguchi, A., Akasaka, T., Kimura, T., Sakai, T., Adachi, Y., and Sawai, T. Role of the conserved quartets of residues located in the N-terminal and C-terminal halves of the transposon-Tn10-encoded metal tetracycline/H$^+$ antiporter of *Escherichia-Coli*. *Biochemistry* **32** (1993) 5698–5704.

CHAPTER 8

Neurotransmitter Transporter Proteins

Posttranslational Modifications

Amrat P. Patel

Introduction

The neurotransmitter transporter protein or reuptake carrier is the most important component in the termination of the synaptic activity. In the past 5 yr, several of these neurotransmitter transporters have been cloned (1). The cloned transporters contain consensus sequences for multiple N-linked glycosylation sites in the large extracellular loop between transmembrane regions 3 and 4. Consensus sites for phosphorylation by several protein kinases are located in the putative cytosolic domains.

It is widely accepted that proteins undergo several forms of posttranslational modifications, for example, glycosylation and phosphorylation. This chapter addresses the role of posttranslational modifications of neurotransmitter transporter proteins, especially the effects of glycosylation on transporter function and stability, when expressed in foreign host-cell systems as well as in native state.

Glycosylation

Glycosylation is a major cotranslational and posttranslational modification undergone by a nascent polypeptide. The two major forms of glycosylations are N-linked and O-linked, and a third form is an attachment of a glycolipid anchor to the C-terminus of the protein (Fig. 1). The N-linked glycosylation is a covalent modification catalyzed by specific glycosyltransferases, at the side chain nitrogen atom of asparagine residues. Similarly, O-linked glycosylation is a covalent oligosaccharide modification of the hydroxyl group of ser-

Neurotransmitter Transporters: Structure, Function, and Regulation
Ed. M. E. A. Reith Humana Press Inc., Totowa, NJ

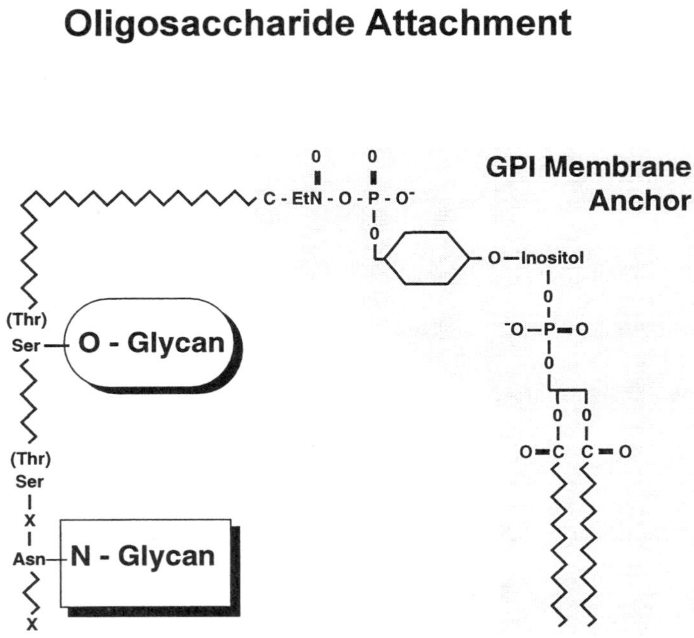

Oligosaccharide Attachment

Fig. 1. The three main forms of eukaryotic protein glycosylation.

ine, threonine, or, sometimes, hydroxylysine. The complex glycosylation machinery involved in the formation of various oligosaccharide structures for protein glycosylation has been reviewed (*21,35,42,43,48,60*). The initial core of oligosaccharide structure transferred onto the asparagine residue is made up of two N-acetylglucosamine (GlcNAc), nine mannose, and three glucose residues (Fig. 2). The assembly of the core oligosaccharide starts in the cytoplasm with a lipid carrier, dolichol pyrophosphate, and phosphorylated N-acetylglucosamine as the substrate catalyzed by N-acetylglucosamine phosphate transferase (*34*). Tunicamycin prevents glycosylation by inhibiting the N-acetylglucosamine phosphate transferase (*45*). The dolichol-PP-GlcNAc in the endoplasmic reticulum (ER) enters a cycle of elongation of the oligosaccharide in the presence of specific glycosyltransferases and substrates. The entire oligosaccharide core is transferred from a dolichol carrier to an asparagine on the emerging nascent polypeptide, a cotranslational modification. In the ER, posttranslational modification of the oligosaccharide takes place with sequential removal of three glucose residues and a mannose residue. Further processing of the glycoprotein takes place in the Golgi appa-

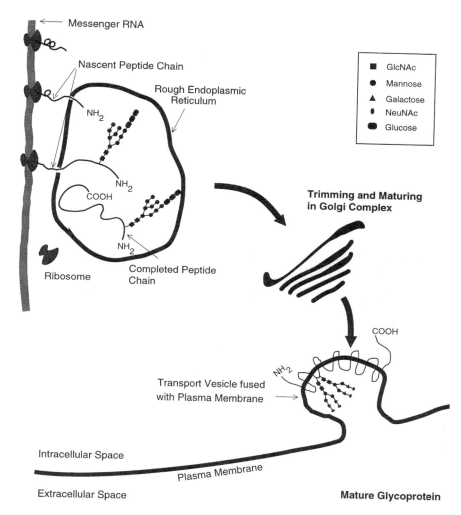

Fig. 2. Biosynthesis of N-linked oligosaccharides.

ratus (35). In the ER and Golgi, the precursor oligosaccharide core is processed, analogous to an assembly line with different stations modifying the core to achieve the final product.

Potential Glycosylation Sites

The consensus sequence for potential N-glycosylation includes the asparagine residue followed by any amino acid except proline, followed in turn by either serine or threonine (Asn-Xaa-Ser/Thr). Not all potential glycosylation sites are necessarily glycosylated in the native state. Furthermore, the pattern of glycosylation of a protein may differ when it is expressed in foreign cell systems (*see* Cell). Glycosylation is affected by the presence of certain amino acids, disulphide bonds, protein folding regions, and proximity to the amino or carboxy terminus (*60*). The O-linked glycosylation sequence motif is not well defined. The hydroxyl group of the serine and threonine can accept GlcNAc as the starting sugar residue in an oligosaccharide. Examples of the O-linked glycoproteins include human chorionic gonadotrophin hormone, mucins, and O-fucosylated blood coagulation factor proteins, in which the glycan is O-linked to hydroxylysine in the sequence gly-gly-OHlys-Xaa (*48,60*).

To date, all of the cloned neurotransmitter transporter cDNAs encode two or more potential N-glycosylation sites. One of the potential N-glycosylation sites is conserved in dopamine, norepinephrine, and serotonin transporter. The transporter proteins are heavily glycosylated, with sugars representing 15–50% of the molecular mass.

Detection of Glycosylated Transporter Proteins

Over the last decade, the study of glycoproteins has escalated, with breakthroughs in analytical technology, detection of minute quantities of oligosaccharides, and the availability of contamination-free recombinant glycosidases. Carbohydrate detection kits are available from commercial sources to detect gross and specific oligosaccharides by chemical and enzymatic methods. The details of the detection and analysis of carbohydrates can be found in texts of carbohydrate analysis (*12,42,48*). The glycosylation nature of a protein can also be assessed from the purification schemes of solubilized protein over a variety of commercially available lectin affinity columns. Commonly used lectins used in columns are wheat germ agglutinin, concanavalin A, and lentil lectin agarose. Purification afforded by lectin affinity chromatography rarely exceeds 10%; however, it is a useful technique to enhance purification and separation of glycosylated peptides from nonglycosylated peptides. Lectin columns have been used in partial purification of dopamine, GABA, glutamate, and serotonin transporters (*16,44,58,69,73*). [^{125}I]-labeled lectins are also used as an overlay for proteins blotted onto membranes to detect glycosylated polypeptides. Specific glycosidases are used for the removal of terminal residues, such as sialic acid, for complete N- and O-deglycosylation and for the removal of the glycophosphatidylinositol (GPI) anchor with phosphatidylinositol-specific phospholipase-C (*49*).

The complement of sugars attached to a potential glycosylation site on a single polypeptide may vary from site to site during the glycosylation process. This variance produces glycoforms with heterogeneous sugar composition, yielding a distinct, broad band in a denaturing gel, and multiple bands in two-dimensional gels. Upon complete deglycosylation, the broad band appears as a sharp band. However, for the dopamine and other neurotransmitter transporter proteins, the enzymatic N-deglycosylated polypeptide is not a sharp band. This result can be caused by O-linked glycosylation, charged moieties on the polypeptide, such as sulphates or phosphates, or N-glycosylation resistant to N-deglycosylation enzymes. A chemical deglycosylation with trifluoromethanesulphonic acid that removes both N- and O-glycosylation and charged species from the polypeptide (23) may resolve this discrepancy.

Some proteins in denaturing polyacrylamide gels display anomalous mobilities, i.e., a discrepancy between predicted and observed molecular mass. The deglycosylated glucose transporter in sodium dodecyl sulphate polyacrylamide denaturing gels has anomalous mobility, in that the electrophoretic molecular mass is higher than that predicted from amino acid sequence (32). Similar findings have been observed with the neurotransmitter transporters (described in Glycosylation Pattern of Native Neurotransmitter Transporters) and other proteins, including basic proteins, such as histones (31). The difference in the reported molecular mass of 68–90 kDa for the dopamine transporter is a result of both the source and concentration of acrylamide and the use of certain prestained protein molecular weight standards. Also, the mobility of the prestained protein standards varies with the difference in dye content between batches.

Differences in Glycosylation Pattern

Glycosylation Pattern of Native Neurotransmitter Transporters
Dopamine Transporter

The dopamine transporter (DAT) is a heavily glycosylated protein with a molecular mass of ≈80 kDa on denaturing polyacrylamide gels (4,27,46,61,71). A modest level of partially purified DAT has been achieved with DEAE ion-exchange and wheat germ lectin affinity chromatography (73). The DAT has been photoaffinity-labeled with GBR12935 derivatives (4,27,46,61,62,71) and the cocaine analog, RTI-82 (61). The photoaffinity ligands have been valuable in the characterization of the glycosylation state of the transporter protein. The rat striatal

DAT has a molecular mass of 80 kDa (*4,47,61*); treatment with neuraminidase and N-glycanase suggested the presence of terminal sialic acid residues and N-linked sugar cores, respectively (*27,46,62,71*). The molecular mass of N-deglycosylated DAT polypeptides from the caudate of canine, human, rat, and rat DAT expressed from a cDNA transfected into COS-7 cells is ≈50 kDa (*62*). The presence of O-linked glycosylation in the native rat DAT or rDAT cDNA expressed in COS-7 cells was not detectable (*62*). The rDAT cDNA expressed in COS-7 cells appeared not to contain sialic acid residues (*62*). The differential glycosylation pattern of the DAT is dependent on the cell, tissue, species, and developmental state, described later.

Norepinephrine Transporter

The human norepinephrine transporter (NET) is a glycoprotein and its properties have been studied by stable expression of hNET cDNA in LLC-PKI, a porcine kidney epithelial cell line (*6,50*). The molecular mass of the native NET in the brain has not been determined to date. Unlike the situation with dopamine or serotonin transporters, photoaffinity ligands for hNET are not available. Western blotting of hNET with NET-specific antibodies is currently employed to address these issues.

Serotonin Transporter

Launay et al. (*44*) purified the serotonin transporter (SERT) from human platelet membranes to homogeneity using affinity chromatography. The SERT protein in one- and two-dimensional denaturing polyacrylamide gels migrated with a molecular mass of 68 kDa and an acidic pI value of 5.2–6.2. The glycoprotein nature of the transporter protein was shown by its adsorption to a wheat germ agglutinin agarose column, and its specific elution with N-acetylglucosamine. A 68-kDa glycoprotein from human platelet membranes also was identified by specific photoaffinity labeling with paroxetine and cyanoimipramine (*44*). In human platelet and rat brain membranes [^{3}H]2-nitroimipramine photolabeled a 30–35 kDa band (*78*). The smaller size of this polypeptide could be the tricyclic binding domain of the SERT or a degradation product. Qian et al. (*68*) reported cell-specific N-linked glycosylation of native SERT proteins from rat brain (76 kDa), lung (80 kDa), platelet (94 kDa), and rSERT expressed from a cDNA transfected in HeLa cells (61 kDa). The human platelet SERT protein was sensitive to neuraminidase, decreasing [^{3}H]5HT binding to the desialated transporter. This possibly suggests a role for the sialic acid residues in substrate recognition.

GABA Transporter

The GABA transporter, an 80-kDa heavily glycosylated protein, was one of the first neurotransmitter transporters to be purified to homogeneity from rat brain (*38,69*). The transporter protein could be adsorbed and specifically eluted from a wheat germ agglutinin agarose column. Enzymatic N-deglycosylated transporter protein has a molecular mass of 60 kDa in a denaturing polyacrylamide gel. Peptide sequence information from the purified protein resulted in successful cloning of the rat and human brain GABA (GAT1) transporters with predicted molecular masses of 67 kDa (*29,56*).

Glutamate Transporter

The glutamate transporter protein has been purified to homogeneity from the rat brain of glial origin. In denaturing polyacrylamide gel, the protein migrated with molecular mass of 73–80 kDa and an acidic pI value of 6.2. Enzymatic N-deglycosylation of the purified protein yielded an apparent molecular mass of 63 kDa, with sugars representing 14% of the mass (*18–20*). In the rat brain, two glycosylated glutamate transporters (GLAST-1) with molecular masses of 64 and 70 kDa have been detected that could be separated by lectin specific-affinity chromatography. The 64 and 70 kDa forms of the glycoproteins were separated by lentil and wheat germ agglutinin lectin columns, respectively (*16*). As yet, splice variants of GLAST-1 have not been reported; the transporter protein is probably differentially glycosylated. It would be of interest to determine whether GLAST-1 transporters with varying sugar components show functional differences.

Glycine Transporter

A glycoprotein of 100 kDa has been purified to homogeneity from pig brain stems (*58*). There are four potential N-linked glycosylation sites on the large extracellular loop between transmembrane domains 3 and 4, two sites of which are glycosylated. The protein might not be O-glycosylated, since enzymatic O-deglycosylation with O-glycanase in the presence of neuraminidase failed to alter the mobility of the band in a denaturing polyacrylamide gel. Neuraminidase also failed to alter the mobility of the transporter protein, compared with untreated transporter protein, suggesting very low sialic acid content (*58*). Complete N-deglycosylation inhibited transporter activity. The loss in activity of the glycine transporter following N-deglycosylation may be caused by failure of the transporter protein to reach the plasma membrane, or increased turnover of the protein.

Cell, Tissue, and Species-Specific Glycosylation

Cell

Insight from the expression and processing of the glycosylated proteins in foreign host cells is now readily available with the success of cloning and expression of candidate genes in amphibian, insect, and mammalian cell systems. Cloned transporter genes, transiently or stably expressed in foreign cell systems, are used for understanding the biochemistry, physiology, and pharmacology of transport mechanisms, and as model systems to screen for potential therapeutic agents. The transporter protein genes cloned from brain cells have been successfully expressed in foreign, nonneuronal cells. There is evidence of some differences in the functional properties of the expressed DAT proteins in different mammalian cells. The difference, for example, in the K_m of [^{3}H]dopamine uptake may be attributed to the posttranslational processing, and in particular, the glycosylation of the transporter protein (61). The molecular mass of rat DAT expressed in LLC-PK1, a porcine kidney epithelial cell line, is 100 kDa, and that expressed in the COS-7 monkey kidney cell line is 110 kDa (62,64). The human DAT expressed in transfected Chinese hamster ovary (CHO) cells has a molecular mass of 93 kDa (64) (Fig. 3).

Olivares et al. (59) studied the properties of the glycine (GLYT1) transporter when expressed in COS-7 cells. The GLYT1 protein migrates in denaturing polyacryiamide gels as a broad band of 80–100 kDa and another band of 57 kDa. The glycine transporter antipeptide antibodies also detected a single band of 47 kDa on Western blots from COS-7 cells expressing GLYT1 transporters grown in the presence of tunicamycin. A similar result was obtained by expressing a GLYT1 mutant with all four potential asparagine glycosylation sites conservatively replaced with glutamine. These results suggest that the 80–100-kDa band is fully glycosylated, the 57-kDa band corresponds to the partially glycosylated form, and the 47-kDa band is the nonglycosylated polypeptide (59). Additional mutagenesis experiments of the glycosylation sites suggested that all four potential glycosylation sites are glycosylated in the COS cell system (59). The author has found from site-directed mutagenesis experiments that all four potential N-glycosylation sites are utilized in rDAT expressed in transfected COS-7 cells (Wang, Patel, and Uhl, submitted).

Because there is a cell-specific difference in the glycosylation pattern, usage of all four potential N-glycosylation sites in the

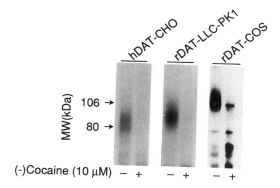

Fig. 3. Cell-specific glycosylation of dopamine transporters. [^{125}I]DEEP-labeled DAT proteins from hDAT-CHO, rDAT-LLC-PK1, and rDATCOS-7 are shown. The cells were labeled with [^{125}I]DEEP in the absence (−) and in the presence (+) of 10 µM (−)-cocaine, as described previously (*62*). The cells were solubilized with SDS-PAGE buffer, resolved in 10% polyacrylamide gels, dried, and exposed to Kodak XAR-5 film. Prestained protein standards (Bio-Rad, Hercules, CA) were electrophoresed on the same gels to estimate the mass of DAT. Human DAT expressed in CHO cells has a molecular mass of 93 kDa. The rat DAT has a molecular mass of 100 and 110 kDa, when expressed in LLC-PK1 and COS-7 cells, respectively.

brain should not be assumed, based on the COS-7 cell results. The usage of potential N-glycosylation sites in the native state of the dopamine and other transporter proteins must be empirically determined. Culture conditions for mammalian and sf9 insect cells can influence the N-glycosylation process, leading to glycan heterogeneity (*37*).

Cell-specific differences in the glycosylation pattern of other neurotransmitter transporter proteins have also been observed. The cell-specific N-linked glycosylation of native SERT protein yields a molecular mass of 76, 80, and 94 kDa in rat brain, lung, and platelets, respectively (*68*); in HeLa cells, rat and human glycosylated SERT proteins have a molecular mass of 61 kDa and the deglycosylated transporter protein has a molecular mass of 56 kDa (*68*). The glycosylated SERT protein in sf9 insect cells has a molecular mass of 60 kDa and the deglycosylated or unglycosylated transporters have a molecular mass of 54 kDa (*74*).

The human NET is a glycoprotein and its properties have been studied by stable expression of hNET in LLC-PK1, porcine kidney epithelial cell line, and LLC-hNET (6,50). The biosynthesis of the hNET protein was detected with anti-hNET antibodies, following metabolic labeling and labeled membranes resolved in denaturing polyacrylamide gels. The antibodies reacted with two proteins with molecular masses of 54 and 80 kDa in the control cells and with a 46-kDa polypeptide in cells grown in the presence of tunicamycin. The enzymatic N-deglycosylated hNET has a molecular mass of 46 kDa. The results show that the unglycosylated polypeptide has a molecular mass of 46 kDa. The 54-kDa band is the partially glyco-sylated intermediate product, and the 80-kDa band is the fully glycosylated polypeptide. Bruss et al. (10) detected hNET with mol-ecular mass of 50 and 58 kDa, using antipeptide antibodies in hNET-COS-7 cells.

Conradt et al. (16) studied the glycosylation properties of rat glial GLAST-1 transporters expressed in *Xenopus* oocytes. The rat GLAST-1 expressed in *Xenopus* oocytes have a monomeric molecular mass of 65 kDa, reduced to 56 kDa on deglycosylation. The glutamate trans-porter formed homodimers in *Xenopus* oocytes with a molecular mass of ≈100 kDA (16).

Tissue

Differences in tissue and species-related processing of native DAT is shown in Figs. 4 and 5. Previously, Lew et al. (47) had shown that the molecular mass of rat DAT in striatum was lower than that in nucleus accumbens. The difference was caused by core oligosaccha-ride and not the terminal sialic acid residues (46). However, labeling with [^{125}I]DEEP (Fig. 4B) or [^{125}I]RTI-82 did not show any apparent difference in the human DAT glycosylated molecular mass between caudate and nucleus accumbens (Patel et al., in preparation). Also, no apparent difference in the molecular mass of the glycosylated human DAT from caudate and putamen was found (Patel et al., unpublished data; 57).

Differences in the tissue-specific N-linked glycosylation of native SERT protein have been reported between rat brain (76 kDa), lung (80 kDa), and platelet (94 kDa) (68). Since there is only a single gene described for the SERT protein, the size variance is probably due to differences in glycosylation similar to that described above for the DAT protein. Glucose transporter proteins GLUT1 and GLUT3 from various rat brain regions also show no changes in the glycosylation pattern from embryonic 19 through postnatal d 30 and adult (77).

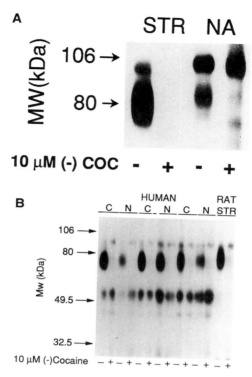

Fig. 4. (A) [^{125}I]DEEP-labeled dopamine transporters from rat nucleus accumbens (NA) and striatum (STR). This figure shows differences in molecular mass of rat dopamine transporters from nucleus accumbens and striatal membranes labeled with [^{125}I]DEEP. The membranes were labeled with [^{125}I]DEEP, as described in Fig. 3. **(B).** [^{125}I]DEEP-labeled human and rat dopamine transporter. The figure shows [^{125}I]DEEP-labeled caudate (C) and nucleus accumbens (N) membranes from human subjects with postmortem intervals (PMI) of 22, 11, and 36 h (from left to right) and rat striatal (RAT STR) membranes with PMI of 0 h. Molecular mass of DAT from the caudate and the nucleus accumbens from individuals with PMI of 2 and 4 h (data not shown) was not different from those shown in this figure. The membranes were labeled as described in Fig. 3. The positions of the prestained protein markers are shown with an arrow.

Species

A difference in the glycosylation of DATs from different species has been observed, with less variability between individuals of the same species (*62*). The molecular mass of photoaffinity-labeled canine caudate DAT is 78 kDa, the human caudate 62–74 kDa, and the rat striatum 80 kDa (*57,62*) (Fig. 5). The deglycosylated size of the

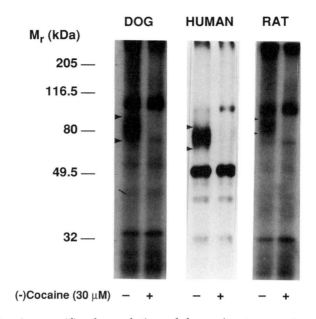

Fig. 5. Species-specific glycosylation of dopamine transporters. [^{125}I]DEEP-labeled DAT proteins from the dog caudate, human caudate, and rat striatal membranes are shown. The membranes were labeled with [^{125}I]DEEP in the absence (–) and in the presence (+) of 30 μ*M* (–)-cocaine as described in Fig. 3. Specifically labeled broad DAT bands are shown between arrowheads. The molecular mass of the dog, human, and rat DATs are ≈78, 74, and 80 kDa, respectively.

DAT from canine, human, and rat caudate/striatum is ≈50 kDa in a denaturing polyacrylamide gel (*62*).

Developmentally Regulated Glycosylation

The DAT protein in the rat brain undergoes differential glycosylation as determined by photoaffinity labeling during postnatal development (*63*). The changes in the molecular mass of rat striatal DAT from postnatal d 4, 14, and 60 (adult) were significantly different (Fig. 6). The DAT molecular mass was slightly higher in older (24 mo) rats, compared with adult rats, and there was no apparent difference in DAT molecular mass between postnatal d 0 (birth) and d 4 (*63*). The difference in DAT molecular mass was caused by glycosylation and, in particular, by the oligosaccharide core, and was not caused by the terminal sialic acid content or the protein backbone as determined by glycosidases and DAT antibodies, respectively (*63*). There are examples in the literature for the differential glycosylation of glycoproteins

DAT DEGLYCOSYLATION

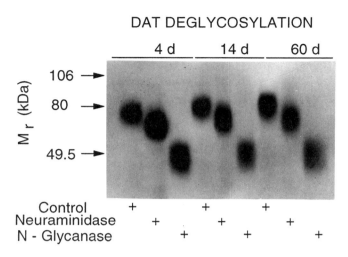

Fig. 6. Developmentally regulated glycosylation of rat striatal dopamine transporters. DAT protein from 4, 14, and 60 d-old rats were labeled with [125I]DEEP and electrophoresed in SDS-polyacrylamide gels, as described in Fig. 3. This figure shows changes in molecular mass of control, after neuraminidase and N-glycanase enzyme treatments. The deglycosylation of the [125I]DEEP-labeled band was carried out as described previously (63). The difference in molecular mass of DAT during early postnatal development persisted after desialation, but not after N-deglycosylation. Reprinted with permission from ref. 63.

during development. The rat pituitary thyrotropin hormone (30), human erythrocyte band-3 protein (24), and chick embryo fibroblast glycopeptides (15) undergo developmentally related differential glycosylation.

In contrast, some glycosylated proteins do not show any changes in their glycosylation pattern during development. A 60-kDa rat brain somatostatin receptor, an N-linked glycoprotein with terminal sialic acid residues (70) shows no glycosylation difference from embryonic d 13 through postnatal d 18 (75). Similarly, glucose transporter proteins GLUT1 and GLUT3 from various brain regions also show no changes in the glycosylation pattern from embryonic d 19 through postnatal d 30 and adult (77). The differences in glycosylation patterns or lack thereof can be explained in the availability of different glycosyltransferases during ontogenesis, as shown previously in the rat intestinal mucosa (5). N-acetylglucosaminyltransferase-IV enzyme-mediated modification of glycoprotein processing may also account for the differences in glycosylation patterns (25).

Role of Glycosylation:
Functional and Structural Implications

The roles of sugars associated with proteins and lipids are diverse in their contribution to structure, function, and disease states (21,22,25,35,42,48,60,65). The cloned transporter genes have been expressed in amphibian, insect, and mammalian cell systems. The expressed protein is cell-specifically processed with varying glycosylation, as described in the section entitled Cell. The difference in glycosylation, however, has not appreciably affected the functioning of the SERT transporter protein expressed in sf9 insect cells, compared with that expressed in rat brain (74). Neither uptake of [^{3}H]5HT nor the [^{125}I]RTI-55 ligand binding to the SERTs in sf9 insect cells requires glycosylation for function. Similarly, the functional properties of hNET or GLYT1 transporters were not compromised by varying degrees of glycosylation, from unglycosylated to fully-glycosylated transporter proteins (16,50,58).

The DAT protein expressed in COS-7 cells is insensitive to neuraminidase, suggesting either a reduced number or the absence of sialic acid residues (62). Such differences in posttranslational processing may account for the differences in the K_m for [^{3}H]dopamine uptake in COS-7 and other mammalian cell expression systems, compared with that in the native state (62). The removal of sialic acid residues from the rat striatal DAT and human platelet SERT affected [^{3}H]dopamine uptake and [^{3}H]5HT binding, respectively (44,80). However, the desialation of the rat striatal membranes did not affect the binding of [^{3}H]CFT to the DAT (46) or the functioning of the glycine and serotonin transporters (50,58). The stability and trafficking/targeting of the glycine, norepinephrine, and serotonin transporter, were greatly dependent on the glycosylation state (16,50,58,74). The turnover of the unglycosylated proteins is faster than that of the glycosylated proteins. This is because the oligosaccharide, N- and O-linked, structures hinder access of cytosolic proteases and thereby decrease the turnover of proteins.

The glucose transporters, GLUT1–GLUT5 (66), have a single potential N-linked glycosylation site in the extracellular loop between transmembranes 1 and 2, except the GLUT2 isoform. The GLUT2 glucose transporter lacks the N-glycosylation motif. Furthermore, enzymes targeted against N-linked and O-linked glycosylation, and against sialic acid linkages, failed to affect the mobility of GLUT2 polypeptide in denaturing polyacrylamide gels

(9). However, the transport function of GLUT2 appears uncompromised, and the transport activity of the deglycosylated red blood cell glucose transporter is also unaffected (79). In contrast, Asano et al. (2) showed that glycosylation is important for the GLUT1 glucose transporter protein expressed in CHO cells for intracellular targeting and protein stability. Similarly, N-glycosylation in human erythrocyte band 3 anion transport protein is not necessary for anion transport function, but plays a role in correct folding of the protein (28).

Other Posttranslational Modifications

Fatty Acid Acylation

The regulatory proteins, particularly the guanine nucleotide binding proteins and the receptors interacting with them, are modified mostly by myristoylation, palmitoylation and prenylation (14). The fatty acyl modification plays an important role in signal transduction and regulation of cell activity. The acylation–deacylation process is analogous to the well-described role of phosphorylation–dephosphorylation in the regulation of cellular activity. Modification of cysteine residues by palmitate is a posttranslational modification (72) described for cellular proteins, including receptors (8,53). Such fatty acid acylation of neurotransmitter transporters has not been described yet. However, there is a recent report of palmitoylation of glucose transporters and its significance to glucose transport regulation in blood–brain barrier capillaries (67).

Myristoylation

Fatty acid acylation as a form of posttranslational modification of a variety of cellular proteins has been described (14). The enzyme responsible for myristoylation is N-myristoyltransferase, which catalyzes the transfer of myristic acid from myristoyl-CoA. In regulatory guanine nucleotide binding protein (G-protein), myristoylation of the N-terminal glycine of alpha subunits of G-proteins (Gi, Go, and Gq) have been shown (11). The function of this acylation of soluble cellular proteins is to allow their anchoring to the cell membranes in close proximity to receptors or effectors with which they interact.

Palmitoylation

Recently, glucose transporters in the blood–brain barrier capillaries were shown to be palmitoylated (67). There are a variety of cellular proteins which are palmitoylated and involved in signal transduction and in membrane trafficking (*8,53,55*). The well-known regulatory α-G-protein subunits, several nonreceptor tyrosine kinase family members, and receptors interacting with G-proteins are palmitoylated (*8,53*). The potential acylation sequence upstream of the acylated cysteine has been suggested for receptor and G-proteins (*8,53*). The significance of myristoylation or palmitoylation of receptors and G-proteins, apart from the anchoring of the subunits to plasma membrane, is in protein–protein interactions, either allowing or preventing access to phosphorylation sites by specific kinases (*8*).

Prenylation

The prenylation of G-protein gamma subunits plays a crucial role in receptor-specific signal transduction (*14,54*). The various isoforms of G-protein gamma subunits are isoform-specific acylated with different chain lengths of fatty acids, isoprenyl, farnesyl, and geranylgeranyl. The acylation is at the C-terminal cystine residues with a motif CAAX (C = cystine, A = aliphatic amino acid, and X = any amino acid) forming a thioester bond. The acylated gamma subunits can form any membrane attachment with the receptor and other G-protein subunits (*54*).

Phosphorylation

Phosphorylation is one of the most widely known forms of post-translational reversible modification of many proteins regulating a variety of physiological functions. Specific sequences within the polypeptide have been identified as potential phosphorylation sites as substrates for specific kinases. The consensus sequence motifs for many protein kinase and phosphatase substrates have been described (*39,40*). The regulation of neurotransmitter transporter protein activity by phosphorylation has been reviewed (*7*). Recent reports on phosphorylation of the GABA (*76*), glycine (*26*), and glutamate (*13*) transporter protein, with activation of protein kinase A and C, lend direct evidence for the role of phosphorylation in the transporter activity. [³H]dopamine uptake by the DAT can be inhibited via activation of protein kinase C (PKC) enzyme in rat synaptosomes (*17*), in COS-7 cells expressing rDAT (*36,41*) and in stably expressing rDAT-LLC-PK1 cells (Patel et al., unpublished data; *36*). However, [¹²⁵I]RTI-55 binding to the dopamine transporter in rDAT-LLC-PK1 cells was not affected by PKC activator phorbol 12-myristate 13-acetate (Patel et al., unpublished data).

Ubiquitination

Cellular proteins destined for degradation are conjugated with ubiquitin, a posttranslational modification via the epsilon amino of lysine (*33*). Some synaptic proteins are conjugated with ubiquitin and they play a role in the stability of the synapses, and are also components of occlusion bodies in neurodegenerative diseases, such as Alzheimer's and Parkinson's diseases (*3*). Neurotransmitter transporter protein activity is modulated by anti-ubiquitin antibodies in rat brain synaptosomes (*51,52*). These experiments show that either the transporter protein or associated protein(s) is ubiquitinated, and that the transporter activity can be modulated. However, whether this has any physiological significance is not clear.

Concluding Comments

Glycosylation of the neurotransmitter transporter proteins is cell-, tissue-, and species-specific, and varies during development and aging. The results on different transporters expressed in various host cell systems show that glycosylation is important for the stability and targeting of the transporter to the plasma membrane. Partial or complete N-deglycosylation has less effect on the transporter function. Modulation of the transporter activity by phosphorylation is intensely studied, and the role of fatty acid acylation and ubiquitination in the transporter function requires further investigation.

Acknowledgments

The author is appreciative of Arlene A. Patel for her assistance in the preparation of this manuscript and thanks Oxford GlycoSystem for providing Figs. 1 and 2.

References

1. Amara, S. G. and Kuhar, M. J. Neurotransmitter transporters: recent progress. *Annu. Rev. Neurosci.* **16** (1993) 73–93.
2. Asano, T., Takata, K., Katagiri, H, Ishihara, H., Inukai, K., Anal, M., Hirano, H., Yazaki, Y., and Oka, Y. The role of N-glycosylation in the targeting and stability of GLUT1 glucose transporter. *FEBS Lett.* **324** (1993) 258–261.
3. Beesley, P. W., Mummery, R., Tibaldi, J., Chapman, A. P., Smith, S. J., and Rider, C. C. The post-synaptic density: putative involvement in synapse stabilization via cadherins and covalent modification by ubiquitination. *Biochem. Soc. Trans.* **23** (1995) 59–64.

4. Berger, P., Martenson, R., Laing, P., Thurcauf, A., DeCosta, B., Rice, K. C., and Paul, S. M. Photoaffinity labeling of the dopamine reuptake carrier protein with 3-azido[3H]GBR-12935. *Mol. Pharmacol.* **39** (1991) 429–435.

5. Biol, M. C., Martin, A., Richard, M., and Louisot, P. Developmental changes in intestinal glycosyl-transferase activities. *Pediatr. Res.* **22** (1987) 250–256.

6. Blakely, R. D, DeFelice, L. J., and Hartzeli, H. C. Molecular physiology of nor-epinephrine and serotonin transporters. *J. Exp. Biol.* **196** (1994) 263–281.

7. Boja, J. B., Vaughan, R. A., Patel, A., Shaya, E., and Kuhar, M. J. The dopamine transporter. In Niznik, H. B. (ed.), *Dopamine Receptors and Transporters*, Dekker, New York, (1994), pp. 611–644.

8. Bouvier, M., Loisel, T. P., and Hebert, T. Dynamic regulation of G-protein cou-pled receptor palmitoylation: potential role in receptor function. *Biochem. Soc. Trans.* **23** (1995) 577–581.

9. Brant, A. M., Gibbs, M. E., and Gould, G. W. Examination of the glycosidation state of five members of the human facilitative glucose transporter family. *Biochem. Soc. Trans.* **20** (1992) 235S.

10. Bruss, M., Hammermann, R., Brimijoin, S., and Bonisch, H. Antipeptide anti-bodies confirm the topology of the human norepinephrine transporter. *J. Biol. Chem.* **270** (1995) 9197–9201.

11. Buss, J. E., Mumby, S. M., Casey, P. J., Gilman, A. G., and Sefton, B. M. Myristoylated alpha subunits of guanine nucleotide-binding regulatory pro-teins. *Proc. Natl. Acad. Sci. U.S.A.* **84** (1987) 7493–7497.

12. Caplin, M. F. and Kennedy, J. F. (eds.) *Carbohydrate Analysis: A Practical Approach.* IRL, Oxford, UK, 1986.

13. Casado, M., Bendahan, A., Zafara, F., Danbolt, N. C., Aragon, C., Gimenez, C., and Kanner, B. I. Phosphorylation and modulation of brain glutamate trans-porters by protein kinase C. *Biol. Chem.* **268** (1993) 27,313–27,317.

14. Casey, P. J. and Buss, J. E. (eds.) *Lipid Modifications of Proteins, Methods in Enzymology*, Vol. 250 Academic, New York (1995).

15. Codogno, P., Botti, J., Font, J., and Aubery, M. Modification of the N-linked oligosaccharides in cell surface glycoproteins during chick embryo develop-ment. *Eur. J. Biochem.* **149** (1985) 453–460.

16. Conradt, M., Storck, T., and Stoffel, W. Localization of N-glycosylation sites and functional role of the carbohydrate units of GLAST-1, a cloned rat brain L-glutamate/L-aspartate transporter. *Eur. J. Biochem.* **229** (1995) 682–687.

17. Copeland, B. J., Neff, N. H., and Hadjiconstantinou, M. Protein kinase C activa-tors decrease dopamine uptake into striatal synaptosomes. *Soc. Neurosci.* **21** (1995) 1381.

18. Danbolt, N. C. The high affinity uptake system for excitatory amino acids in the brain. *Prog. Neurobiol.* **44** (1994) 377–396.

19. Danbolt, N. C., Pines, G., and Kanner, B. I. Purification and reconstitution of the sodium- and potassium-coupled glutamate transport glycoprotein from rat brain. *Biochemistry* **29** (1990) 6734–6740.

20. Danbolt, N. C., Storm-Mathisen, J., and Kanner, B. I. A [Na^+–K^+] coupled L-glu-tamate transporter purified from rat brain is located in glial cell processes. *Neuroscience* **51** (1992) 295–310.

21. Dwek, R. A. Glycobiology: Towards understanding the function of sugars. *Biochem. Soc. Trans.* **23** (1995) 1–25.

22. Dwek, R. A. Glycobiology: more functions for oligosaccharides. *Science* **269** (1995) 1234–1235.

23. Edge, A. S. B., Faltynek, C. R., Hof, L., Reichert, Jr., L. E., and Weber, P. Deglycosylation of glycoprotein by trifluoromethanesulfonic acid. *Anal. Biochem.* **118** (1981) 131–137.

24. Fukuda, M., Fukuda, M. N., and Hakomori, S. Developmental change and defect in the carbohydrate structure of band 3 glycoprotein of human erythrocyte membrane. *J. Biol. Chem.* **254** (1979) 3700–3703.

25. Goldberg, D. E. and Kornfeld, S. Evidence for extensive subcellular organization of asparagine-linked oligosaccharide processing and lysosomal enzyme phosphorylation. *J. Biol. Chem.* **258** (1983) 3159–3165.

26. Gomeza, J., Zafara, F., Olivares, L., Gimenez, C., and Aragon, C. Regulation by phorbol esters of the glycine transporter (GLYT1) in glioblastoma cells. *Biochim. Biophys. Acta.* **1233** (1995) 41–46.

27. Grigoriadis, D. E., Wilson, A. A., Lew, R., Sharkey, J. S., and Kuhar, M. J. Dopamine transporter sites selectively labeled by a novel photoaffinity probe: [^{125}I]DEEP. *J. Neurosci.* **9** (1989) 2664–2670.

28. Groves, J. D. and Tanner, M. J. Role of N-glycosyiation in the expression of human band 3-mediated anion transport. *Mol. Membr. Biol.* **11** (1994) 31–38.

29. Guastella, J., Nelson, N., Nelson, H., Czyzyk, L., Keynan, S., Miedel, M. C., Davidson, N. C., Lester, H. A., and Kanner, B. I. Cloning and expression of a rat brain GABA transporter. *Science* **249** (1990) 1303–1306.

30. Gyves, P. W., Gesundheit, N., Stannard, B. S., DeCherney, G. S., and Weintraub, B. D. Alterations in the glycosylation of secreted thyrotropin during ontogenesis. *J. Biol. Chem.* **264** (1989) 6104–6110.

31. Hames, B. D. An introduction to polyacrylamide gel electrophoresis. In Hames, B. D. and Rickwood, D. (eds.), *Gel Electrophoresis of Protein–A Practical Approach*, IRL, Oxford UK, 1981, pp. 1–91.

32. Haspel, H. C., Revillame, J., and Rosen, O. M. Structure, biosynthesis, and function of the hexose transporter in Chinese hamster ovary cells deficient in N-acetylglucosaminyl transferase 1 activity. *J. Cell Physiol.* **136** (1988) 361–366.

33. Hershko, A. and Ciechanover, A. The ubiquitin system for protein degradation. *Annu. Rev. Biochem.* **61** (1992) 761–807.

34. Hirschberg, C. B. and Snider, M. D. Topography of glycosylation in the rough endoplasmic reticulum and Golgi apparatus. *Ann. Rev. Biochem.* **56** (1987) 63–87.

35. Hubbard, S. C. and Ivatt, R. J. Synthesis and processing of asparagine-linked oligosaccharides. *Ann. Rev. Biochem.* **50** (1981) 555–583.

36. Huff, R. A., Vaughan, R. A., Kuhar, M. J., and Uhl, G. R. Protein kinase activity modulates dopamine transporter function. *Soc. Neurosci.* **21** (1995) 1380.

37. Jenkins, N. Monitoring and control of recombinant glycoprotein heterogeneity in animal cell cultures. *Biochem. Soc. Trans.* **23** (1995) 171–175.

38. Kanner, B. I. Sodium-coupled neurotransmitter transport: Structure, function and regulation. *J. Exp. Biol.* **196** (1994) 237–249.

39. Kemp, B. E. and Pearson, R. B. Protein kinase recognition sequence motifs. *Trends Biochem. Sci.* **15** (1990) 342–346.

40. Kennely, P. J. and Krebs, E. G. Consensus sequences as substrate specificity determinants for protein kinases and protein phosphatases. *J. Biol. Chem.* **266** (1991) 15,555–15,558.

41. Kitayama, S., Dohi, T., and Uhl, G. R. Phorbol esters alter functions of the expressed dopamine transporter. *Eur. J. Pharmacol.* **268** (1994) 115–119.
42. Kobata, A. Structures and function of the sugar chains of glycoproteins. *Eur. J. Biochem.* **209** (1992) 483–501.
43. Kornfeld, R. and Kornfeld, S. Assembly of asparagine-linked oligosaccharides. *Ann. Rev. Biochem.* **54** (1985) 631–664.
44. Launay, J.-M., Geoffroy, C., Mutel, V., Buckel, M., Cesura, A., Alouf, J. E., and Da Prada, M. One-step purification of the serotonin transporter located at the human platelet plasma membrane. *J. Biol. Chem.* **267** (1992) 11,344–11,351.
45. Lehrman, M. A. Biosynthesis of N-acetylglucosamine-P-P-dolichol, the committed step of asparagine-linked oligosaccharide assembly. *Glycobiology.* **1** (1991) 553–562.
46. Lew, R., Patel, A., Vaughan, R. A., Wilson, A., and Kuhar, M. J. Microheterogeneity of dopamine transporters in rat striatum and nucleus accumbens. *Brain Res.* **584** (1992) 266–271.
47. Lew, R., Vaughan, R., Simantov, R., Wilson, A., and Kuhar, M. J. Dopamine transporters in the nucleus accumbens and the striatum have different apparent molecular weights. *Synapse,* **8** (1991) 152–153.
48. Lis, H. and Sharon, N. Protein glycosylation, structural and functional aspects. *Eur. J. Biochem.* **218** (1993) 1–27.
49. Low, M. G. Glycosyl-phosphatidylinostiol: a versatile anchor for cell surface proteins. *FASEB J.* **3** (1989) 1600–1608.
50. Melikian, H. E., McDonald, J. K., Gu, H., Rudnick, G., Moore, K. R., and Blakely, R. D. Human norepinephrine transporter, biosynthetic studies using a site-directed polyclonal antibody. *J. Biol. Chem.* **269** (1994) 12,290–12,297.
51. Meyer, E. M., West, C. M., and Chau, V. Antibodies directed against ubiqintin inhibit high affinity [^{3}H]choline uptake in rat cerebral cortical synaptosomes. *J. Biol. Chem.* **261** (1986) 14,365–14,368.
52. Meyer, E. M., West, C. M., Stevens, B. R., Chau, V., Nguyen, M-T., and Judkins, J. H. Ubiquitin-directed antibodies inhibit neuronal transporters in rat brain synaptosomes. *J. Neurochem.* **49** (1987) 1815–1819.
53. Milligan, G., Parenti, M., and Magee, A. I. The dynamic role of palmitoylation in signal transduction. *Trends Biochem. Sci.* **20** (1995) 181–186.
54. Muller, S. and Lohse, M. J. The role of βγ subunits in signal transduction. *Biochem. Soc. Trans.* **23** (1995) 141–148.
55. Mundy, D. I. Protein palmitoylation in membrane trafficking. *Biochem. Soc. Trans.* **23** (1995) 572–576.
56. Nelson, H., Mandiyan, S., and Nelson, N. Cloning of the human brain GABA transporter. *FEBS Lett.* **269** (1990) 181–184.
57. Niznik, H. B., Fogel, E. F., Fasso, F. F., and Seeman, P. The dopamine transporter is absent in Parkinsonian putamen and reduced in the caudate nucleus. *J. Neurochem.* **56** (1991) 192–198.
58. Nunez, E. and Aragon, C. Structural analysis and functional role of the carbohydrate component of glycine transporter. *J. Biol. Chem.* **269** (1994) 16,920–16,924.
59. Olivares, L., Aragon, C., Gimenez, C., and Zafra, F. The role of N-glycosylation in the targeting and activity of the GLYT1 glycine transporter. *J. Biol. Chem.* **270** (1995) 9437–9442.

60. Opdenakker, G., Rudd, P. M., Ponting, C. P., and Dwek, R. A. Concepts and principles of glycobiology. *FASEB J.* **7** (1993) 1330–1337.

61. Patel, A., Boja, J. W., Lever, J., Lew, R., Simantov, R., Carroll, F. I., Lewin, A. H., Phillip, A., Gao, Y., and Kuhar, M. J. A cocaine analog and a GBR analog label the same protein in rat striatal membranes. *Brain Res.* **576** (1991) 173,174.

62. Patel, A., Uhl, G., and Kuhar, M. J. Species differences in dopamine transporters: postmortem changes and glycosylation differences. *J. Neurochem.* **61** (1993) 496–500.

63. Patel, A. P., Cerruti, C., Vaughan, R. A., and Kuhar, M. J. Developmentally regulated glycosylation of dopamine transporter. *Dev. Brain Res.* **83** (1994) 53–58.

64. Patel, A. P., Martel, I.-C., Vandenbergh, D. J., Uhl, G. R., and Kuhar, M. J. Cell lines expressing human and rat dopamine transporter cDNAs: different ligands yield different radiolabeling patterns. *Soc. Neurosci.* **21** (1995) 781.

65. Paulson, J. C. Glycoproteins: what are the sugars chains for? *Trends Biochem. Sci.* **14** (1989) 272–276.

66. Pessin, J. E. and Bell, G. I. Mammalian facilitative glucose transporter family: Structure and molecular regulation. *Annu. Rev. Physiol.* **54** (1992) 911–930.

67. Poulit, J-F. and Beliveau, R. Palmitoylation of the glucose transporter in blood-brain barrier capillaries. *Biochim. Biophys. Acta* **1234** (1994) 191–196.

68. Qian, Y., Melikian, H. E., Rye, D. B., Levey, A. I., and Blakely, R. D. Identification and characterization of antidepressant-sensitive serotonin transporter proteins using site-specific antibodies. *J. Neurosci.* **15** (1995) 1261–1274.

69. Radian, R., Bendahan, A., and Kanner, B. I. Purification and identification of the functional sodium- and chloride-coupled y-aminobutyric acid transport glycoprotein from rat brain. *J. Biol. Chem.* **261** (1986) 15,437–15,441.

70. Rens-Domiano, S. and Reisine, T. Structural analysis and functional role of the carbohydrate component of somatostatin receptors. *J. Biol. Chem.* **266** (1991) 20,094–20,102.

71. Sallee, F. R., Fogel, E. L., Schwartz, E., Choi, S. M., Curran, D. P., and Niznik, H. B. Photoaffinity labeling of the mammalian dopamine transporter. *FEBS Lett.* **256** (1989) 219–224.

72. Saltiel, A. R., Ravetch, A. R., and Aderem, A. A. Functional consequences of lipid-mediated protein-membrane interactions. *Biochem. Pharmacol.* **42** (1991) 1–11.

73. Simantov, R., Vaughan, R., Lew, R., Wilson, A., and Kuhar, M. J. Dopamine transporter cocaine receptor characterization and purification. *Adv. Biosci.* **82** (1991) 151–154.

74. Tare, C. G. and Blakely, R. D. The effect of N-linked glycosylation on activity of the Na$^+$ Cl$^-$ dependent serotonin transporter expressed using recombinant baculovirus in insect cells. *J. Biol. Chem.* **269** (1994) 26,303–26,310.

75. Theveniau, M. and Reisine, T. Developmental changes in expression of a 60 kDa somatostatin receptor immunoreactivity in the rat brain. *J. Neurochem.* **60** (1993) 1870–1875.

76. Tian, Y., Kapatos, G., Granneman, J. G., and Bannon, M. J. Dopamine and gamma-aminobutyric acid transporters: differential regulation by agents that promote phosphorylation. *Neurosci. Lett.* **173** (1994) 143–146.

77. Vannucci, S. Developmental expression of GLUT1 and GLUT3 glucose transporters in rat brain. *J. Neurochem.* **62** (1994) 240–246.

78. Wennogle, L. P., Ashton, R. A., Schuster, D. I., Murphy, R. B., and Meyerson, L. R. 2-Nitroimipramine: a photoaffinity probe for the serotonin uptake/tricyclic binding site complex. *EMBO J.* **4** (1985) 971–977.

79. Wheeler, T. J. and Hinkel, P. C. Kinetic properties of the reconstituted glucose transporter from human erythrocytes. *J. Biol. Chem.* **256** (1981) 8907–8914.

80. Zaleska, M. M. and Erecinska, M. Involvement of sialic acid in high-affinity uptake of dopamine by synaptosomes from rat brain. *Neurosci. Lett.* **82** (1987) 107–112.

CHAPTER 9

Dopamine Transporter Uptake Blockers

Structure–Activity Relationships

F. Ivy Carroll, Anita H. Lewin, and Michael J. Kuhar

Introduction

The dopamine transporter (DAT), a protein located on presynaptic nerve terminals (*43,44,61*), plays a major role in the reuptake of released dopamine. Uptake of DA is sodium- and chloride ion-, as well as temperature- and time-dependent, and is inhibited by a variety of compounds, including cocaine. Even though cocaine binds to several sites in the brain, only binding potencies at the DA site have been shown to correlate with the reinforcing properties of cocaine in animal models, which are the primary factors in its abuse. Thus, the DAT has been called a cocaine receptor (*11,81*) and may be the initial site responsible for producing cocaine's drug reinforcement. The cDNA for the DAT has been cloned from rat (*39,51,85*), bovine (*88*), and human (*91*) brains. The hydrophobicity profile indicates 12 possible membrane-spanning regions with the amino and carboxy termini located intracellularly. The protein from human and rat brains contains three and four extracellular N-glycosylation sites, respectively (Fig. 1).

Since changes in DA neuron density and/or DAT sites are involved in a number of neurological disorders, as well as in drug abuse, probes for the DAT may be useful as a marker for dopaminergic terminals in some diseases (*see* Chapter 10). For example, cocaine congeners have been used as binding ligands to detect reduced densities of the DAT in Parkinson's-diseased brains. In order to develop potent and selective

Neurotransmitter Transporters: Structure, Function, and Regulation
Ed.: M. E. A. Reith Humana Press Inc., Totowa, NJ

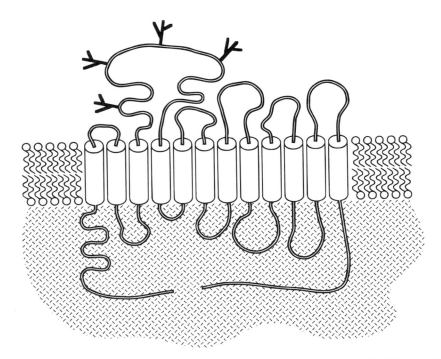

Fig. 1. Schematic representation of the cloned DAT. Reprinted with permission from ref. *85.*

probes for the DAT, an understanding of the structure–activity relationship (SAR) of the binding site(s) is required. This may be accomplished experimentally by correlation of structural variations with inhibition of dopamine uptake, or, more conveniently, with the inhibition of radioligand binding at the DAT. The latter approach also has the potential for identifying structures capable of blocking the binding of cocaine without inhibiting dopamine transport. Such compounds are considered dopamine-transport-sparing cocaine antagonists and are yet to be identified (*see* section on cocaine antagonists).

Compounds capable of inhibiting DA transport and of binding at the DAT display remarkable variations in structure. The compound classes for which SARs are discussed in this chapter are: tropane analogs, 1,4-dialkylpiperazine analogs, mazindol analogs, phencyclidine analogs, and methylphenidate analogs. With the exception of the 1,4-dialkylpiperazine class of compounds, the SARs discussed in this chapter are based on the inhibition of radioligand binding at the

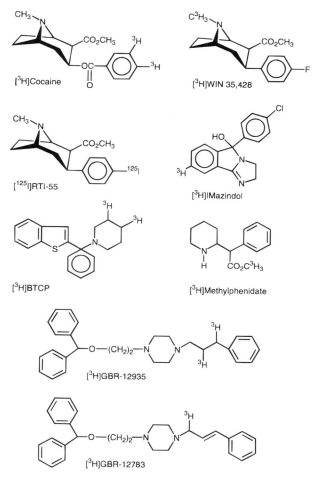

Scheme 1. Radioligands used for inhibition of binding to the DAT.

DAT. For the 1,4-dialkylpiperazines, the SAR is based on inhibition of [³H]dopamine uptake.

Assay Conditions

To conduct an SAR study for a binding site requires a radioligand that shows specific, saturable binding that is linear with increasing tissue content. Several suitable radioligands for the DAT have been developed. Scheme 1 shows the radioligands that have been used for the SAR studies that are presented in this chapter. Some of the ligands bind only one site, but others, like [³H]cocaine, bind a high- and a low-affinity site. There are conflicting reports whether the various radioligands are binding to the same site(s) or different site(s) or possibly to the same site in structurally and/or biochemically different ways. Most SAR studies have been conducted using rat brain striata; however, some studies have used monkey caudate or putamen. In either case, the buffer used, as well as the incubation temperature and time, can have effects on the assay results. Nevertheless, there is evidence for mutually exclusive binding of the ligands (*78*), and there is remarkable consistency in most of the reported SAR studies. Thus, unless there are gross differences, no distinctions are made in this chapter as to the exact assay conditions. Recently, a few SAR studies have been reported using cloned rat or human DATs (Uhl, personal communication). Because of the limited amount of data on cloned DATs and possible posttranslational differences, these studies are not included.

Classes of Compounds

Tropane Class

Tropane, 8-methyl-8-azabicyclo[3.2.1]octane, provides the backbone for three distinct classes of compounds whose SARs for binding the DAT have been investigated. For the purpose of this chapter, these classes have been termed cocaine analogs, WIN 35,065-2 analogs, and benztropine analogs. Cocaine analogs are characterized by possession of a benzoyloxy or similar group at the 3-position of the tropane ring. The WIN 35,065-2 and benztropine analogs have an aryl and diphenylmethylether group, respectively, at this position.

Cocaine Analogs

Structurally, natural (–)-cocaine (**1a**) is [1*R*-(exo,exo)]-3-benzoyloxy-8-methyl-8-azabicyclo[3.2.1]octane-2-carboxylic acid methyl ester. Since this structure has three sites of asymmetry, there are eight possible isomers. Only (–)-cocaine (**1a**), with an IC_{50} value of 89–150 nM, has appreciable affinity for the DAT; other isomers are 60–600 times weaker (*23*). SAR studies of cocaine have included variations in the 3-benzoyloxy, 2-carbomethoxy, and N-methyl groups. Each is addressed separately. Since stereochemistry plays an important part in the potency of cocaine analogs, results from substrates that are mixtures of isomers are not included in this chapter.

MODIFICATION OF THE 3β-BENZOYLOXY GROUP

Substitution of the aromatic ring with electron-releasing, as well as electron-donating groups (**1b**), results in a small to large loss of affin-

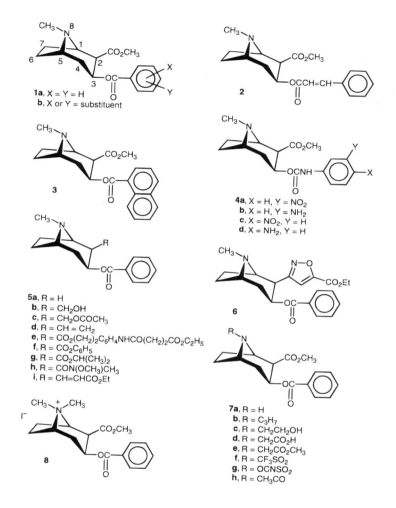

1a, X = Y = H
b, X or Y = substituent

2

3

4a, X = H, Y = NO$_2$
b, X = H, Y = NH$_2$
c, X = NO$_2$, Y = H
d, X = NH$_2$, Y = H

5a, R = H
b, R = CH$_2$OH
c, R = CH$_2$OCOCH$_3$
d, R = CH = CH$_2$
e, R = CO$_2$(CH$_2$)$_2$C$_6$H$_4$NHCO(CH$_2$)$_2$CO$_2$C$_2$H$_5$
f, R = CO$_2$C$_6$H$_5$
g, R = CO$_2$CH(CH$_3$)$_2$
h, R = CON(OCH$_3$)CH$_3$
i, R = CH=CHCO$_2$Et

6

7a, R = H
b, R = C$_3$H$_7$
c, R = CH$_2$CH$_2$OH
d, R = CH$_2$CO$_2$H
e, R = CH$_2$CO$_2$CH$_3$
f, R = CF$_3$SO$_2$
g, R = OCNSO$_2$
h, R = CH$_3$CO

8

ity for the DAT (*38,72,80,96*). Large losses in affinity result from changing the 3β-benzoyloxy group to a cinnamoyloxy (**2**) or to a naphthoyloxy (**3**) group (*16*). Replacement of the 3β-benzoyloxy group of cocaine with an *m*-nitrophenylcarbamoyloxy (*see* **4a**) group has little effect on binding potency; however, the *m*-amino, as well as *p*-nitro and *p*-amino analogs **4b-d** have reduced potency (*53*).

MODIFICATION OF THE 2-POSITION

Early SAR studies showed that the presence and nature of a 2β-substituent contributed substantially to binding affinities (*23,63,79,80*). The substantial reduction in binding potency observed on replacement of the 2β-carbomethoxy group in cocaine (**1a**) by a hydrogen atom (**5a**) or by a methylenehydroxy group (**5b**), and the partial restoration of binding potency with a methyleneacetoxy group (**5c**), suggested that one or more heteroatoms might be required for high potency, and that some type of electrostatic interaction with the DAT was involved (*63*). Later studies revealed that the 2β-vinyl analog **5d** possessed good affinity for the DAT, showing that a heteroatom in the 2β-group was not an essential feature for high-potency binding (*57*).

A number of 2β-alkyl and aryl ester analogs of cocaine have been evaluated (*13,17,25,63*). In general, only minor effects on binding affinity at the DAT were observed (*63*), even when the 2β-carbomethoxy methyl group in cocaine was replaced by very large groups. For example, compound **5e**, which possesses a 2β-[p-(ethylsuccinamido)phenyl]ethyl ester group, has an IC_{50} value of 86 nM, which is essentially identical to that of cocaine (*63*). The most interesting finding in this group of compounds is that the phenyl and isopropyl esters **5f** and **5g**, respectively, are similar to cocaine in their affinity for the DAT, but show much lower potencies at the serotonin (5-HT) and norepinephrine (NE) transporters (*13,15,20*).

There are a number of 2β-substituted analogs of cocaine with wide variation in size, shape, hydrophobicity, and other physical parameters that show binding affinity equal to or slightly less than that of cocaine. However, there are only a few compounds in this class of analogs, such as the 2β-amide **5h** (*20*), the β-carbethoxyvinyl analog **5i** (*60*), and the 2β-isoxazole **6**(*60*), that possess binding potencies exceeding that of cocaine.

MODIFICATION OF THE N-METHYL GROUP

The syntheses and binding affinities of a variety of N-nor-N-substituted cocaine analogs have been described (*3,57,79,87*). Replacement of the N-methyl group with a hydrogen atom, or with allyl, 2-hydroxyethyl, carboxymethyl, carbomethoxymethyl, trifluorosulfonyl, or isocyanatosulfonyl groups (compounds **7a–g**) has only a small effect on binding potency. In contrast, replacement of the N-methyl group by an acetyl moiety to give the amide **7h**, or addition of a methyl group to create the quaternary salt **8**, reduces binding potency by factors of 33 and 111, respectively.

WIN 35,065-2 Analogs

The structure of WIN 35,065-2 (**9**) differs from that of cocaine (**1a**) by having an aromatic ring with β-stereochemistry connected directly to the 3-position of the tropane ring. Analogs in this series

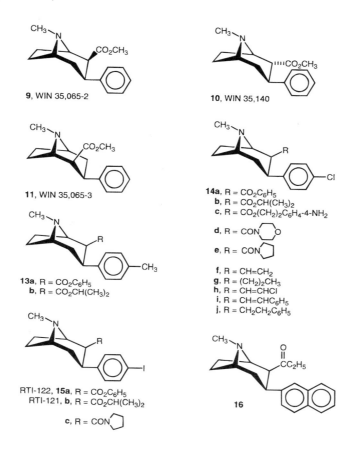

9, WIN 35,065-2

10, WIN 35,140

11, WIN 35,065-3

13a, R = CO₂C₆H₅
b, R = CO₂CH(CH₃)₂

RTI-122, **15a**, R = CO₂C₆H₅
RTI-121, **b**, R = CO₂CH(CH₃)₂

c, R = CON

14a, R = CO₂C₆H₅
b, R = CO₂CH(CH₃)₂
c, R = CO₂(CH₂)₂C₆H₄-4-NH₂

d, R = CON O

e, R = CON

f, R = CH=CH₂
g, R = (CH₂)₂CH₃
h, R = CH=CHCl
i, R = CH=CHC₆H₅
j, R = CH₂CH₂C₆H₅

16

possess potencies to bind the DAT that are more than 100 times that of cocaine and its analogs. Like cocaine (**1a**), WIN 35,065-2 (**9**) has three sites of asymmetry and eight possible isomers. The 2α-isomer (WIN 35,140, **10**) and the enantiomer (WIN 35,065-3, **11**) both have much lower affinity for the DAT than WIN 35,065-2 (**9**), showing that the orientation at the 2-position and the absolute stereochemistry are important contributors to high potency (*66,79,80*). Binding properties for the other five isomers have not been reported. SAR studies of WIN 35,065-2 analogs have followed a pattern much like that described for cocaine and include variation in the 3β-phenyl, 2β-carbomethoxy, and N-methyl groups. In the first subsection of this part of the chapter, the effect of changes in the 3β-phenyl ring is addressed. For the most part, the SAR studies addressing changes in the 2β-carbomethoxy and N-methyl group have been carried out on 3β-(substituted phenyl) WIN 35,065-2 analogs. For the purpose of this chapter, we have assumed that the SAR observed for changes in the 2β-carbomethoxy and N-methyl groups are not significantly affected by the substituent on the 3β-phenyl group.

MODIFICATION OF THE 3β-PHENYL GROUP

Removal of the ester linkage between the phenyl and tropane rings of cocaine results in the compound designated WIN 35,065-2 (27). This compound demonstrates a fivefold higher affinity for the DAT than cocaine. SAR studies from several laboratories have shown that, unlike cocaine, binding affinity in this series is dependent upon the substituents and their positions on the 3β-phenyl ring (*15,18,22,25,54, 66,69,79,80*). The results from some of the studies (Table 1) revealed that over half of the compounds have IC_{50} values <12 nM. The 4'-methyl, 4'-chloro, 4'-bromo, and 4'-iodo (**12a–d**) and the 4'-amino-3'-iodo, 3',4'-dichloro, and 4'-chloro-3'-methyl analogs (**12e–g**) possess IC_{50} values of less than 2 nM, as does the 3β-naphthyl analog **12h** (*16*). Strikingly, **12j**, with an electron withdrawing 4'-nitro substituent and **12k–m**, which possess a 4'-amino, a 4'-hydroxy, and a 4'-methoxy group, respectively, all have IC_{50} values in the same range. Compounds **12x–aa**, with large substituents, such as 4'-acetylamino, 4'-propionylamino, 4'-ethoxycarbonylamino, and 4'-trimethylstannyl, possess relatively low affinity for the DAT. However, even these compounds have IC_{50} values in the same range as cocaine. It is surprising that the potency of the 4'-ethyl analog **12bb**, with an IC_{50} value of 55 nM, is so different from that of the 4'-methyl derivative **12a** (*25*). Substituents in the 3'-position show somewhat inconsistent results. The 3'-chloro, 3'-bromo, and 3'-iodo analogs (**12n, 12o**, and **12w**) have lower affinity than the corresponding 4'-substituted analogs, **12b-d**, the 3'-and 4'-fluoro analogs (**12t** and **12u**, respectively) fall into the same IC_{50} range. It is interesting to note that addition of a 3'-chloro or 3'-methyl group to analog **12b** to give the 3',4'-dichloro, and 4'-chloro-3'-methyl analogs, **12f** and **12g**, respectively, have only a minor effect on potency. By contrast, the addition of a 3'-methyl group to the 4'-fluoro analog **12u** or of a 3'-iodo substituent to the 4'-amino analog **12k**, to give **12q** and **12e**, respectively, increases potency relative to the 4'-substituted analogs.

Quantitative structure–activity relationship (QSAR) and comparative molecular field analysis (CoMFA) models were initially reported for 12 (*18*), and then for 25 (*24*), of the compounds listed in Table 1. The classical QSAR models suggest that distribution properties (hydrophobicity) are important contributors to binding at the DAT. The CoMFA

Table 1

DAT Binding Potency of 3β-(Substituted Phenyl)Tropane-2β-Carboxylic Acid Methyl Esters

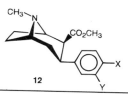

Com-pound	< 2 nM X, Y	Com-pound	2 to 12 nM X, Y	Com-pound	12 to 30 nM X, Y	Com-pound	30 to 200 nM X, Y
a	CH_3, H	i	N_3, H	s (**9**)	H, H	x	$NHCOCH_3$, H
b	Cl, H	j	NO_2, H	t	H, F	y	$NHCOC_2H_5$, H
c	Br, H	k	NH_2, H	u	F, H	z	$NHCO_2C_2H_5$, H
d	I, H	l	HO, H	v	CF_3, H	aa	$Sn(CH_3)_3$, H
e	NH_2, I	m	CH_3O, H	w	H, I	bb	CH_3CH_2, H
f	Cl, Cl	n	H, Cl				
g	Cl, CH_3	o	H, Br				
h	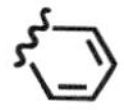 (thiophene)	p	N_3, I				
		q	F, CH_3				
		r	NH_2, Br				

IC$_{50}$ Values

models show that some steric bulk extending from and above the 4′-position contributes to enhanced potency, although excessive bulk leads to reduced potency. In addition, the model suggests that electrostatic forces account for approximately one-quarter of the binding affinity and thus may make a significant contribution to potency.

MODIFICATION OF THE 2-POSITION

Since WIN 35,065-2 (**9**) is considerably more potent than its 2α-isomer WIN 35,140 (**10**), it appears that, as for cocaine (**1a**), a 2β-substituent is required for high affinity at the DAT (*66,79,80*). A number of 2β-alkyl and aryl ester analogs of **12a**, **12b**, and **12d** have been studied (*13,15,20*). As in the cocaine series, the phenyl and isopropyl esters

(**13a**, **13b**, **14a**, **14b**, **15a**, and **15b**) are highly potent and more selective for the DAT relative to binding at the 5-HT and NE transporters (*15,20,21*). Also as in the cocaine series, replacement of the methyl group of **12b** with a large group, such as a 2-(4'-aminophenyl)ethyl group (**14c**), has only small effects on the IC$_{50}$ value for binding of the DAT (*17*).

Several amide analogs of **12a**, **12b**, and **12d** were evaluated for their affinity and selectivity at the DAT (*20,21*). Tertiary amides are more potent than primary and secondary amide analogs. In particular, 3β-(4'-chlorophenyl)tropane-2β-N-morpholinocarboxamide (**14d**), as well as 3β-(4'-chlorophenyl)- and 3β-(4'-iodophenyl)tropane-2β-N-pyrrolidinocarboxamides (**14e** and **15c**), possess high affinity and selectivity for the DAT.

The binding affinity of the 2β-acetyl, 2β-propanoyl, and 2β-isopropanoyl analogs of **12s** (**9**, WIN 35,065-2), **12u** (WIN 35,428), **12a**, **12h**, and of **12bb** have been reported (*8,31,32*). The most potent compound in this series, 3β-(2-naphthyl)-2β-propanoyltropane (**16**), with an IC$_{50}$ of 0.043 nM for the DAT, is the most potent compound thus far reported.

The binding affinity of a number of other 2-substituted analogs of **12s** (**9**, WIN 35,065-2) and **12b** have been reported. Compounds with the 2β-substituent equal to vinyl (**14f**), propyl (**14g** or **17a**), chlorovinyl (**14h**), phenylvinyl (**14i**), phenylethyl (**14j**), carbomethoxyvinyl (**17b**), hydroxymethylvinyl (**17c**), 2-carbomethoxyethyl (**17d**), and 3-hydroxypropyl (**17e**) all show potencies similar to their parent 2β-carbomethoxy analog **12s** (**9**) and **12b** (*50,57,59*). The SAR of this set of compounds has been interpreted to suggest a hydrophobic pocket for the 2β-substituent (*50,57,59*). However, no correlation with the hydrophobicity of the various 2β-substituents was reported (*50,57,59*).

In another study (*56*), the potency of 3β-(4'-chloropheny)-2β-(3'-phenyl-isoxazol-5'-yl)tropane (**18**) for the DAT was reported to be 15-times greater than that of the isomeric 2β-heterocyclic analog 3β-(4'-chlorophenyl)-2β-(5'-phenyloxazole-2'-yl)tropane (**19**). An analysis of the molecular electrostatic potential (MEP) of these two compounds suggests an electrostatic interaction between the 2β-heterocyclic group and the cocaine binding site on the DAT. In addition to being highly potent at the DAT, compound **18** is also highly selective for the DAT relative to the 5-HT and NE transporters.

The binding properties of all four stereoisomers of the (1*R*,5*S*)-3-phenyl-2-(3'-methyl-1',2',4'-oxadiazol-5',-yl)-tropane (**20a–d**) bioisosteres of WIN 35,065-2 (**9**) have been reported (*19*). As expected, the

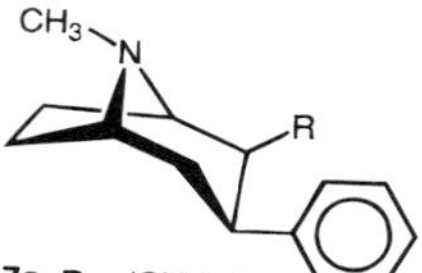

17a, R = (CH₂)₂CH₃
 b, R = CH=CHCO₂CH₃
 c, R = CH=CHCH₂OH
 d, R = CH₂CH₂CO₂CH₃
 e, R = CH₂CH₂CH₂OH

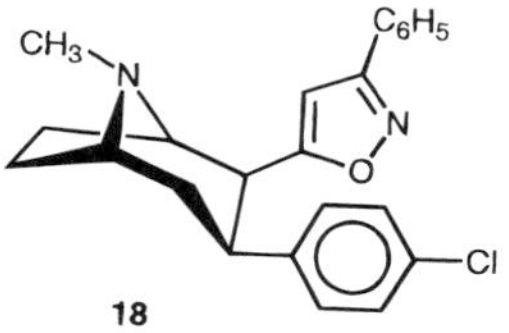

18

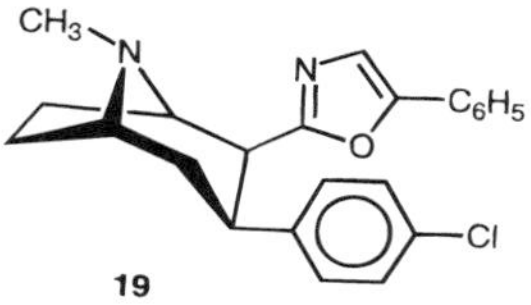

19

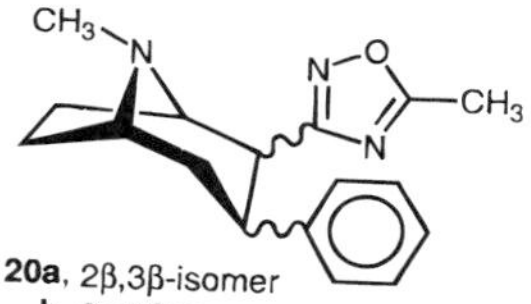

20a, 2β,3β-isomer
 b, 2α,3β-isomer
 c, 2β,3α-isomer
 d, 2α,3α-isomer

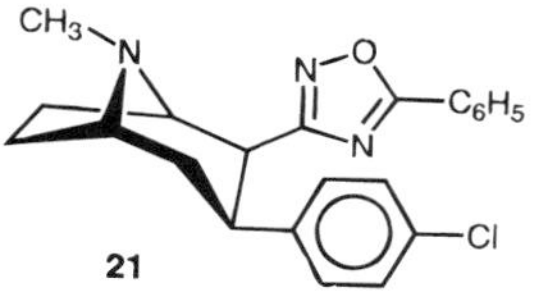

21

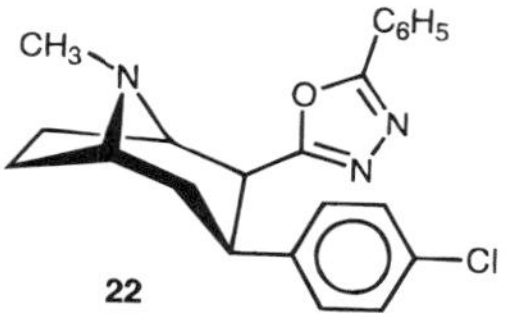

22

2β,3β-isomer, which has the WIN 35,065-2 (**9**) stereochemistry, possesses the greatest potency for the DAT. However, the IC_{50} values of the 2β,3α- and 2α,3α-isomers are only slightly higher than those of the 2β,3β-isomer. Several other 2β-(1′,2′,4′-oxadiazole) bioisosteres of the corresponding 3β-(4′-chlorophenyl)tropane-2β-carboxylic acid esters show potencies for the DAT similar to those of their parent esters. 3β-(4′-Chlorophenyl)-2β-(3′-phenyl-1′,2′,4′-oxadiazole-5′-yl) tropane (**21**) has a potency eight times greater than the isomeric 3β-(4′-chlorophenyl)-2β-(5′-phenyl-1′,3′,4′-oxadiazole-2′-yl)tropane (**22**) (*19,56*). Comparison of MEP again suggests an electrostatic interaction with the DAT.

MODIFICATION OF THE N-METHYL GROUP

Only a few compounds in this class have been reported. Removal of the N-methyl group to give the corresponding N-nor analogs (**23a–f**) has little effect on potency at the DAT, but increases potency at the 5-HT transporter (*12,64,69,73,80*). Replacement of the N-methyl group of **12u** with allyl, propyl, or iodopropenyl groups (**24a–c**) or of the N-methyl group of **12d** with ethyl, propyl, butyl, fluoroethyl, or fluoropropyl groups (**24d–h**) has minor effects on binding potency (*1,36,64,73,75*).

23a, X = Y = H (WIN 35,981)
b, X = F, Y = H
c, X = Cl, Y = H
d, X = I, Y = H
e, X = C₂H₅, Y = H
f, X = Y = Cl

24a, X = F, R = CH₂CH=CH₂
b, X = F, R = CH₂CH₂CH₃
c, X = F, R = CH₂CH=CHI
d, X = I, R = CH₂CH₃
e, X = I, R = CH₂CH₂CH₃
f, X = I, R = CH₂(CH₂)₂CH₃
g, X = I, R = CH₂CH₂F
h, X = I, R = CH₂CH₂CH₂F

Benztropine Analogs

Benztropine (**25a**) binds the DAT with a potency about one-half to one-third that of cocaine (*70,71,76,77*). Since the structure of **25a** contains a tropane and a diphenylmethoxy moiety, it bears resemblance to both cocaine and the 1,4-dialkylpiperazine (GBR) series of dopamine inhibitors (*see* 1,4-Dialkylpiperazine, below). The binding affinity of a series of 4′- and 4′,4″-substituted analogs of **25a** has been reported (*76,77*). The 4′,4″-difluoro analog (**25b**), which is 10 times more potent than **25a**, is the most potent analog. The 4′,4″-substituted analogs **25c–h** have binding potencies 3.1–6.2 greater than **25a**. All of the analogs, including **25a**, show weak affinity at the 5-HT and NE transporters. Benztropine (**25a**) shows high affinity for both the m_1 and m_2 muscarinic receptors. The analogs **25b–h** show potency at the m_1 receptor similar to those at the DAT, but are weaker at the m_2 receptor as compared to **25a**.

The addition of a 2-carbomethoxy group to the benzotropine structure creates three centers of asymmetry and, like cocaine, eight possible diastereoisomers. An SAR study of the eight possible diastereoisomers of 2-carbomethoxy-4′,4″-difluorobenztropine reveals that only the S-isomer **26a** with potency 28.6-times greater than **25a** possess high affinity for the DAT (*71*). An SAR study of other 4′,4″,-substituted analogs of **26a** revealed that analogs **26b–e** have potencies 5.6–23.6-times greater than **25a**.

1,4-Dialkylpiperazine Class

The 1,4-dialk(en)ylpiperazines had been found to be potent and selective inhibitors of dopamine transport (*90*) and to label the DAT (*6,10,14*). However, although the binding of cocaine and analogs in

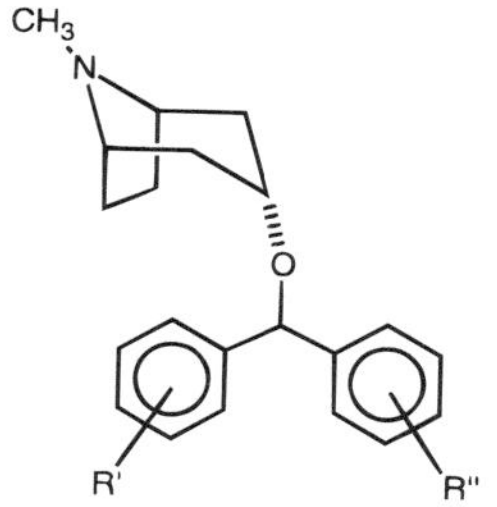

25a, R' = R" = H
   b, R' = 4'-F, R" = 4"-F
   c, R' = 4'-Cl, R" = 4"-Cl
   d, R' = 4'-F, R" = H
   e, R' = 4'-Cl, R" = H
   f, R' = 4'-Br, R" = H
   g, R' = 4'-Cl, R" = 3"-Cl
   h, R' = 4'-F, R" = 3",4"-diCl

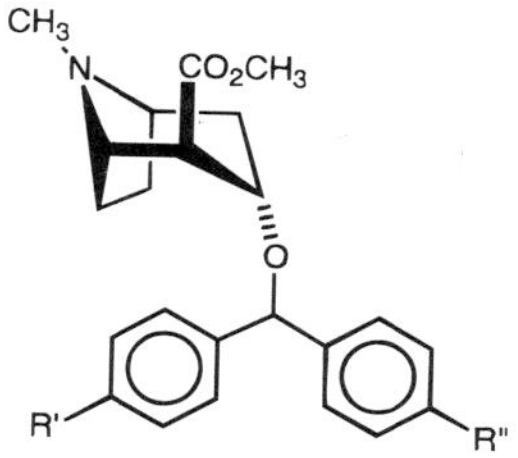

26a, R' = R" = F
   b, R' = F, R" = H
   c, R' = Cl, R" = H
   d, R' = CH₃, R" = H
   e, R' = I, R" = H

the tropane class (*see* Tropane, *above*) has two components, the compounds in the 1,4-dialk(en)ylpiperazine class label only one component (*66*). Furthermore, ligands in the 1,4-dialk(en)ylpiperazine class do not fully displace ligands in the tropane class from binding at the dopamine transporter, and vice versa (*37,66*). Finally, in addition to binding the dopamine transporter, 1,4-dialk(en)ylpiperazines bind a piperazine-acceptor site (*6*). Structural changes have been made in the benzhydryl moiety, in the six-membered heterocycle, and in the 4-substituent (*see* **27**).

Modifications of the Benzhydryl Moiety

Most of the modifications to the benzhydryl group have been carried out using the GBR 12783 skeleton (**27a**). No significant effects on potency to inhibit dopamine uptake have been noted with either symmetrically or unsymmetrically 3- and 4-substituted analogs (*33,89,90*). Introduction of a 3-isothiocyanato group (**27b**) (*33,34*), 2,4-dichloro substituents (**27c**) (*90*), or of maleimide groups at positions 3 or 4 (**27d**) (*33,34*), were exceptions, leading to 4- to 100-fold decreases in potency. For the isothiocyanato and maleimide substituted compounds, this has been interpreted to indicate that the domain recognized by the benzhydryl portion of the ligand may be a small cleft that is sensitive to steric effects (*34*). It has also been proposed that the fact that unsymmetrical substitution can lead to substantial changes in potency indicates that both phenyl rings are involved in binding (*34*).

27a, X = Y = N R$_1$ = R$_2$ = H R$_3$ = CH$_2$CH=CHPh
  b, X = Y = N R$_1$ = 3-NCS R$_2$ = H R$_3$ = CH$_2$CH=CHPh
  c, X = Y = N R$_1$ = 2,4-Cl$_2$ R$_2$ =F R$_3$ = CH$_2$CH=CHPh

  d, X = Y = NR$_1$ = 3- or 4- —N(succinimidyl) R$_2$ = H R$_3$ = CH$_2$CH=CHPh

  e, X = Y = N R$_1$ = R$_2$ =H R$_3$ = (CH$_2$)$_3$Ph
  f, X = Y = N R$_1$ = R$_2$ = 4-F R$_3$ = (CH$_2$)$_3$Ph
  g, X = Y = N R$_1$ = R$_2$ = 4-F R$_3$ = H
  h, X =N Y = C R$_1$ = R$_2$ = 4-F R$_3$ = (CH$_2$)$_3$Ph
  i, X = C Y = N R$_1$ = R$_2$ = 4-F R$_3$ = (CH$_2$)$_3$Ph
  j, X = Y = N R$_1$ = R$_2$ = 4-F R$_3$ = CH$_2$CH=CHPh
  k, X = Y = N R$_1$ = R$_2$ = 4-F R$_3$ = CH$_3$

28a, R = R = H, R$_1$ = (CH$_2$)$_3$Ph, W = Z = CH$_2$
  b, R = R = H, R$_1$ = (CH$_2$)$_3$Ph, W = CH$_2$, Z = (CH$_2$)$_2$
  c, R = R = F, R$_1$ = (CH$_2$)$_3$Ph, W = CH$_2$, Z = (CH$_2$)$_2$
  d, R = R = F, R$_1$ = H, W = Z = CHCH$_3$
  e, R = R = F, R$_1$ = (CH$_2$)$_3$Ph, W = Z = CHCH$_3$

Modifications of the Heterocycle

The effects of modifications of the heterocyclic moiety of 1,4-dialk(en)ylpiperazines have been carried out using the 1-(2-diphenyl-methoxy)ethyl-4-(3-propylphenyl)piperazine skeleton (**28a**).

Expansion of the piperazine ring of GBR 12935 (**27e**) and GBR 12909 (**27f**) to give the seven-membered ring analogs **28b** and **28c**, respectively, does not significantly affect potency at the DAT, although selectivity for the DAT, relative to the serotonin and norepinephrine transporters, is enhanced by a factor of 4000 (*83*).

Introduction of methyl groups, *trans* to each other, at positions 2 and 5 of the piperazine ring of GBR 11513 (**27g**) and GBR 12909 (**27f**) affords the chiral compounds **28d** and **28e** (*67*). Though no improvements in potency are obtained by this modification, the enantioselectivity observed in the binding of the 2S,5R enantiomers of these compounds suggests the operation of a receptor-mediated mechanism for the inhibition of dopamine reuptake by this class of compounds (*67*).

To determine whether both amino groups are required for binding the DAT site, the piperazine ring of 1-[2-*bis*(4-fluorophenyl)-methoxy]ethyl-4-(3-propylphenyl)piperazine (GBR 12909, **27f**) was replaced by a piperidine ring with nitrogen atom either proximal (**27h**) or distal (**27i**) to the benzhydryl moiety (*65*). Based on the relative potencies to displace [^{3}H]WIN 35,428 and [^{3}H]GBR 12935 binding, it was concluded that only the distal nitrogen (**27i**) is required for binding to the DAT. Potencies to displace [^{3}H]citalopram binding indicated only a slight (factor of 2) decrease in affinity for the ligand with only a proximal nitrogen (**27h**). Experiments in the presence of mazindol to inhibit binding to the DAT demonstrated that removal of the proximal nitrogen (**27i**) substantially decreases potency at the piperazine acceptor site, making **27i** more selective for the DAT than the parent compound GBR 12909 (**27f**)(*65*).

Modifications of the 4-Substituent

Most of the modifications of the 4-substituent have been carried out on the 1-[2-*bis*(4-fluorophenyl)methoxy]ethyl-4-piperazine skeleton (GBR 11513, **27g**) (*74,89,90*). Highest potencies were achieved with 3-phenylpropyl and 3-phenyl-2-propenyl substituents (GBR 12909 and GBR 12879, **27f** and **27j**, respectively). Though replacement of the 4-position hydrogen in GBR 11513 (**27g**), by a 3-phenylpropyl substituent to give GBR 12909 (**27f**), increases potency to inhibit dopamine uptake by a factor of 70 (*89,90*), the analogous replacement of the 4-position hydrogen in the *trans*-2,5-dimethylpiperazine analog **28d**, by a 3-phenylpropyl group to give **28e**, only increases potency by a factor of 2.4 in both the racemate and the more potent enantiomer (*67*); a decrease in potency is observed for the less active enantiomer (*67*). Substituents on the phenyl portion of the 3-phenylpropenyl group of GBR 12789 (**27j**) do not lead to significant changes in potency, although electron donating substituents have a slightly adverse effect on potency (*90*). An important compound in this series is the 4-methyl analog **27k** (NNC12-0722) (*74*). Although not highly

enol   Mazindol, **29**   keto

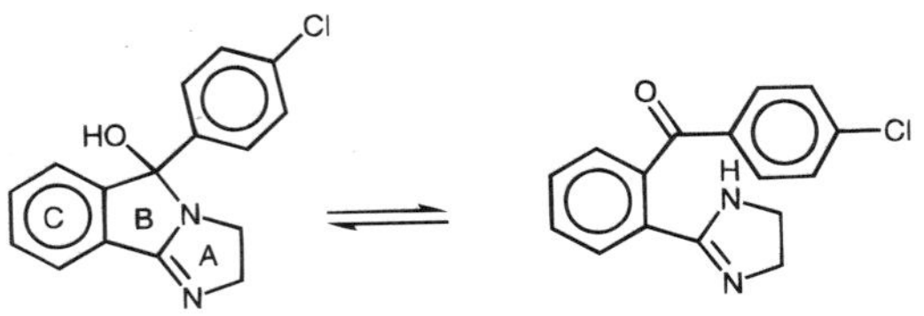

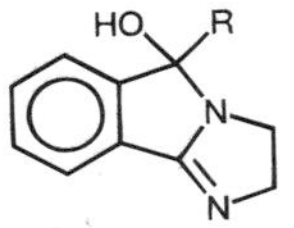

30a, R = CH₃
b, R = (CH₃)₃C

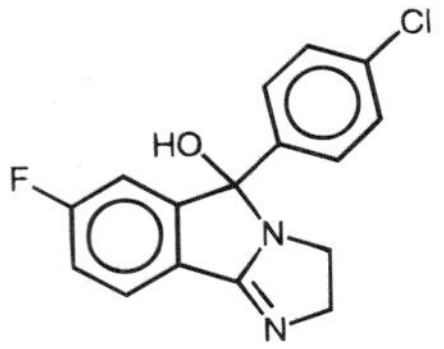

32

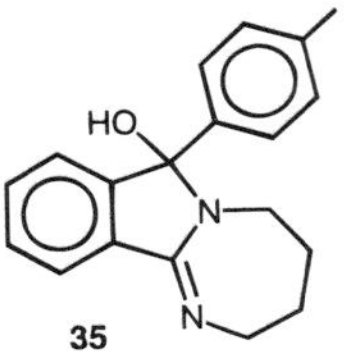

35

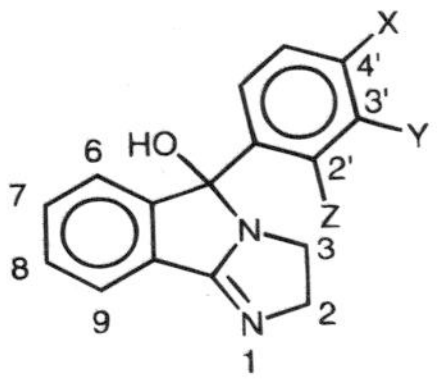

31a, X = F, Y = Z = H
b, X = Br, Y = Z = H
c, X = OCH₃, Y = Z = H
d, X = Y = Cl, Z = H
e, Z = Y = Z = H
f, Z = Y = H, X = I
g, X = Z = Cl, Y = H
h, X = Z = H, Y = Cl
i, X = Y = H, Z = Cl

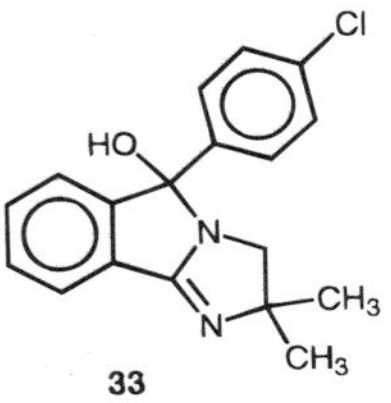

33

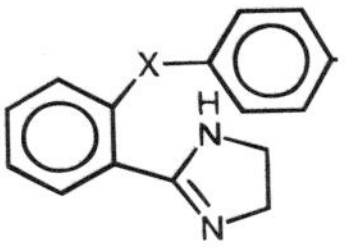

34

36a, X = CH₂
b, X = O
c, X = S
d, X = SO₂

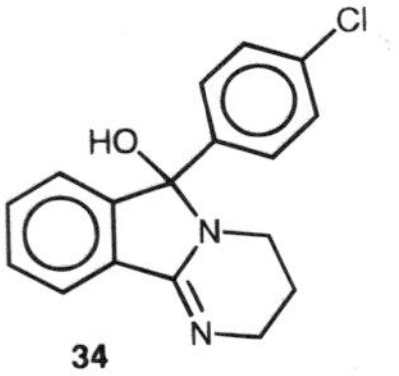

potent, this compound could be a useful imaging ligand for the dopamine transporter, when labeled with carbon-11.

Mazindol Class

Mazindol (**29**) (Sanoxex or Mazanor) (*2,4,5*) is a clinically utilized appetite suppressant that is reported to be abuse-free and shows reduced craving for cocaine abusers (*9,26*). It potently inhibits monoamine uptake (*48*). [³H]Mazindol labels the DAT in the striatum and the NE transporter in the cerebral cortex with K_D values of 18 and 4 nM, respectively (*48*). Mazindol (**29**) has been reported to exist exclusively in the enol form in the solid state (*7*). However, it can be present in either the enol or keto form in solution, depending on the pH of the solution (*4*). There have been no reports whether both forms or, if not, which form can bind the DAT. For convenience, all mazindol analogs in this chapter are drawn in the enol form.

The DAT binding and/or uptake properties of only a limited number of mazindol analogs have been reported (45–47). The studies show that replacement of the p-chlorophenyl ring, with either a methyl or a t-butyl group (**30a–b**), causes a large loss of binding affinity, indicating that the aromatic ring is needed for potent binding at the DAT. The studies also show that replacement of the 4′-chloro group on the 4′-chlorophenyl ring of mazindol with a fluoro, bromo, and methoxy group (**31a–c**), or the addition of a 3′-chloro substituent (**31d**), increase potency by two-to fivefold, and replacement of the 4′-chloro with a hydrogen or iodine (**31e** or **31f**, respectively), or the addition of a 2′-chloro group (**31g**), results in a two- to ninefold loss in potency. Adding a fluoro to the 7-position (**32**) has very little effect on potency. The replacement of the hydrogen atoms at the 2′-position by methyl groups results in a six-fold loss of potency (**33**). Moving the 4′-chloro group to the 3′-position (**31h**) causes a twofold increase in potency, but moving the 4′-chloro to the 2′-position (**31i**) causes a 36-fold reduction in potency. Expansion of the imidazole ring-A to a pyrimido or diazepino ring system (**34** and **35**, respectively) gives analogs that are five times more potent than mazindol. The carbinol group appears to be important for high potency, since replacement of this moiety group with a methylene group, oxygen or sulfur atom, or by a sulfone group (**36a–d**) results in loss of potency.

Phencyclidine Class

PCP (**37a**) has been observed to induce generalization to cocaine in rats trained to discriminate cocaine solutions from saline (30). In addition, the PCP class of compounds had been found to inhibit synaptosomal dopamine uptake (93), and it has been suggested that the complex nature of the behaviors associated with PCP abuse is a result of the interaction of PCP with both the NMDA receptor complex and the DAT (92). Since the reinforcing properties of cocaine have been correlated with its ability to increase dopamine levels in the synapse by virtue of its effectiveness in inhibiting dopamine uptake (62), the interaction of PCP (**37a**) and its congeners with the DAT (55) may involve the cocaine binding site.

A comparison of the effects of substitution on the potency of phencyclidine analogs to inhibit the binding of [³H]PCP and to inhibit dopamine uptake revealed that the effects were not correlated (92).

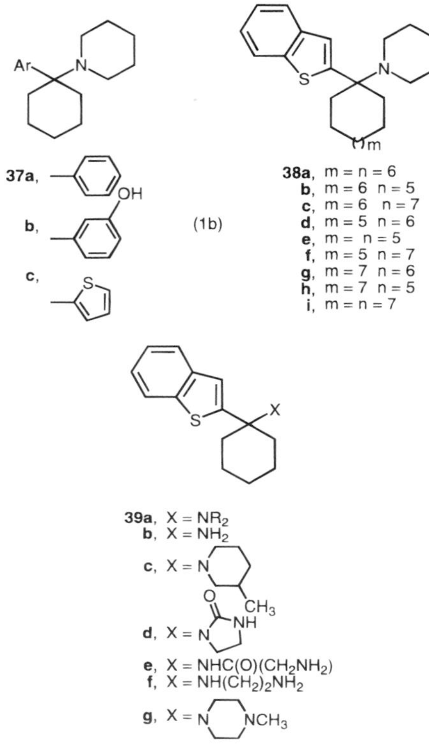

37a,

b,

c,

(1b)

38a, m = n = 6
b, m = 6 n = 5
c, m = 6 n = 7
d, m = 5 n = 6
e, m = n = 5
f, m = 5 n = 7
g, m = 7 n = 6
h, m = 7 n = 5
i, m = n = 7

39a, X = NR₂
b, X = NH₂

c, X = N

d, X = N

e, X = NHC(O)(CH₂NH₂)
f, X = NH(CH₂)₂NH₂

g, X = N

For example, though the substitution of the phenyl group in PCP (**37a**) by an *m*-hydroxy group (to give **37b**) increased the potency to inhibit [³H]PCP binding by an order of magnitude, it decreased the potency to inhibit DA uptake by a factor of three, and replacement of the phenyl group by a 2-thienyl group (to give **37c**) increased potency to displace [³H]PCP by more than an order of magnitude, while decreasing the potency to inhibit DA uptake by a factor of 3. Conversely, replacement of the phenyl group in PCP (**37a**) by a 2-benzothienyl group (to give BTCP, **38a**) decreased potency to displace [³H]PCP by a factor of 30, while increasing the potency to inhibit DA uptake by a factor of 60. Eventually, it was demonstrated that the binding of the radiolabeled form of this ligand, [³H]BTCP, was directly displaced by cocaine (*94*). Further similarity to cocaine is suggested by the identification of two [³H]BTCP binding sites, with affinities 0.9 and 20 n*M* and B_max values of 3.5 and 7.5 pmol/mg protein, respectively (*92*).

Modifications of the Carbocyclic Ring

Analogs and derivatives of BTCP have been investigated over the past few years, but no significant improvements in potency have been achieved. Structures in which the cyclohexyl ring was either decreased (to cyclopentyl, as in **38d–f**), or enlarged (to cycloheptyl, as in **38g–i**), have potencies 2–11-times lower than the parent compound (*41*).

Modifications of the Amino Group

Modifications in the size of the nitrogen heterocycle lead to modest increases in potency with the largest (threefold) observed for the pyrrolidine analog (**38b**) of BTCP (*41*). A threefold decrease in potency is observed when both the carbocyclic and the heterocyclic rings are seven-membered (**38i**). The detrimental effects of steric bulk at the amino group are even more apparent from a study in which numerous replacements of the amino group were investigated (*42*). In general, analogs with tertiary amino groups (**39a**) are more potent than their primary amine counterparts (**39b**), but compounds with large sub-stituents ($>C_6$) exhibit pronounced decreases in potency. On the other hand, introduction of a methyl substituent at the 3'-position of the piperidine ring of **38a**, to give **39c**, has been found to increase potency by a factor of 2.5 (*28*). Strikingly, and somewhat surprisingly, although slight enantioselectivity (factor of 3) was found for (–)-(S)-1-[1-(2-benzo[b]thiophenyl)cyclohexyl]-3-methylpiperidine over the (+)-(R)-enantiomer, the potency of the racemate was the same as that of the more potent of the optical antipodes.

Replacement of the amino group by an imidazoline-2-one (**39d**) leads to total loss of potency (*42*), demonstrating the need for an amino functionality. Replacement by a β-aminoacetamido group (**39e**) restores some potency, but reduction of the carbonyl group to a methylene, i.e., replacement of the amino group by an ethylenedi-amine group (**39f**), increases potency by a factor of 5 (*42*). Replacement by a cyclic diamine, i.e., by a piperazino group (**39g**), improves potency by an additional factor of 2 (*29*).

Methylphenidate

Methylphenidate (Ritalin, **40**) is a drug used for the treatment of hyperactive children (*1*). Since **40** has two centers of asymmetry, four isomers are possible. Methylphenidate is the (±)-*threo*-isomer (**40a**). It possesses an IC_{50} value of 83–390 nM for radioligand displacement at the DAT, depending on the radioligand used in the assay (*35,81,84*). In a comparison of the potency of the stereoisomers to displace

40a, (±)-threo
b, (±)-erythro

41a, R = H
b, R = group larger
than CH₃

42a, Y = Cl, X = Z = H
b, Y = Br, X = Z = H
c, X = Br, Y = Z = H
d, X = Y = Cl, Z = H
e, X = OH, Y = Z = H
f, X = NH₂, Y = Z = H
g, X = Z = H, Y = OH
h, X = Z = H, Y = NH₂
i, X = Y = H, Z = CH₃O
j, X = Y = H, Z = F

[³H]methylphenidate binding, it was found that the *threo* diastere-omer (**40a**) is about 80 times more potent than the *erythro* diastereomer (**40b**) (*84*); within the more active *threo* diastereomer, the (+)-enantiomer is 13.6 and 2.4 times more potent than the (–)-enantiomer and the racemate, respectively (*84*).

Replacement of the carbomethoxy methyl group by a hydrogen to give **41a** leads to total loss of potency (*84*). Similarly, alkyl groups other than methyl afford inactive compounds (**41b**); losses in potency appear to be associated with increasing mass of the alkyl group, but not necessarily with steric bulk (*84*).

Investigation of the effect of aromatic substitution on binding potency in (±)-*threo*-**40** revealed all 2-substituted analogs to have greatly reduced potencies, but, in general, electron withdrawing sub-stituents in positions 3- and 4- are linked to increased potency, and electron donating groups in the 3- and 4-positions had little effect or decreased potency (*35*). The most potent compounds are the 3-chloro, 3- and 4-bromo, and 3,4-dichloro analogs **42a–d**, which are 12- to 20-times more potent than **40a**. Analogs **42e** and **42f**, which are 4-hydroxy-and 4-amino-substituted, have slightly reduced and enhanced potencies, respectively; the 3-hydroxy- and 3-amino-analogs **42g** and **42h** show 3- to 4-fold decreases in potency relative to **40a**. The most deactivating substituent is a methoxy group in the 2-position (1200-fold lower potency, **42i**), but even the 2-fluoro ana-log **42j** shows a 17-fold decrease in potency.

Cocaine Antagonists

The function of the DAT is to transport (move) the neurotransmit-ter dopamine from the synaptic gap back into the cytoplasm of the presynaptic neuron. The uptake of dopamine is coupled to the flow of sodium and chloride ions and, as indicated in this chapter, is inhibited by many structurally different compounds. Considerable effort has been devoted to the biochemical characterization of the site(s) where these inhibitors bind (24). Some studies suggest a competitive mechanism for the inhibition of DA by cocaine and other inhibitors, while other studies suggest an allosteric, or more complex, mechanism (24). Uncompetitive inhibition of DA uptake by cocaine was observed in a multisubstrate study of analogs of dopamine that used rotating disk voltametry to measure DA uptake in striatal suspension (*see* Fig. 2); in the same study cocaine was found to competitively inhibit the binding of both sodium and chloride ions (68). Furthermore, based on the differential effects on [^{3}H]DA uptake and [^{3}H]WIN 35,428 binding in mutants prepared by site-directed mutagenesis of cloned DAT(s), as compared to the wild-type clones, it was concluded that aspartate 79, in the first hydrophobic region, and serine 356 and 359, in the seventh hydrophobic region, are more instrumental in DA transport than in WIN 35,428 binding (52). It follows that the DA and the WIN 35,428 binding sites may not be identical (52). Dissociation of DA uptake and cocaine binding has also been concluded from investigations of chimeras of DAT and NET (40). Other investigations have demonstrated that cocaine is substantially better than DA in protecting the DAT to reaction with sulfhydryl reagents, suggesting that the sites are different (49). Thus, the data from several studies, which show that there are differences between the cocaine binding site(s) on the DAT and the site(s) for DA uptake, suggest that some compounds might inhibit cocaine binding without inhibiting the translocation of DA. Such a compound has been referred to as a cocaine antagonist or, perhaps preferably, as a dopamine-transport-sparing cocaine antagonist (52) (*see* Fig. 3). A recent study has shown that, when measured under identical conditions, the potencies of a group of compounds to inhibit [^{3}H]DA uptake is 2.3 times greater than to inhibit [^{3}H]WIN 35,428 binding (95). In other words, only one-half of the binding sites must be occupied in order to completely inhibit DA transport. However, a few of the compounds, RTI-121, WF-29, GBR 12909, **25b**, and **44a–d**, presented in previous sections of this chapter, as well as the racemate **43**, have shown four- to ninefold greater potencies to inhibit radioligand binding to the cocaine binding site than to inhibit DA uptake, when evaluated under the usual binding and uptake assay conditions (*see* p. 286) (8,20,33,35,76,86). If future studies con-

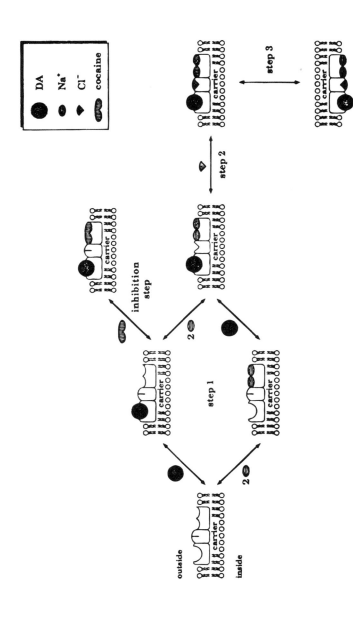

Fig. 2. Schematic illustration of the partially random, sequential multisubstrate mechanism of dopamine uptake in striatal tissue and how it may be influenced by cocaine. The sequence proceeds from left to right. In step 1, dopamine or Na$^+$ binds to the uptake carrier in random order, followed by Cl$^-$ binding in step 2. In step 3, the carrier transports dopamine across the membrane. If cocaine is present, the process is inhibited by cocaine binding at the Na$^+$-binding site as illustrated in the *inhibition step*. The illustration is highly schematic and is not intended to represent the structure of the carrier protein and its mechanism of translocation. Reprinted with permission from ref. *68*.

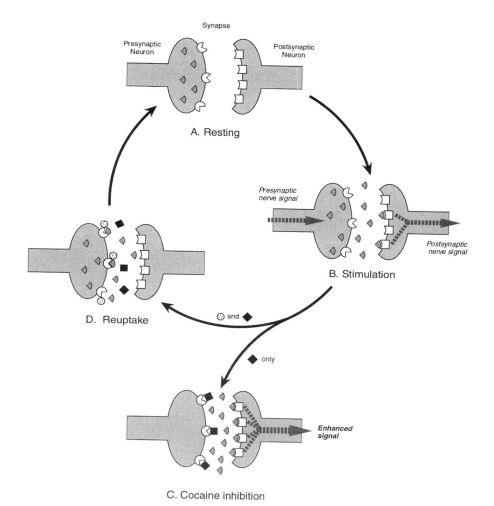

Fig. 3. Schematic representation of a dopamine-transport-sparing cocaine antagonist within the context of the dopamine hypothesis *(62)*. Stimulation of a resting neuron (**A**) releases dopamine (◀) from the presynaptic terminal into the synapse where it may bind dopamine receptors (▭) on the postsynaptic terminal, resulting in transmission of the signal (**B**). Reuptake of dopamine (◀) by its transporter (⊂) is inhibited by cocaine (◆) binding to its recognition site (**C**) but a dopamine-transport-sparing cocaine antagonist (◉) compromises the ability of cocaine (◆) to bind to its recognition site without inhibiting dopamine (◀) reuptake (**D**).

firm the reported differences between binding and uptake potencies for the compounds shown, then one or more of these structures could serve as lead compounds for the development of a dopamine-transport-sparing cocaine antagonist. On the other hand, it is important to note that when binding and uptake for several of the compounds, for which potency ratios for inhibition of DA uptake to radioligand binding different than 2 had been reported, were measured under nearly identical conditions, these differences disappeared (*8,82,95*; Reith, personal communication).

Summary

The important role of the DAT in several neurological disorders and in cocaine abuse has prompted investigations aimed at a better understanding of the mechanism of dopamine uptake and of its inhibition. The short-range goal of identifying ligands with high potency and selectivity for the DAT by and large has been met. Thus, compounds with potency to inhibit radioligand binding at the cocaine site at the DAT <2 n*M*, and with selectivities greater than two orders of magnitude for binding at the DAT relative to the norepinephrine or serotonin transporter, have been identified (*see* WIN35,065-2 Analogs section). Some of these compounds have been used successfully as biological markers, in particular, in imaging.

In addition, some progress has been made in the identification of specific molecular features associated with potency and selectivity at the DAT; most of this has been associated with compounds in the tropane class (*see* Tropane). On the other hand, attempts to correlate molecular features of compounds in different compound classes have met with complete failure. In fact, the only important conclusion that can be drawn from examination of the various compound classes that bind the so-called cocaine receptor at the DAT is that the protein may be quite adaptable to the several compound classes, assuming different conformations and possibly utilizing different amino acid residues to bind compounds in the different compound classes. The differences in binding properties (e.g., B_{max}; number of binding sites, Hill coefficients) associated with the different compound classes may also be accounted for in this manner. This hypothesis may be confirmed experimentally by investigations with cloned wild-type receptors and cloned mutants (*see* Cocaine Antagonist section). The observations that, in the tropane class, high potency ligands can be obtained when the 2β-substituent is capable of hydrogen bonding, or of electrostatic interaction, with the binding site, but also when it is incapable of such interactions, may similarly be accommodated because the protein is so readily adaptable. These problems have also prevented the definition of a specific pharmacophore for the cocaine site at the DAT. Progress has been made within subsets of the tropane class of compounds, but it appears that definition of a generalized pharmacophore may not be a realistic goal.

A very important goal that has not been met so far is the determination as to whether dopamine-transporter-sparing cocaine antagonism may be feasible. Since, in general, it appears that occupancy of only half of the cocaine receptor sites at the DAT is required for complete inhibition of DA-transport, it may be possible that DAT oligomers (dimers?) may be involved. In principle, it would seem that the state of aggregation and the nature of the oligomers (e.g., homo- or heterodimers) may be related to the state of occupancy of the receptor, and, if the protein is indeed very adaptable, DA transport may or may not be inhibited by occupancy of the receptor site. Unfortunately, this theoretical possibility has not been either confirmed or refuted (Cocaine Antagonists). The question may be answered when the mechanism of DA transport is elaborated. Since very important research tools, e.g., potent and selective ligands, irreversible ligands, radio-isotopically labeled ligands, as well as wild-type cloned DAT protein and mutagens thereof, are now available, this goal may be soon accomplished. Until then, the quest for a ligand capable of blocking cocaine binding but sparing DA transport remains an important research objective.

Acknowledgments

The authors express their appreciation to Howard M. Deutsch, William J. Houlihan, J.-M. Kamenka, Peter Meltzer, Amy Hauck Newman, and Kenner C. Rice for supplying articles submitted for publication or in press, as well as detailed information from papers presented at scientific meetings.

References

1. *Physicians' Desk Reference*, 49th ed., Medical Economics Data, Montvale, NJ, 1995, pp. 309, 897.
2. *Physicians' Desk Reference*, 49th ed., Medical Economics Data, Montvale, NJ, 1995, pp. 2190–2191, 269.
3. Abraham, P., Pitner, J. B., Lewin, A. H., Boja, J. W., Kuhar, M. J., and Carroll, F. I. N-Modified analogues of cocaine: synthesis and inhibition of binding to the cocaine receptor. *J. Med. Chem.* **35** (1992) 141–144.
4. Aeberli, P., Eden, P., Gogerty, J. H., Houlihan, W. J., and Penberthy, C. 5-Aryl-2,3-dihydro-5*H*-imidazo[2-1-α]isoindol-5-ols. A novel class of anorectic agents. *J. Med. Chem.* **18** (1975) 177–182.
5. Aeberli, P., Eden, P., Gogerty, J. H., Houlihan, W. J., and Penberthy, C. Anorectic agents. 2. Structural analogs of 5-(*p*-chlorophenyl)-2,3-dihydro 5*H*-imdazo[2,1-α]isoindol-5-ol. *J. Med. Chem.* **18** (1975) 182–185.
6. Anderson, P. H. Biochemical and pharmacological characterization of [³H]GBR-12935 binding in vitro to rat striatal membranes: labeling of the dopamine uptake complex. *J. Neurochem.* **48** (1987) 1887–1896.
7. Barcza, S. and Houlihan, W. J. Structure determination of the anorexic agent Mazindol. *J. Pharm. Sci.* **64** (1975) 829–831.
8. Bennett, B. A., Wichems, C. H., Hollingsworth, C. K., Davies, H. M. L., Thornley, C., Sexton, T., and Childers, S. R. Novel 2-substituted cocaine analogs: uptake and ligand binding studies at dopamine, serotonin and norepinephrine transport sites in the rat brain. *J. Pharmacol. Exp. Ther.* **272** (1995) 1176–1186.
9. Berger, P., Gawin, F., and Koster, T. R., Treatment of cocaine abuse with mazindol. *Lancet* **II** (1989) 283.
10. Berger, P., Janowsky, A., Vocci, F., Skolnick, P., Schweri, M. M., and Paul, S. M. [³H]GBR-12935: a specific high affinity ligand for labeling the dopamine transport complex. *Eur. J. Pharmacol.* **107** (1985) 289, 290.

11. Bergman, J., Madras, B. K., Johnson, S. E., and Spealman, R. D. Effects of cocaine and related drugs in nonhuman primates. III. Self-administration by squirrel monkeys. *J. Pharmacol. Exp. Ther.* **251** (1989) 150–155.

12. Boja, J. W., Kuhar, M. J., Kopajtic, T., Yang, E., Abraham, P., Lewin, A. H., and Carroll, F. I. Secondary amine analogues of 3β-(4'-substituted phenyl)tropane-2β-carboxylic acid esters and *N*-norcocaine exhibit enhanced affinity for serotonin and norepinephrine transporters. *J. Med. Chem.* **37** (1994) 1220–1223.

13. Boja, J. W., McNeill, R. M., Lewin, A. H., Abraham, P., Carroll, F. I., and Kuhar, M. J. Selective dopamine transporter inhibition by cocaine analogs. *NeuroReport* **3** (1992) 984–986.

14. Bonnet, J.-J., Protais, P., Chagraoui, A., and Costentin, J. High-affinity [³H]GBR 12783 binding to a specific site associated with the neuronal dopamine uptake complex in the central nervous system. *Eur. J. Pharmacol.* **126** (1986) 211–222.

15. Carroll, F. I., Abraham, P., Lewin, A. H., Parham, K. A., Boja, J. W., and Kuhar, M. J. Isopropyl and phenyl esters of 3β-(4-substituted phenyl)tropan-2β-carboxylic acids. Potent and selective compounds for the dopamine transporter. *J. Med. Chem.* **35** (1992) 2497–2500.

16. Carroll, F. I. and Lewin, A. H. (1996) (unpublished).

17. Carroll, F. I., Gao, Y., Abraham, P., Lewin, A. H., Lew, R., Patel, A., Boja, J. W., and Kuhar, M. J. Probes for the cocaine receptor. Potentially irreversible ligands for the dopamine transporter. *J. Med. Chem.* **35** (1992) 1813–1817.

18. Carroll, F. I., Gao, Y., Rahman, M. A., Abraham, P., Lewin, A. H., Boja, J. W., and Kuhar, M. J. Synthesis, ligand binding, QSAR, and CoMFA study of 3β-(p,substituted phenyl)tropan-2β-carboxylic acid methyl esters. *J. Med. Chem.* **34** (1991) 2719–2927.

19. Carroll, F. I., Gray, J. L., Abraham, P., Kuzemko, M. A., Lewin, A. H., Boja, J. W., and Kuhar, M. J. 3-Aryl-2-(3'-substituted-1',2',4'-oxadiazol-5'-yl)tropane analogues of cocaine: affinities at the cocaine binding site at the dopamine, serotonin, and norepinephrine transporters. *J. Med. Chem.* **36** (1993) 2886–2890.

20. Carroll, F. I., Kotian, P., Dehghani, A., Gray, J. L., Kuzemko, M. A., Parham, K. A., Abraham, P., Lewin, A. H., Boja, J. W., and Kuhar, M. J. Cocaine and 3β-(4'-substituted phenyl)tropane-2β-carboxylic acid ester and amide analogues. New high-affinity and selective compounds for the dopamine transporter. *J. Med. Chem.* **38** (1995) 379–388.

21. Carroll, F. I., Kotian, P., Gray, J. L., Abraham, P., Kuzemko, M. A., Lewin, A. H., Boja, J. W., and Kuhar, M. J. 3β-(4'-Chlorophenyl)tropan-2β-carboxamides and cocaine amide analogues: new high affinity and selective compounds for the dopamine transporter. *Med. Chem. Res.* **3** (1993) 468–472.

22. Carroll, F. I., Kuzemko, M. A., Gao, Y., Abraham, P., Lewin, A. H., Boja, J. W., and Kuhar, M. J. Synthesis and ligand binding of 3β-(3-substituted phenyl)- and 3β-(3,4-disubstituted phenyl)tropane-2β-carboxylic acid methyl esters. *Med. Chem. Res.* **1** (1992) 382–387.

23. Carroll, F. I., Lewin, A. H., Abraham, P., Parham, K., Boja, J. W., and Kuhar, M. J. Synthesis and ligand binding of cocaine isomers at the cocaine receptor. *J. Med. Chem.* **34** (1991) 883–886.

24. Carroll, F. I., Lewin, A. H., Boja, J. W., and Kuhar, M. J. Cocaine receptor: Biochemical characterization and structure-activity relationships for the dopamine transporter. *J. Med. Chem.* **35** (1992) 969–981.

25. Carroll, F. I., Mascarella, S. W., Kuzemko, M. A., Gao, Y., Abraham, P., Lewin, A. H., Boja, J. W, and Kuhar, M. J. Synthesis, ligand binding, and QSAR (CoMFA and classical) study of 3β-(3′-substituted phenyl)-, 3β-(4′-substituted phenyl)-, and 3β-(3′,4′-disubstituted phenyl)tropane-2β-carboxylic acid methyl esters. *J. Med. Chem.* **37** (1994) 2865–2873.

26. Chait, L. D., Uhlenhuth, E. H., and Johansen, C. E. Reinforcing and subjective effects of several anorectics in normal human volunteers. *J. Pharmacol. Exp. Ther.* **242** (1987) 777–783.

27. Clarke, R. L., Daum, S. J., Gambino, A. J., Aceto, M. D., Pearl, J., Levitt, M., Cumiskey, W. R., and Bogado, E. F. Compounds affecting the central nervous system. 4. 3β-Phenyltropane-2-carboxylic esters and analogs. *J. Med. Chem.* **16** (1973) 1260–1267.

28. Coderc, E., Cerruti, P., Vignon, J., Rouayrenc, J. F., and Kamenka, J.-M. PCP receptor and dopamine uptake sites are discriminated by chiral TCP and BTCP derivatives of opposite configuration. *Eur. J. Med. Chem.* **30** (1995) 463–470.

29. Coderc, E., Martin-Fardon, R., Vignon, J., and Kamenka, J.-M. New compounds resulting from structural and biochemical similarities between GBR 12783 and BTCP, two potent inhibitors of dopamine uptake. *Eur. J. Med. Chem—Chim. Thera.* **28** (1993) 893–898.

30. Colpaert, F. C., Niemegeers, C. J. E., and Janssen, P. A. J. Discriminative stimulus properties of cocaine. Neuropharmacological characteristics as derived from stimulus generalization experiments. *Pharmacol. Biochem. Behav.* **10** (1978) 535–546.

31. Davies, H. M. L., Saikali, E., Huby, N. J. S., Gilliat, V. J., Matasi, J. J., Sexton, T., and Childers, S. R. Synthesis of 2β-Acyl-3β-aryl-8-azabicyclo[3.2.1]octanes and their binding affinities at dopamine and serotonin transport sites in rat striatum and frontal cortex. *J. Med. Chem.* **37** (1994) 1262–1268.

32. Davies, H. M. L., Saikali, E., Sexton, T., and Childers, S. R. Novel 2-substituted cocaine analogs: binding properties at dopamine transport sites in rat striatum. *Eur. J. Pharmacol.—Mol. Pharmacol. Sec.* **244** (1993) 93–97.

33. Deutsch, H. M., Schweri, M., M., Culbertson, C. T., and Zalkow, L. H. Synthesis and pharmacology of irreversible affinity labels as potential cocaine antagonists: aryl 1,4-dialkylpiperazines related to GBR-12783. *Eur. J. Pharmacol.* **220** (1992) 173–180.

34. Deutsch, H. M. and Schweri, M. M. Can stimulant binding and dopamine transport be differentiated? Studies with GBR 12783 derivatives. *Life Sci.* **55** (1994) PL 115–120.

35. Deutsch, H. M., Shi, Q., Kowalik, E., and Schweri, M. M. Synthesis and pharmacology of potential cocaine antagonists. 2. Structure-activity relationship studies of aromatic ring substituted methylphenidate analogs. *J. Med. Chem.* **39** (1996) 1201–1209.

36. Elmaleh, D. R., Madras, B. K., Shoup, T. M., Byon, C., Hanson, R. N., Liang, A. Y., Meltzer, P. C., and Fischman, A. J. Radiosynthesis and evaluation of E and Z-[^{125}I]-2β-carbomethoxy-3β-(4-fluorophenyl)-N-(iodoprop-1-en-3-yl)nortropane (Altropane): a selective SPECT agent for imaging DA reuptake sites. *J. Nucl. Chem.* in press.

37. Fahey, M. A., Canfield, D. A., Spealman, R. D., and Madras, B. K. Comparison of [^{3}H]GBR 12935 and [^{3}H]cocaine binding sites in monkey brain. *Soc. Neurosci. Abstracts* **515** (1989) 252.

38. Gatley, S. J., Yu, D.-W., Fowler, J. S., MacGregor, R. R., Schlyer, D. J., Dewey, S. L., Wolf, A. P., Martin, T., Shea, C. E., and Volkow, N. D. Studies with differentially labeled [^{11}C]cocaine, [^{11}C]norcocaine, [^{11}C]benzoylecgonine, and [^{11}C]- and 4'-[^{18}F]fluorococaine to probe the extent to which [^{11}C]cocaine metabolites contribute to PET images of the baboon brain. *J. Neurochem.* **62** (1994) 1154–1162.

39. Giros, B., el Mestikawy, S., Bertrand, L., and Caron, M. G. Cloning and functional characterization of a cocaine-sensitive dopamine transporter. *FEBS Lett.* **295** (1991) 149–154.

40. Giros, B., Wang, Y.-M., Suter, S., McLeskey, S. B., Pifl, C., and Caron, M. G. Delineation of discrete domains for substrate, cocaine, and tricyclic antidepressant interactions using chimeric dopamine-norepinephrine transporters. *J. Biol. Chem.* **269** (1994) 15,985–15,988.

41. He, X.-S., Raymon, L. P., Mattson, M. V., Eldefrawi, M. E., and de Costa, B. R. Synthesis and biological evaluation of 1-[1-(2-benzo[b]-thienyl)cyclohexyl]piperidine homologues at dopamine-uptake and phencyclidine-and σ-binding sites. *J. Med. Chem.* **36** (1993) 1188–1193.

42. He, X.-S., Raymon, L. P., Mattson, M. V., Eldefrawi, M. E., and de Costa, B. R. Further studies of the structure-activity relationships of 1-[1-(2-benzo[*b*]thienyl)cyclohexyl]piperidine. Synthesis and evaluation of 1-(2-benzo[*b*]thienyl)-*N,N*-dialkylcyclohexylamines at dopamine uptake and phencyclidine binding sites. *J. Med. Chem.* **36** (1993) 4075–4081.

43. Horn, A. S. In Roberts, P. J., Woodruff, G. N., and Iversen, L. L. (eds.), *Dopamine. Advances in Biochemical Psychopharmacology*, vol. 19, Raven, New York, 1978, pp. 25–34.

44. Horn, A. S. Dopamine uptake: a review of progress in the last decade. Prog. Neurobiol. **34** (1990) 387–400.

45. Houlihan, W. J., Boja, J. W., Kuhar, M. J., Kopajtic, T. A., and Parrino, V. A. Mazindol analogs as potential inhibitors of the cocaine binding site. Structure activity relationships. *Abstracts of College on Problems of Drug Dependence*, Scottsdale, AZ, June 10–15, 1995, pp. 66.

46. Houlihan, W. J., Boja, J. W., Parrino, V. A., Kuhar, M. J., and Kopajtic, T. A. Halogenated mazindol analogs as potential inhibitors of the cocaine binding site at the dopamine transporter. *208th American Chemical Society National Meeting, Abstr. No. 173*, Washington, DC, August 21–25, 1994.

47. Houlihan, W. J., Heikkila, R. E., and Babington, R. G. Pharmacological studies with several analogs of mazindol: correlation between effects on dopamine uptake and various in vivo responses. *Eur. J. Pharmacol.* **71** (1981) 277–286.

48. Javitch, J. A., Blaustein, R. O., and Snyder, S. H. [^{3}H] Mazindol binding associated with neuronal dopamine and norepinephrine uptake sites. *Mol. Pharmacol.* **26** (1984) 35–44.

49. Johnson, K. M., Bergmann, J. S., and Kozikowski, A. P. Cocaine and dopamine differentially protect [^{3}H]mazindol binding sites from alkylation by N-ethylmaleimide. *Eur. J. Pharmacol.* **227** (1992) 411–415.

50. Kelkar, S. V., Izenwasser, S., Katz, J. L., Klein, C. L., Zhu, N., and Trodell, M. L. Synthesis, cocaine receptor affinity, and dopamine uptake inhibition of several new 2β-substituted 3β-phenyltropanes. *J. Med. Chem.* **37** (1994) 3875–3877.

51. Kilty, J. E., Lorang, D., and Amara, S. G. Cloning and expression of a cocaine-sensitive rat dopamine transporter. *Science* **254** (1991) 528,529.

52. Kitayama, S., Shimada, S., Xu, H., Markham, L., Donovan, D. M., and Uhl, G. R. Dopamine transporter site-directed mutations differentially alter substrate transport and cocaine binding. *Proc. Natl. Acad. Sci. USA* **89** (1992) 7782–7785.

53. Kline, R. H., Jr., Wright, J., Fox, K. M., and Eldefrawi, M. E. Synthesis of 3-arylecgonine analogues as inhibitors of cocaine binding and dopamine uptake. *J. Med. Chem.* **33** (1990) 2024–2027.

54. Kline, R. H., Jr., Wright, J., Eshleman, A. J., Fox, K. M., and Eldefrawi, M. E. Synthesis of 3-carbamoylecgonine methyl ester analogues as inhibitors of cocaine binding and dopamine uptake. *J. Med. Chem.* **34** (1991) 702–705.

55. Koek, W., Colpaert, F. C., Woods, J. H., and Kamenka, J.-M. The phencyclidine (PCP) analog N-[1-(2-benzo(*B*)thiophenyl)cyclohexyl]-piperidine shares cocaine-like but not other characteristic behavioral effects with PCP, ketamine and MK-801. *J. Pharmacol. Exp. Ther.* **250** (1989) 1019–1027.

56. Kotian, P., Abraham, P., Lewin, A. H., Mascarella, S. W., Boja, J. W., Kuhar, M. J., and Carroll, F. I. Synthesis and ligand binding study of 3β-(4′-substituted phenyl)-2β-(heterocyclic)tropanes. *J. Med. Chem.* **38** (1995) 3451–3453.

57. Kozikowski, A. P., Roberti, M., Xiang, L., Bergmann, J. S., Callahan, P. M., Cunningham, K. A., and Johnson, K. M. Structure–activity relationship studies of cocaine: replacement of the C-2 ester group by vinyl argues against H-bonding and provides an esterase-resistant, high-affinity cocaine analogue. *J. Med. Chem.* **35** (1992) 4764–4766.

58. Kozikowski, A. P., Saiah, M. K. E., Bergmann, J. S., and Johnson, K. M. Structure–activity relationship studies of N-sulfonyl analogs of cocaine: role of ionic interaction in cocaine binding. *J. Med. Chem.* **37** (1994) 3440–3442.

59. Kozikowski, A. P., Saiah, M. K. E., Johnson, K. M., and Bergmann, J. S. Chemistry and biology of the 2β-alkyl-3β-phenyl analogues of cocaine: subnanomolar affinity ligands that suggest a new pharmacophore model at the C-2 position. *J. Med. Chem.* **38** (1995) 3086–3093.

60. Kozikowski, A. P., Xiang, L., Tanaka, J., Bergmann, J. S., and Johnson, K. M. Use of nitrile oxide cycloaddition *(NOC)* chemistry in the synthesis of cocaine analogues: mazindol binding and dopamine uptake studies. *Med. Chem. Res.* **1** (1991) 312–321.

61. Kuhar, M. J. Neurotransmitter uptake: a tool in identifying neurotransmitter-specific pathways. *Life Sci.* **13** (1973) 1623–1634.

62. Kuhar, M. J., Ritz, M. C., and Boja, J. W. The dopamine hypothesis of the reinforcing properties of cocaine. *Trends Neurosci.* **14** (1991) 299–302.

63. Lewin, A. H., Gao, Y., Abraham, P., Boja, J. W., Kuhar, M. J., and Carroll, F. I. 2β-Substituted analogues of cocaine. Synthesis and inhibition of binding to the cocaine receptor. *J. Med. Chem.* **35** (1992) 135–140.

64. Madras, B. K., Kamien, J. B., Fahey, M. A., Canfield, D. R., Milius, R. A., Saha, J. K., Neumeyer, J. L., and Spealman, R. D. N-Modified fluorophenyltropane analogs of cocaine with high affinity for cocaine receptors. *Pharmacol. Biochem. Behav.* **35** (1990) 949–953.

65. Madras, B. K., Reith, M. E. A., Meltzer, P. C., and Dutta, A. K. O-526, a piperidine analog of GBR 12909, retains high affinity for the dopamine transporter in

monkey caudate-putamen. *Eur. J. Pharmacol.-Mol. Pharmacol. Sec.* **267** (1993) 167–173.

66. Madras, B. K., Spealman, R. D., Fahey, M. A., Neumeyer, J. L., Saha, J. K., and Milius, R. A. Cocaine receptors labeled by [³H]2β-carbomethoxy-3β-(4-fluorophenyl)tropane. *Mol. Pharmacol.* **36** (1989) 518–524.

67. Matecka, D., Rice, K. C., Rothman, R. B., de Costa, B. R., Glowa, J. R., Wojnicki, F. H., Becketts, K. M., and Partilla, J. S. Synthesis and absolute configuration of chiral piperazines related to GBR 12909 as dopamine uptake inhibitors. *Med. Chem. Res.* **5** (1994) 43–53.

68. McElvain, J. S. and Schenk, J. O. A multisubstrate mechanism of striatal dopamine uptake and its inhibition by cocaine. *Biochem. Pharmacol.* **43** (1992) 2189–2199.

69. Meltzer, P. C., Liang, A. Y., Brownell, A.-L., Elmaleh, D. R., and Madras, B. K. Substituted 3-phenyltropane analogs of cocaine: synthesis, inhibition of binding at cocaine recognition sites, and positron emission tomography imaging. *J. Med. Chem.* **36** (1993) 855–862.

70. Meltzer, P. C., Liang, A. Y., and Madras, B. K. 2-Carbomethoxy-3-(diarylmethoxy)-1αH,5αH-tropane analogs: synthesis and inhibition of binding at the dopamine transporter and comparison with piperazines of the GBR series. *J. Med. Chem.* **39** (1996) 371–379.

71. Meltzer, P. C., Liang, A. Y., and Madras, B. K. The discovery of an unusually selective and novel cocaine analog: difluoropine. Synthesis and inhibition of binding at cocaine recognition sites. *J. Med. Chem.* **37** (1994) 2001–2010.

72. Metwally, S. A. M., Gatley, S. J., Wolf, A. P., and Yu, D.-W. Synthesis and binding to striatal membranes of no carrier added I-123 labeled 4'-iodococaine. *J. Label. Compd. Radiopharm.* **XXXI** (1992) 219–225.

73. Milius, R. A., Saha, J. K., Madras, B. K., and Neumeyer, J. L. Synthesis and receptor binding of N-substituted tropane derivatives. High-affinity ligands for the cocaine receptor. *J. Med. Chem.* **34** (1991) 1728–1731.

74. Muller, L., Halldin, C., Farde, L., Karlsson, P., Hall, H., Swahn, C. G., Neumeyer, J., Gao, Y., and Milius, R. [11C]β-CIT, a cocaine analogue. Preparation, autoradiography and preliminary PET investigations. *Nucl. Med. Biol.* **20** (1993) 249–255.

75. Neumeyer, J. L., Wang, S., Gao, Y., Milius, R. A., Kula, N. S., Campbell, A., Baldessarini, R. J., Zea-Ponce, Y., Baldwin, R. M., and Innis, R. B. N-ω-Fluoroalkyl analogs of (1R)-2β-carbomethoxy-3β-(4-iodophenyl)-tropane (β-CIT): radiotracers for positron emission tomography and single photon emission computed tomography imaging of dopamine transporters. *J. Med. Chem.* **37** (1994) 1558–1561.

76. Newman, A. H., Allen, A. C., Izenwasser, S., and Katz, J. L. Novel 3α-(diphenylmethoxy)tropane analogs: potent dopamine uptake inhibitors without cocaine-like behavioral profiles. *J. Med. Chem.* **37** (1994) 2258–2261.

77. Newman, A. H., Kline, R. H., Allen, A. C., Izenwasser, S., George, C., and Katz, J. L. Novel 4'- and 4',4"-substituted-3α-(diphenylmethoxy)tropane analogs are potent and selective dopamine uptake inhibitors. *J. Med. Chem.* **38** (1995) 3933–3940.

78. Reith, M. E. A., de Costa, B., Rice, K. C., and Jacobson, A. E. Evidence for mutually exclusive binding of cocaine, BTCP, GBR 12935, and dopamine to the

dopamine transporter. *Eur. J. Pharmacol.—Mol. Pharmacol. Sec.* **227** (1992) 417–425.

79. Reith, M. E. A., Meisler, B. E., Sershen, H., and Lajtha, A. Structural requirements for cocaine congeners to interact with dopamine and serotonin uptake sites in mouse brain and to induce stereotyped behavior. *Biochem. Pharmacol.* **35** (1986) 1123–1129.

80. Ritz, M. C., Cone, E. J., and Kuhar, M. J. Cocaine inhibition of ligand binding at dopamine, norepinephrine and serotonin transporters: a structure–activity study. *Life Sci.* **46** (1990) 635–645.

81. Ritz, M. C., Lamb, R. J., Goldberg, S. R., and Kuhar, M. J. Cocaine receptors on dopamine transporters are related to self-administration of cocaine. *Science* **237** (1987) 1219–1223.

82. Rothman, R. B., Becketts, K. M., Radesca, L. R., de Costa, B. R., Rice, K. C., Carroll, F. I., and Dersch, C. M. Studies of the biogenic amine transporters. II. A brief study on the use of [^{3}H]DA-uptake-inhibition to transporter-binding-inhibition ratios for the in vitro evaluation of putative cocaine antagonists. *Life Sci.* **53** (1993) PL267–PL272.

83. Rothman, R. B., Lewis, B., Dersch, C., Xu, H., Radesca, L., de Costa, B. R., Rice, K. C., Kilburn, R. B., Akunne, H. C., and Pert, A. Identification of a GBR 12935 homolog LR1111 which is over 4,000-fold selective for the dopamine transporter, relative to serotonin and norepinephrine transporters. *Synapse* **14** (1993) 34–39.

84. Schweri, M. M., Skolnick, P., Rafferty, M. F., Rice, K. C., Janowsky, A. J., and Paul, S. M. [^{3}H]Threo-(±)-methylphenidate binding to 3,4-dihydroxyphenylethylamine uptake sites in corpus striatum correlation with the stimulant properties of ritalinic acid esters. *J. Neurochem.* **45** (1985) 1062–1070.

85. Shimada, S., Kitayama, S., Lin, C.-L., Patel, A., Nanthakumar, E., Gregor, P., Kuhar, M., and Uhl, G. Cloning and expression of a cocaine-sensitive dopamine transporter complementary DNA. *Science* **254** (1991) 576–578.

86. Simoni, D., Stoelwinder, J., Kozikowski, A. P., Johnson, K. M., Bergmann, J. S., and Ball, R. G. Methoxylation of cocaine reduces binding affinity and produces compounds of differential binding and dopamine uptake inhibitory activity: discovery of a weak cocaine "antagonist". *J. Med. Chem.* **36** (1993) 3975–3977.

87. Stoelwinder, J., Roberti, M., Kozikowski, A. P., Johnson, K. M., and Bergmann, J. S. Differential binding and dopamine uptake activity of cocaine analogues modified at nitrogen. *Bioorg. Med. Chem. Lett.* **4** (1994) 303–308.

88. Usdin, T. B., Mezey, E., Chen, C., Brownstein, M. J., and Hoffman, B. J. Cloning of the cocaine-sensitive bovine dopamine transporter. *Proc. Natl. Acad Sci.* **88** (1991) 11,168–11,171.

89. Van der Zee, P., and Hespe, W. Interactions between substituted 1-[2-(diphenylmethoxy)ethyl]piperazines and dopamine receptors. *Neuropharmacology* **24** (1985) 1171–1174.

90. Van der Zee, P., Koger, H. S., Gootjes, J., and Hespe, W. Aryl 1,4-dialk(en)ylpiperazines as selective and very potent inhibitors of dopamine uptake. *Eur. J. Med. Chem.* **15** (1980) 363–370.

91. Vandenbergh, D. J., Persico, A. M., Hawkins, A. L., Griffin, C. A., Li, X., Jabs, E. W., and Uhl, G. R. Human dopamine transporter gene (DAT1) maps to chromosome 5p15.3 and displays a VNTR. *Geomomics* **14** (1992) 1104–1106.

92. Vignon, J., Cerruti, C., Chaudieu, I., Pinet, V., Chicheportiche, M., Kamenka, J.-M., and Chicheportiche, R. Interaction of molecules in the phencyclidine series with the dopamine uptake system. Correlation with their binding properties to the phencyclidine receptor. Binding properties of ^{3}H-BTCP, a new PCP analog, to the dopamine uptake complex. In Domino, E. F., and Kamenka, J.-M. (eds.), *Sigma and Phencyclidine-Like Compounds as Molecular Probes in Biology*, NPP Books, Ann Arbor, MI, 1988, pp. 199–208.

93. Vignon, J. and Lazdunski, M. Structure–function relationships in the inhibition of synaptosomal dopamine uptake by phencyclidine and analogues: Potential correlation with binding sites identified with [^{3}H]phencyclidine. *Biochem. Pharmacol.* **33** (1984) 700–702.

94. Vignon, J., Pinet, V., Cerruti, C., Kamenka, J.-M., and Chicheportiche, R. [^{3}H]N-[1-(2-Benzo(b)thiophenyl)cyclohexyl]piperidine ([^{3}H]BTCP): a new phencyclidine analog selective for the dopamine uptake complex. *Eur. J. Pharmacol.* **148** (1988) 427–436.

95. Xu, C., Coffey, L. L., and Reith, M. E. A. Translocation of dopamine and binding of 2β-carbomethoxy-3β-(4-fluorophenyl)tropane (WIN 35,428) measured under identical conditions in rat striatal synaptosomal preparations. Inhibition by various blockers. *Biochem. Pharmacol.* **49** (1995) 339–350.

96. Yu, D. W., Gatley, S. J., Wolf, A. P., MacGregor, R. R., Dewey, S. L., Fowler, J. S., and Schlyer, D. J. Synthesis of carbon-11 labeled iodinated cocaine derivatives and their distribution in baboon brain measured using positron emission tomography. *J. Med. Chem.* **35** (1992) 2178–2183.

CHAPTER 10

Imaging Transporters for Dopamine and Other Neurotransmitters in Brain

Michael J. Kuhar, F. Ivy Carroll, Anita H. Lewin, John W. Boja, Ursula Scheffel, and Dean F. Wong

Introduction

There has been substantial progress in the imaging of dopamine transporters. The earliest positron emission tomography (PET) experiments used carbon-11 labeled nominfensine (*1,44*); whereas recent investigations by both PET and single photon emission computed tomography (SPECT) utilize a variety of ligands with a variety of properties and address many biological questions (*see below*). The earliest ligands utilized, [^{11}C]nomifensine and [^{11}C]cocaine, were somewhat limited because of low signal-to-noise ratios. Nevertheless, [^{11}C]cocaine as a ligand continues to be popular, because it is the same authentic substance that is abused around the world. The best, current 3-substituted phenyltropane ligands, such as RTI-55, have vastly improved signal-to-noise ratios. These successes are in no small part because of the development of the chemistry of cocaine analogs and other analogs of inhibitors for transporters (Fig. 1) (*4,8*). Despite this progress, several important things remain to be achieved. We need to develop methods to carry out rigorous calculations of B_{max}, instead of relying on more inexact but easier measures of relative occupancy and binding potential. We also need useful ligands for all transporters in brain.

Why image transporters? There are several answers to this question. Transporters are involved in the reuptake of released neurotransmitter and are therefore physiologically significant because they terminate the process of synaptic transmission. Thus, transporters are key proteins in the functioning brain. Transporters can also be considered

Neurotransmitter Transporters: Structure, Function, and Regulation
Ed.: M. E. A. Reith Humana Press Inc., Totowa, NJ

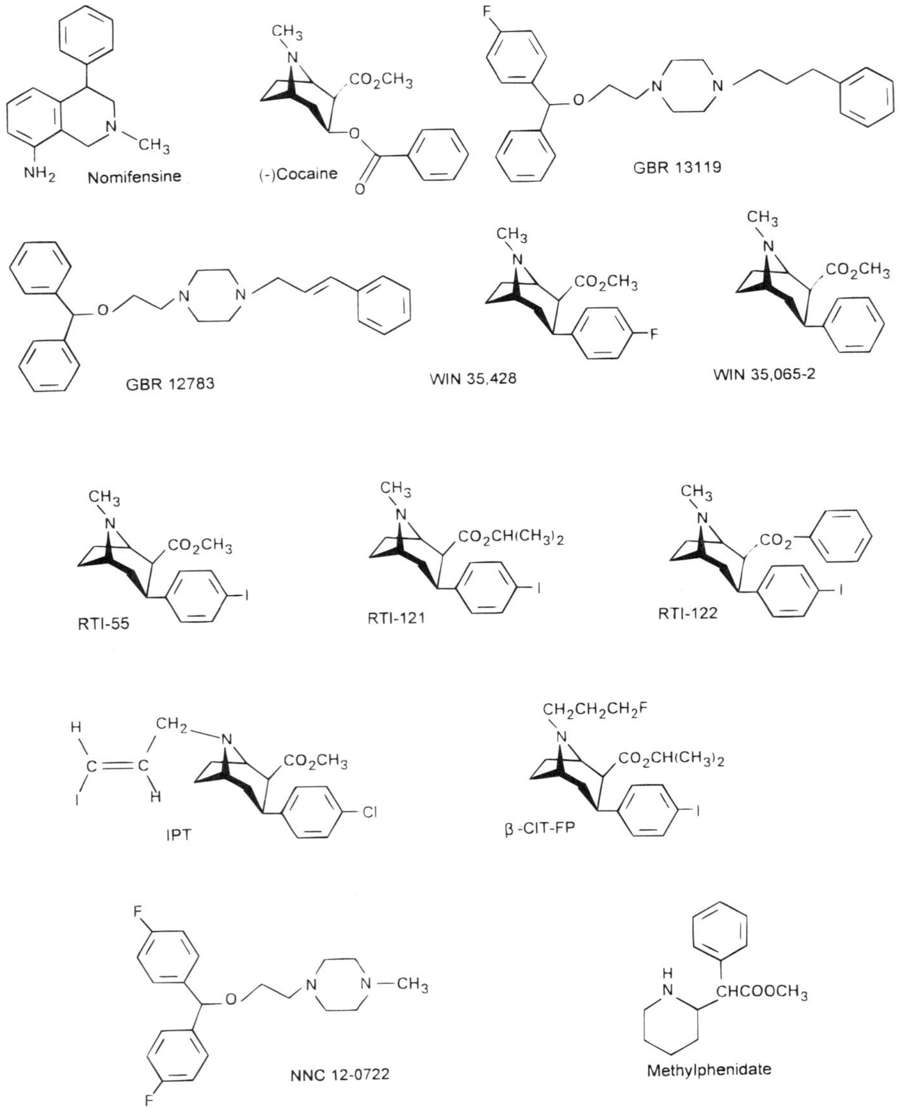

Fig. 1. Structures of commonly used ligands for the dopamine transporter. Courtesy of J. W. Boja.

markers for neurons (*38*). Some transporters, such as the dopamine transporter, are selectively localized to neurons utilizing that neurotransmitter. Given this characteristic of being markers for specific neurons, they are useful for studying either regulatory or drug-induced changes in transporter levels, or loss of neurons in brain caused by neurodegenerative diseases, such as Parkinson's. In addition, transporters are important drug targets. The involvement of dopamine transporters in psychostimulant action is well established and the role of serotonin and norepinephrine transporters in antidepressant drug action is also well known. Neurotoxins, such as MPTP, are also thought to require the presence of a transporter for their ultimate neurotoxic action.

At the outset, let us consider some limitations of imaging transporters. Both PET and SPECT imaging have limitations in resolution. This creates difficulties when areas of interest are relatively small in size, like the nucleus accumbens, when compared to the caudate nucleus and putamen; the nucleus accumbens is thought to be an especially critical area for the action of psychostimulant drugs, but it is not easy to image. Low levels of resolution also create problems with interpretation. Cellular structures cannot be resolved and therefore correlative microscopic studies are needed to complement PET and SPECT images. Recent immunohistochemical successes with antibodies against the transporter (*11,21,45,54,55*) will enhance our ability to interpret these images. Also, there are several potential confounding factors in imaging measurements. One of these is the possible inhibition of ligand binding by endogenous substances. If levels of dopamine in the synaptic area are high, for example, and if the ligand used has a relatively low affinity, then dopamine could effectively compete for binding with the radioligand. This would result in an erroneously small number in the calculation of transporters. This issue has been the subject of recent experiments and information will begin to accumulate on this topic. Specificity of the binding ligand can be another problem, although binding ligands can be characterized quite thoroughly and there are many selective ligands that are available for use. Nevertheless, despite these problems and shortcomings, transporter imaging has progressed quite well. This chapter summarizes progress in the field and focuses on the dopamine transporter, where, perhaps, progress has been the greatest.

In many instances, we include preimaging data obtained, for example, in mice, because such data are routinely used to assess the usefulness of compounds as ligands in PET and SPECT imaging. These studies usually involve measuring regional ligand binding by dissection and scintillation counting, although autoradiography can also be used. For example, as the striatum contains high densities of dopamine transporters and the cerebellum, by comparison, contains none, the ratio of striatal radioactivity to cerebellar radioactivity is a measure of total to nonspecific binding. This ratio is universally used to evaluate almost all ligands for dopamine transporters; higher ratios indicate higher signal-to-noise ratios and are therefore desirable.

Another important factor is the kinetics of binding. In the calculations of numbers of sites, it is useful to have a ligand that reaches equilibrium relatively soon with respect to the half-life of the isotope used. Carbon-11 has a half-life of 22 min and therefore a ligand that needs 10 h to reach equilibrium will preclude equilibrium measurements. The great variety of structures and properties of potential ligands for the dopamine transporter enhances the opportunity to develop ligands with desirable properties.

Early Imaging Studies and Ligand Development

Perhaps the first ligand used for PET imaging of dopamine transporters was [^{11}C]nomifensine (1,44,67). The extraordinarily high concentration of dopamine transporters in the basal ganglia permitted the successful imaging of dopamine transporters with this compound, which has a very low ratio of specific to nonspecific binding (39). [^{11}C]cocaine was also used successfully, but it has an equally low ratio (20). In addition, it was realized that GBR compounds had utility and were among the first ligands noted for improved specific to nonspecific binding ratios (10,32). Because of the high concentration of dopamine transporters in dopaminergic nerve terminals, and because of the early success using receptor binding as a neuropathological tool (71), the possibilities of using PET imaging of dopamine transporters as a means of detecting degeneration of dopaminergic neurons, such as in Parkinson's disease, was addressed in these very early studies. For example, Aquilonius et al. (1) showed that dopamine transporter binding was reduced on the side of a lesion in a hemi-Parkinsonian patient. These early successes fueled the movement for better imaging ligands and procedures.

Discovery of Phenyltropane Ligands and Other Compounds

An important advance in imaging dopamine transporters occurred when investigators utilized 3(substituted phenyl)tropane analogs of

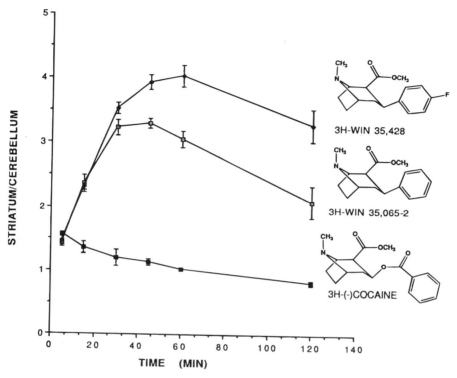

Fig. 2. Time-course of striatal to cerebellar ratios for [³H]WIN 35,428; [³H]WIN 35,065-2; and [³H] (–)cocaine in mice. Data are expressed as means ± SEM, n = 4. The structures of the compounds utilized are shown next to their respective data. It is clear that the phenyltropane compounds, WIN 35,428 and WIN 35,065-2, provide higher levels of specific binding compared to cocaine. (Reproduced with permission from ref. *59*.)

cocaine as binding ligands. Radiolabeled WIN 35,428, developed by Madras et al. (*46*) and WIN 35,065-2, developed by Ritz et al. (*56,57*), were utilized in in vivo labeling studies along with radiolabeled cocaine. These studies in mice clearly showed that the specific to nonspecific binding ratios for the phenyltropane compounds were substantially improved over that of cocaine (Fig. 2). Both compounds showed striatal to cerebellar ratios of approx 4, whereas the maximal striatal to cerebellar ratio obtained for cocaine was about 1.5.

Several compounds from the GBR class also showed enhanced in vivo binding. [¹⁸F]GBR 13119 exhibited striatal to cerebellar ratios of about 3 (*12,34,36,37*). Another compound from this group, radiolabeled

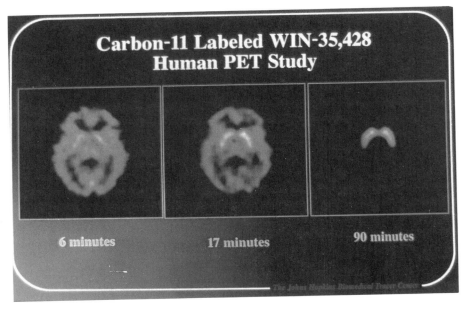

Fig. 3. Images of [¹¹C]WIN 35,428 binding to dopamine transporters in human brain by PET. (Reproduced with permission from ref. *72*.)

GBR 12783, was shown to have a comparable ratio of approximately 2 (*68*), compared to less than 2 for [¹¹C]cocaine and [¹¹C]nomifensine.

Following its successful utilization in preimaging studies in mice, WIN 35,428 has been useful in imaging dopamine transporters in animals and humans by PET. For example, the in vivo binding of [¹¹C]WIN 35,428 in animals and humans (Fig. 3) has been characterized (*25,31,72*), and the feasibility of using dopamine transporter imaging for diagnosing Parkinson's disease (*22,73*) has been shown. Other investigators also have pursued this idea as well (*see next section*).

Iodinated Ligands and SPECT Imaging

RTI-55 (also known as β-CIT) is an important compound, because of its very high striatal to cerebellar ratios obtained in preimaging studies (*4,13*). However, one difficulty with RTI-55 is that it is not a highly selective compound for the dopamine transporter and has a lesser, but still significant, affinity for serotonin transporters. This has not been a significant hindrance, because there are few serotonin transporters in basal ganglia compared to dopamine transporters, and dopamine transporter imaging in the basal ganglia is not a problem. Second, the affinity of RTI-55 for serotonin transporters has been exploited in a positive sense, because the same compound can also be used to image serotonin transporters, albeit in different brain regions, where there are few or no dopamine transporters, such as the cerebral cortex (*3,62*). [^{123}I]RTI-55 was the first SPECT ligand for imaging dopamine reuptake sites in vivo (*9,27,62*). Again, the utility for measuring dopamine transporters as a means of assessing neurodegenerative disease was shown in an animal model of Parkinson's disease (*25,62,73*). The unilateral destruction of dopaminergic projections by MPTP was clearly revealed in a baboon utilizing [^{123}I]RTI-55 (Fig. 4). Several groups are using RTI-55 to study Parkinson's disease in humans (*5,19,28,40,41*). Work by Innis et al. (*28*) shows that 2 d after injection of [^{123}I]RTI-55 into controls and Parkinson patients, there are much lower ratios in the Parkinson brain, and that such imaging can be used as a diagnostic measure (Fig. 5).

Analogs of RTI-55, the compounds RTI-121 and RTI-122, which are more specific for dopamine transporters, have also been explored as potential imaging agents (*60*). However, these compounds did not produce striatal to cerebellar ratios that were as great as those obtained with RTI-55, possibly because the lipid solubility of these substances was greater and therefore produced higher nonspecific binding levels. Nevertheless, in situations where lower ratios are acceptable, these compounds offer greater binding selectivity for the dopamine transporter and faster binding kinetics.

Yet other compounds in the 3(substituted phenyl)tropane series have proven interesting. These include fluoro-alkyl N-nor-substituted analogs of RTI-55 and RTI-31 (*2,23,42,52,58*). Some 3(disubstituted phenyl)tropanes are also potent, effective and, therefore, useful (*8,48,49*). NNC12-0722, a benzhydryl substituted piperazine, has also proven useful in imaging (*51*), and radiolabeled methylphenidate, a compound that has a lower affinity for transporters and, therefore, may be useful in studying neurotransmitter and drug competition in vivo, has been utilized as an imaging agent (*18*). Also, compounds with iodinated side chains replacing the methyl group on the nitrogen atom have been proposed as brain-imaging agents (*23*). Other tropane analogs have been synthesized (*53*) but their utility as imaging agents has not yet been demonstrated.

Other Monoamine Transporters

Several compounds have been utilized to image serotonin transporters in brain. The utilization of RTI-55, a compound with a higher

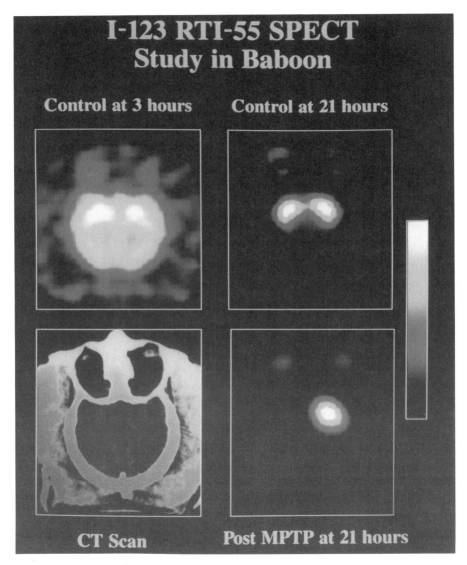

Fig. 4. Top left: [^{123}I]RTI-55 SPECT image at 3 h postinjection, showing symmetrical tracer distribution in striata, eyes, and cortical structures of control baboon. Top right: [^{123}I]RTI-55 SPECT image at 21 h postinjection, showing symmetrical binding in left and right striata and eyes of the control baboon but with lower background because of longer time. Bottom left: CAT scan showing anatomical structures of the imaging plane that was used. Bottom right: [^{123}I]RTI-55 SPECT image at 21 h postinjection, showing lack of tracer accumulation in the right striatum (the side of MPTP pretreatment) and symmetrical accumulation in the eyes. (Reproduced with permission from ref. 62.)

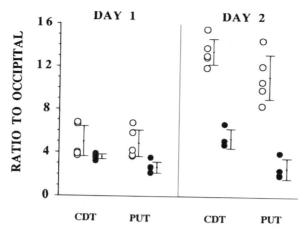

Fig. 5. Ratio of activity in caudate (CDT) and putamen (PUT) to that in occipital lobe in healthy subjects (o) and patients (●) on d 1 (255 ± 2 min) and d 2 (1330 ± 56 min). Error bars indicate means ± 2 SEMs, which approximates a 95% confidence interval. (Reproduced with permission from ref. *28*.)

affinity for dopamine transporters but still with significant affinity for serotonin transporters, has been mentioned above (*3,43*). Pharmacological displacement of radiolabeled 6-nitroquipazine revealed results compatible with serotonin transporter binding (*26*). An analog of the previous compound labeled with iodine-125, [^{125}I]5-iodo-6-nitro-2-piperazinylquinoline, has also been examined (*47*). Scheffel and coworkers (*64,65,66*) have recently utilized [11C]McN5652 and others have used [123I]5-iodo-6-nitroquipazine (*29*).

There are no currently accepted ligands that are effective in labeling norepinephrine transporters. However, nisoxetine showed at least some promise (*24*), although the signal to noise ratio was not very great. Radiolabeled iodobenzylguanidine is a substrate for the norepinephrine transporter and can accumulate inside cells bearing the transporter (*6,63*). However, this compound is useful only for labeling transporters in the periphery, as it does not cross the blood–brain barrier.

[^{18}F]flurodopa is a well-known compound that is thought to be metabolized in the brain to flurodopamine and that is then accumulated by the dopamine transporter with subsequent visualization of the dopaminergic nerve terminal (*7*). This compound has been used in a variety of studies. However, its main drawbacks are its low signal-to-noise ratio, its nonspecificity regarding monoamine trans-

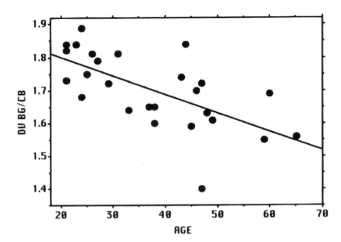

Fig. 6. Dopamine transporters decline with age. Correlation between the ratio of the distribution volume (DV) in the basal ganglia (BG) to that in the cerebellum (CB) and age ($r = -0.65$, $p < 0.0005$). There is a decrease in dopamine transporters with age. (Reproduced with permission from ref. *70*.)

porters, and the need for metabolic conversion, uptake, and storage to provide a signal.

All of the aforementioned discussion refers to neurotransmitter transporters in the nerve terminal membrane, but there are also monoamine transporters in the intracellular organelles, the synaptic vesicles. Carbon-11 labeled tetrabenazine labels monoamine transporters in vesicles. The compound is not selective, since it is thought to bind to many vesicular transporters, including those for norepinephrine, dopamine, and serotonin (*15,16,17,33*).

Analogs of vesamicol have been used as radiotracers for cholinergic neurons. [^{18}F]-labeled fluoroethoxybenzovesamicol has been used as such a radiotracer (*50*), and a methylamino analog has been used as well (*35*). A large number of analogs of vesamicol have also been synthesized and tested (*30*).

Uses of Transporter Imaging

As noted several times, a major role for transporter imaging has been in the identification of losses of neurons bearing the transporter, such as in Parkinson's disease. But imaging studies have also been used to show that transporter density decreases with aging, a feature shared by many biochemicals in the brain (*70*) (Fig. 6). Dopamine

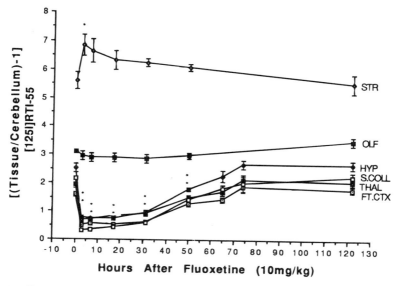

Fig. 7. Time-course of the inhibitory effect of fluoxetine on [^{125}I]RTI-55 binding in different regions of the mouse brain in vivo. Data are mean [(tissue/cerebellum)-1] radioactivity ratios ± SEM; $n = 4$ for each time point. FT.CTX, prefrontal cortex; HYP, hypothalamus; OLF, olfactory tubercle; S COLL, superior colliculus; STR, striatum; THAL, thalamus. Significantly different from controls: *$p < 0.05$; **$p < 0.01$. (Reproduced with permission from ref. *61.*)

transporters begin to decline with age during the second or third decade of life.

Transporter imaging can also be used to measure in vivo occupancy of transporters by various drugs. For example, the important class of antidepressant drugs, the serotonin selective reuptake inhibitors, have a fairly high and selective binding affinity for serotonin transporters. By carrying out in vivo competition studies, it is possible to identify the dose and duration of occupancy of serotonin transporters by antidepressant drugs. For example, a preimaging study in mice utilizing [^{125}I]RTI-55 binding in vivo shows that a single dose of fluoxetine inhibits transporter binding for up to 50 h, indicating a very long occupancy of transporter by these drugs (Fig. 7). These in vivo occupancy measures can be used to relate occupancy to functions or behaviors. For example, it has been shown that high levels of occupancy of dopamine transporters are needed to produce the beginnings of locomotor behavior (*14,69*).

At present, we are quite fortunate in having a variety of binding ligands available for a variety of different approaches and with different advantages. Again considering dopamine transporters as an example, many phenyltropanes can be used with PET scanning ([76]Br-, [18]F-, or ^{11}C-labeled), and some, such as RTI-55, RTI-121, and RTI-122, can be used in SPECT scanning (^{123}I-labeled). We have compounds with a low in vivo and in vitro binding affinity that are thus quite sensitive to competition at the binding site; these include radiolabeled cocaine and methylphenidate. We also have compounds that have a very high affinity for the transporter and therefore exhibit very high binding ratios; compounds in this category include RTI-55, although it takes a long time for the highest ratios to form, for example, 1–2 d. On the other hand, other compounds reach maximal striatal to cerebellar ratios in much earlier times after injection (e.g., WIN 35,428). Overall, it appears that the dopamine transporter has been a success as a target in imaging studies, and our continuing work will contribute to a thorough understanding and knowledge of dopaminergic systems in brain in vivo. Our efforts will also lead to a better exploration of other transporters.

References

1. Aquilonius, S. M., Bergstrom, K., Ecernas, S. A., Hartvig, P., Leenders, K. L., Lundquist, H., Antoni, G., Gee, A., Rimoand, A., Uhlin, J., and Langstrom, B. In vivo evaluation of striatal dopamine reuptake sites using [^{11}C]-nomifensine and positron emission tomography. *Acta Neurol. Scand.* **76** (1987) 283–287.

2. Baldwin, R. M., Zea-Ponce, Y., Al-Tikriti, M. S., Zoghbi, S. S., Seibyl, J. P., Charney, D. S., Hoffer, P. B., Wang, S., Milius, R. A., Neurmeyer, J. L., and Innis, R. B. Regional brain uptake and pharmacokenetics of [^{123}I]N-Fluoroalkyl-2β-carboxy-3β-(4-iodophenyl)nortropane esters in baboons. *Nucl. Med. Biol.* **22** (1995) 211–219.

3. Boja, J. W., Mitchell, W. M., Patel, A., Kopajtic, T. A., Carroll, F. I., Lewin, A. H., Abraham, P., and Kuhar, M. J. High affinity binding of [^{125}I] RTI-55 to dopamine and serotonin transporters in the rat brain. *Synapse* **12** (1992) 27–36.

4. Boja, J. W., Vaughan, R., Patel, A., Shaya, E. K., and Kuhar, M. J. The dopamine transporter. In Niznik H. B. (ed.), *Dopamine Receptors and Transporters*, Dekker, New York, 1994, pp. 611–644.

5. Brücke, T., Kornhuber, J., Angelberger, P., Asenbaum, S., Frassine, H., and Podreka, I. SPECT imaging of dopamine and serotonin transporters with [^{123}I]β-CIT. Binding kinetics in the human brain. *J. Neural. Transm.* **94** (1993) 137–146.

6. Buck, J., Bruchelt, G., Girgert, R., Treuner, J., and Niethammer, D. Specific uptake of m-[^{125}I]iodobenzylguanidine in the human neuroblastoma cell line SK-N-SH. *Canc. Res.* **45** (1985) 6366–6370.

7. Calne, D. B., Langstrom, J. W., Martin, W. R. W., Stoessl, A. J., Ruth, T. J., Adam, M. J., Pate, B. D., and Schulzer, M. Positron emission tomography after MPTP: observations relating to the cause of Parkinson's disease. *Nature* **317** (1985) 246–248.

8. Carroll, F. I., Lewin, A. H., Boja, J. W., and Kuhar, M. J. Cocaine receptor: biochemical characterization and structure-activity relationships of cocaine analogues at the dopamine transporter. *J. Med. Chem.* **35** (1992) 969–981.

9. Carroll, F. I., Rahman, M. A., Abraham, P., Parham, K., Lewin, A. H., Dannals, R. F., Shaya, E., Scheffel, U., Wong, D., Boja, J. W., and Kuhar, M. J. [^{123}I]3β-(4-iodephenyl)tropan-2β-carboxylic acid methyl ester (RTI-55), a unique cocaine receptor ligand for imaging the dopamine and serotonin transporters *in vivo*. *Med. Chem. Res.* **1** (1991) 289–294.

10. Chagraoui, A., Bonnet, J.-J., Protais, P., and Costentin, J. In vivo binding of [^{3}H]GBR 12783, a selective dopamine uptake inhibitor, in mouse striatum. *Neurosci. Lett.* **78** (1987) 175.

11. Ciliax, B. J., Heilman, C., Demchyshyn, L. L., Pristupa, Z. B., Ince, E., Hersch, S. M., Niznik, H. B., and Levey, A. I. The dopamine transporter: immunochemical characterization and localization in brain. *J. Neurosci.* **15** (1995) 1714–1723.

12. Ciliax, B. J., Kilbourn, M. R., Haka, M. S., Penney, J. B. Imaging the dopamine uptake site with ex vivo [^{18}F]GBR 13119 binding autoradiography in rat brain. *J. Neurochem.* **55** (1990) 619–623.

13. Cline, E. J., Scheffel, U., Boja, J. W., Carroll, F. I., Katz, J. L., and Kuhar, M. J. Behavioral effects of novel cocaine analogs: a comparison with in vivo receptor binding potency. *JPET* **3** (1992) 1174–1179.

14. Cline, E. J., Scheffel, U., Boja, J. W., Mitchell, W. M., Carroll, F. I., Abraham, P., Lewin, A. H., and Kuhar, M. J. In vivo binding of [^{125}I]RTI-55 to dopamine transporters: pharmacology and regional distribution with autoradiography. *Synapse* **12** (1992) 37–46.

15. DaSilva, J. N. and Kilbourn, M. R. In vivo binding of [^{11}C]tetrabenazine to vesicular monoamine transporters in mouse brain. *Life Sci.* **51** (1992) 593–600.

16. DaSilva, J. N., Kilbourn, M. R., and Domino, E. F. In vivo imaging of monoaminergic nerve terminals in normal and MPTP-lesioned primate brain using positron emission tomography (PET) and [^{11}C]tetrabenazine. *Synapse* **14** (1993) 128–131.

17. DaSilva, J. N., Kilbourn, M. R., and Mangner, T. J. Synthesis of [^{11}C]tetrabenazine, a vesicular monoamine uptake inhibitor, for PET imaging studies. *App. Radiat. Isot.* **44** (1993) 673–676.

18. Ding, Y.-S., Fowler, J. S., Volkow, N. D., Gatley, S. J., Logan, J., Dewey, S. L., Alexoff, D., Fazzini, E., and Wolf, A. P. Pharmacokinetics and in vivo specificity of [^{11}C]*dl-threo*-methylphenidate for the presynaptic dopaminergic neuron. *Synapse* **18** (1994) 152–160.

19. Farde, L., Halldin, C., Müller, L., Suhara, T., Karlsson, P., and Hall, H. PET study of [^{11}C]β-CIT binding to monoamine transporters in the monkey and human brain. *Synapse* **16** (1994) 93–103.

20. Fowler, J. S., Volkow, N. D., Wolf, A. P., Dewey, S. L., Schlyer, D. J., MacGregor, R. R., Hitzemann, R., Logan, J., Bendriem, B., Gatley, S. J., and Christman, D. Mapping cocaine binding sites in human and baboon brain in vivo. *Synapse* **4** (1989) 371–377.

21. Freed, C., Revay, R., Vaughan, R. A., Kriek, E., Grant, S., Uhl, G. R., and Kuhar, M. J. Dopamine transporter immunoreactivity in rat brain. *J. Comp. Neurol.* **359** (1995) 340–349.

22. Frost, J. J., Rosier, A. J., Reich, S. G., Smith, J. S., Ehlers, M. D., Snyder, S. H., Ravert, H. T., and Dannals, R. F. Positron emission tomographic imaging of the dopamine transporter with [^{11}C]-WIN 35,428 reveals marked declines in mild Parkinson's disease. *Ann. Neurol.* **34** (1993) 423–431.

23. Goodman, M. M., Kung, M.-P., Kabalka, G. W., Kung, H. F., and Switzer, R. Synthesis and characterization of radioiodinated N-(3-iodopropen-1-yl)-2β-carbomethoxy-3β-(4-chlorophenyl)tropanes: potential dopamine reuptake site imaging agents. *J. Med. Chem.* **37** (1994) 1535–1542.

24. Haka, M. S. and Kilbourn, M. R. Synthesis and regional mouse brain distribution of [^{11}C]nisoxetine, a norepinephrine uptake inhibitor. *Nucl. Med. Biol.* **16** (1989) 771–774.

25. Hantraye, P., Brownell, A.-L., Elmaleh, D., Spealman, R. D., Wullner, U., Brownell, G. L., Madras, B. K., and Isacson, O. Dopamine fiber detection by [^{11}C]-CFT and PET in a primate model of parkinsonism. *NeuroReport* **3** (1992) 265–268.

26. Hashimoto, K. and Goromaru, T. 4-bromo-6-nitroquipazine: a new ligand for studying 5-hydroxytryptamine uptake sites in vivo. *Neuropharm.* **31** (1992) 869–874.

27. Innis, R., Baldwin, R., Sybirska, E., Zea, Y., Laruelle, M., Al-Tikriti, M., Charney, D., Zoghbi, S., Smith, E., Wisniewski, G., Hoffer, P., Wang, S., Milius, R., and Neumeyer, J. Single photon emission computed tomography imaging of monoamine reuptake sites in primate brain with [^{123}I]CIT. *Eur. J. Pharm.* **200** (1991) 369–370.

28. Innis, R. B., Seibyl, J. P., Scanley, B. E., Laruelle, M., Abi-Dargham, A., Wallace, E., Baldwin, R. M., Zea-Ponce, Y., Zoghbi, S., Wang, S., Gao, Y., Neumeyer, J. L., Charney, D. S., Hoffer, P. B., and Marek, K. L. Single-photon emission-computed tomography imaging demonstrates loss of striatal dopamine transporters in Parkinson disease. *Proc. Natl. Acad. Sci. USA* **90** (1993) 11,965–11,969.

29. Jagust, W. J., Eberling, J. L., Roberts, J. A., Brennan, K. M., Hanrahan, S. M., VanBrocklin, H., Enas, J. D., Biegon, A., and Mathis C. A. In vivo imaging of the 5-hydroxytryptamine reuptake site in primate brain-using single photon emission computed tomography and [^{123}I]5-iodo-6-nitroquipazine. *Eur. J. Pharmacol.* **242** (1993) 189–193.

30. Jung, Y.-W., Van Dort, M. E., Gildersleeve, D. L., and Wieland, D. M. A radio-tracer for mapping cholinergic neurons of the rain. *J. Med. Chem.* **33** (1990) 2065–2068.

31. Kaufman, M. J. and Madras, B. K. Distribution of cocaine recognition sites in monkey brain: II. Ex vivo autoradiography with [^{3}H]CFT and [^{125}I]RTI-55. *Synapse* **12** (1992) 99–111.

32. Kilbourn, M. R. In vivo binding of [^{18}F]GBR 13119 to the brain dopamine uptake system. *Life Sci.* **42** (1988) 1347–1353.

33. Kilbourn, M. R., DaSilva, J. N., Frey K. A., Koeppe, R. A., and Kuhl, D. E. In vivo imaging of vesicular monoamine transporters in human brain using [^{11}C]tetrabenazine and positron emission tomography. *J. Neurochem.* **60** (1993) 2315–2318.

34. Kilbourn, M. R., Haka, M. S., Mulhollond, G. K., Sherman, P. S., and Pisani, T. Regional brain distribution of [18F]GBR 13119, a dopamine uptake inhibitor, in CD-1 and C57BL/6 mice. *Eur. J. Pharm.* **166** (1989) 331–334.

35. Kilbourn, M. R., Jung, Y.-W., Haka, M. S., Gildersleeve, D. L., Kuhl, D. E., and Wieland, D. M. Mouse brain distribution of a carbon-11 labeled vesamicol derivative: presynaptic marker of cholinergic neurons. *Life Sci.* **47** (1990) 1955–1963.

36. Kilbourn, M. R., Mulholland, G. K., Sherman, P. S., and Pisani, T. In vivo binding of the dopamine uptake inhibitor [18F]GBR 13119 in MPTP-treated C57BL/6 mice. *Nucl. Med. Biol.* **18** (1991) 803–806.

37. Kilbourn, M. R., Sherman, P. S., and Pisani, T. Repeated reserpine administration reduces in vivo [18F]GBR 13119 binding to the dopamine uptake site. *Eur. J. Pharm.* **216** (1992) 109–112.

38. Kuhar, M. J. Neurotransmitter uptake: A tool in identifying neurotransmitter-specific pathways. *Life Sci.* **13** (1973) 1623–1634.

39. Kuhar, M. J., Sanchez-Roa, P. M., Wong, D. F., Dannals, R. F. Grigoriadis, D. E., Lew, R., and Milberger, M. Dopamine transporter: biochemistry, pharmacology and imaging. *Eur. Neurol.* **30**(1) (1990) 15–20.

40. Kuikka, J. T., Bergström, K. A., Ahonen, A., and Länsimies, E. The dosimetry of iodine-123 labelled 2β-carbomethoxy-3β-(4-iodophenyl)tropane. *Eur. J. Nucl. Med.* **21** (1994) 53–56.

41. Kuikka, J. T., Bergström, K. A., Vanninen, E., Laulumaa, V., Hartikainen, P., and Länsimies, E. Initial experience with single-photon emission tomography using iodine-123-labelled 2β-carbomethyoxy-3β-(4-iodophenyl)tropane in human brain. *Eur. J. Nucl. Med.* **20** (1993) 782–786.

42. Kung, M. P., Essman, W. D., Frederick, D., Meegalla, S., Goodman, M., Mu, M., Lucki, I., and Kung, H. F. IPT: a novel iodinated ligand for the CNS dopamine transporter. *Synapse* **20** (1995) 316–324.

43. Laruelle, M., Baldwin, R. M., Malison, R. T., Zea-Ponce, Y., Zoghbi, S. S., Al-Tikriti, M. S., Sybirska, E. H., Zimmermann, R. C., Wisniewski, G., Neumeyer, J. L., Milius, R. A., Wang, S., Smith, E. O., Roth, R. H., Charney, D. S., Hoffer, P. B., and Innis, R. B. SPECT imaging of dopamine and serotonin transporters with [123I] β-CIT: pharmacological characterization of brain uptake in nonhuman primates. *Synapse* **13** (1993) 295–309.

44. Leenders, K. L., Aquilonius, S. M., Bergstrom, K., Bjurling, P., Crossman, A. R., Eckernas, S. A., Gee, A. G., Hartvig, P., Lundquist, H., Langstrom, B., Rimland, A., and Tedroff, J. Unilateral MPTP lesion in a rhesus monkey: effects on the striatal dopaminergic system measured in vivo with PET using various novel tracers. *Brain Res.* **445** (1988) 61–67.

45. Lorang, D., Amara, S. G., and Simerly, R. B. Cell-type-specific expression of catecholamine transporters in the rat brain. *J. Neurosci.* **14** (1994) 4903–4914.

46. Madras, B. K., Spealman, R. D., Fahey, M. A., Neumeyer, J. L., Saha, J. K., and Milius, R. A. Cocaine receptors labeled by [3H] 2β-carbomethoxy-3β-(4-fluorophenyl)tropane. *Mol. Pharmacol.* **36** (1989) 518–524.

47. Mathis, C. A., Biegon, A., Taylor, S. E., Enas, J. D., and Hanrahan, S. M. [125I]5-iodo-6-nitro-2-piperazinylquinoline: a potent and selective ligand for the serotonin uptake complex. *Eur. J. Pharm.* **210** (1992) 103–104.

48. Meltzer, P. C., Lian, A. Y., Brownell, A.-L., Elmaleh, D. R., and Madras, B. K. Substituted 3-phenyltropane analogs of cocaine: synthesis, inhibition of bind-

ing at cocaine recognition sites, and positron emission tomography imaging. *J. Med. Chem.* **36** (1993) 855–862.

49. Meltzer, P. C., Liang, A. Y., and Madras, B. K. The discovery of an unusually selective and novel cocaine analog: difluoropine. Synthesis and inhibition of binding at cocaine recognition sites. *J. Med. Chem.* **37** (1994) 2001–2010.

50. Mulholland, G. K., Jung, Y.-W., Wieland, D. M., Kilbourn, M. R., and Kuhl, D. E. Synthesis of [^{18}F]fluoroethoxy-benzovesamicol, a radiotracer for cholinergic neurons. *J. Lab. Comp. Radiopharm.* **33** (1993) 583–591.

51. Müller, L. K. (ed.) *Development of Radioligands for the Dopamine Transporter*, Stockton Press, Stockholm, 1994.

52. Neumeyer, J. L., Wang, S., Gao, Y., Milius, R. A., Kula, N. S., Campbell, A., Baldessarini, R. J., Zea-Ponce, Y., Baldwin, R. M., and Innis, R. B. (1994) N-fluoroalkyl analogs of (1R)-2β-carbomethoxy-3β-(4-iodophenyl)-tropane (β-CIT): radiotracers for positron emission tomography and single photon emission computed tomography imaging of dopamine transporters. *J. Med. Chem.* **37** (1994) 1558–1561.

53. Newman, A. H., Allen, A. C., Izenwasser, S., and Katz, J. L. Novel 3α-(diphenylmethoxy)tropane analogs: potent dopamine uptake inhibitors without cocaine-like behavioral profiles. *J. Med. Chem.* **37** (1994) 2258–2261.

54. Nirenberg, M. J., Vaughan, R. A., Uhl, G. R., Kuhar, M. J., and Pickel, V. M. The dopamine transporter is localized to dendritic and axonal plasma membranes of nigrostriatal dopaminergic neurons. *J. Neurosci.* **16** (1996) 436–447.

55. Revay, R., Vaughan, R., Grant, S., and Kuhar, M. J. Dopamine transporter immohistochemistry in median eminence, amygdala, and other areas of the rat brain. *Synapse* **22** (1995) 93–99.

56. Ritz, M. C., Boja, J. W., Zaczek, R., Carroll, F. I., and Kuhar, M. J. [^{3}H] WIN 35,065-2: a ligand for cocaine receptors in rat striatum. *Soc. Neurosci.* **15** (1989) 1092.

57. Ritz, M. C., Boja, J. W., Zaczek, R., Carroll, F. I., and Kuhar, M. J. [^{3}H] WIN 35,065-2: A ligand for cocaine receptors in striatum. *J. Neurochem.* **55** (1990) 1556–1562.

58. Scanley, B. E., Al-Tikriti, M. S., Gandelman, M. S., Laruelle, M., Zea-Ponce, Y., Baldwin, R. M., Zoghbi, S. S., Hoffer, P. B., Charney, D. S., Wang, S., Neumeyer, J. L. and Innis, R. B. Comparison of [^{123}I]β-CIT and [^{123}I]IPCIT as single-photon emission tomography radiotracers for the dopamine transporter in nonhuman primates. *Eur. J. Nucl. Med.* **22** (1995) 4–11.

59. Scheffel, U., Boja, J. W., and Kuhar, M. J. Cocoaine receptors: in vivo labeling with [^{3}H]-(-)cocaine, [^{3}H]-WIN 35,065-2, and [^{3}H]-WIN 35,428. *Synapse* **4** (1989) 390–392.

60. Scheffel, U., Dannals, R. F., Wong, D. F., Yokoi, F., Carroll, F. I., and Kuhar, M. J. Dopamine transporter imaging with novel, selective cocaine analogs. *NeuroReport* **3** (1992) 969–972.

61. Scheffel, U., Kims, S., Cline, E. J., and Kuhar, M. J. Occupancy of the serotonin transporter by fluoxetine, paroxetine, and sertraline: in vivo studies with [^{125}I]RTI-55. *Synapse* **16** (1994) 263–268.

62. Shaya, E. K., Scheffel, U., Dannals, R. F., Ricaurte, G. A., Carroll, F. I., Wagner, H. N., and Kuhar, M. J. In vivo imaging of dopamine reuptake sites in the primate brain using single photon emission computed tomography (SPECT) and Iodine-123 labelled RTI-55. *Synapse* **10** (1992) 169–172.

63. Smets, L. A., Loesberg, C., Janssen, M., Metwally, E. A., and Huiskamp, R. Active uptake and extravesicular storage of m-iodobenzylguanidine in human neuroblastoma SK-N-SH cells. *Canc. Res.* **49** (1989) 2941–2944.

64. Suehiro, M., Scheffel, U., Dannals, R. F., Ravert, H. T., Riocaurte, G. A., and Wagner, H. N. A PET radiotracer for studying serotonin uptake sites: carbon-11-McN-5652Z. *J. Nuc. Med.* **34** (1993) 120–127.

65. Suehiro, M., Scheffel, U., Ravert, H. T., Dannals, R. F., and Wagner, H. N. [^{11}C](+)McN5652 as a radiotracer for imaging serotonin uptake sites PET. *Life Sci.* **53** (1993) 883–892.

66. Szabo, Z., Kao, P. F., Scheffel, U., Suehiro, M., Mathews, W. B., Ravert, H. T., Musachio, J. L., Marenco, S., Kim, S. E., Ricaurte, G. A., Wong, D. F., Wagner, H. N., Jr., and Dannals, R. F. Positron emission tomography imaging of serotonin transporters in the human brain using [^{11}C](+)McN5652. *Synapse* **20** (1995) 37–43.

67. Tedroff, J., Aquilonius, S.-M., Hartvig, P., Lundqvist, H., Gee, A. G., Uhlin, J., and Långström, B. Monoamine re-uptake sites in the human brain evaluated in vivo by means of [^{11}C]-nominfensine and positron emission tomography: the effects of age and Parkinson's disease. *Acta Neurol. Scand.* **77** (1988) 192–201.

68. Vaugeois, J.-M., Bonnet, J.-J., and Costentin, J. In vivo labeling of the neuronal dopamine uptake complex in the mouse striatum by [^{3}H]GBR 12783. *Eur. J. Pharm.* **210** (1992) 77–84.

69. Vaugeois, J.-M., Bonnet, J.-J., Duterte-Boucher, D., and Costentin, J. In vivo occupancy of the striatal dopamine uptake complex by various inhibitors does not predict their effects on locomotion. *Eur. J. Pharm.* **230** (1993) 195–201.

70. Volkow, N. D., Fowler, J. S., Wang, G. J., Logan J., Schlyer, D., MacGregor, R., Hitzemann, R., and Wolf, A. P. Decreased dopamine transporters with age in healthy human subjects. *Ann. Neurol.* **36** (1994) 237–239.

71. Whitehouse, P. J., Wamsley, J. K., Zarbin, M. A., Price, D. L., Tourtellotte, W. W., and Kuhar, M. J. Amyotrophic lateral sclerosis: alterations in neurotransmitter receptors. *Ann. Neurol.* **14** (1983) 8–16.

72. Wong, D. F., Yung, B., Dannals, R. F., Shaya, E. K., Ravert, H. T., Chen, C. A., Chan, B., Folio, T., Scheffel, U., Ricaurte, G. A., Neumeyer, J. L., Wagner, H. N., and Kuhar, M. J. In vivo imaging of baboon and human dopamine transporters by positron emission tomography using [^{11}C]WIN 35, 428. *Synapse* **15** (1993) 130–142.

73. Wüllner, U., Pakzaban, P., Brownell, A.-L., Hantraye, P., Burns, L., Shoup, T., Elmaleh, D., Petto, A. J., Spealman, R. D., Brownell, G. L., and Isacson, O. Dopamine terminal loss and onset of motor symptoms in MPTP-treated monkeys: A positron emission tomography study with [^{11}C]-CFT. *Exp. Neurol.* **126** (1994) 305–309.

CHAPTER 11

The Dopamine Transporter in Human Brain

Characterization and Effect of Cocaine Exposure

Deborah C. Mash and Julie K. Staley

Introduction

Deaths involving psychoactive drugs stem not only from overdose, but also from drug-induced mental states that may lead to serious injuries (9). Mortality data have revealed the virulence of the cocaine epidemic, although other indicators, including crime, drug-exposed neonates, drug-related traffic accidents, and drug use by workers, provide a more extensive view of the nature and extent of the problem of cocaine abuse. The arrival of inexpensive smokable crack cocaine has radically changed the nature of the epidemic and revealed the great addictive potential of this drug.

The epidemic of cocaine abuse has led to the search for effective treatments to block or substitute for cocaine. The reinforcing and additive properties of cocaine arise from its ability to block reuptake of the neurotransmitter dopamine (DA) by binding to recognition sites on the DA transport carrier (25,49,70). DA uptake is inhibited with a distinct pharmacological profile by a variety of structurally diverse compounds. Identification and cloning of the gene for the DA transporter has provided insight into the molecular mechanism of DA reuptake inhibition by cocaine binding to the transport carrier (21,30,67,83). Rothman (71) suggested that DA transport inhibitors can be divided into two groups: type 1 DA reuptake inhibitors, such as cocaine, which produce euphoria and addiction in humans, and type 2 inhibitors, such as mazindol and buproprion, which do not

Neurotransmitter Transporters: Structure, Function, and Regulation
Ed.: M. E. A. Reith Humana Press Inc., Totowa, NJ

produce euphoria and have low abuse liability. The underlying assumption is that type 2 inhibitors interact differently than cocaine at sites on the DA transporter. Molecular biological and ligand binding studies have delineated discrete domains within the structure of the DA transporter protein for substrate, cocaine, and antidepressant interactions (31,44,45), raising the possibility that it may be feasible to design cocaine antagonists that are devoid of uptake blockade for the clinical management of cocaine addiction.

The neuronal DA transporter has been identified and studied recently in human brain postmortem by radioligand binding techniques using novel cocaine congeners and transport inhibitors. In vitro binding and autoradiography of radioligands specific for the DA transporter afford systematic visualization of the status of cocaine binding sites on the DA transporter. These studies in postmortem human brain are a counterpart to the rapidly developing noninvasive techniques of in vivo brain imaging, and are important for establishing quantitative and regional neurochemical adaptations resulting from cocaine abuse. Equally important will be studies aimed at determining the long-term neurobiological consequences of chronic cocaine abuse on the DA transporter in aging populations that have abused psychostimulants. Determining how cocaine exposure affects the human DA transporter may disclose the mechanisms responsible for tolerance and sensitization (reverse tolerance), and provide a basis for designing pharmacotherapeutic interventions to treat cocaine dependence.

Ligand-Binding Studies of the Human DA Transporter

The DA transporter is the primary recognition site for cocaine that is related to drug abuse (49,70). DA transporters function to rapidly control the removal of transmitter molecules from the synaptic cleft. Cocaine potentiates DAergic neurotransmission by blocking the reuptake of DA, leading to marked elevations in the levels of neurotransmitter (29,30). Radioligand binding to the DA transporter has been best characterized with the cocaine congeners [^{3}H]WIN 35,428 and [^{125}I]RTI-55, and more recently with [^{125}I]RTI-121 (for review, *see* ref. 4). In contrast to the classic DA transport inhibitors ([^{3}H]mazindol, [^{3}H]GBR 12935, and [^{3}H]nomifensine), the cocaine congeners ([^{3}H]WIN 35,428, [^{125}I]RTI-55, and [^{125}I]RTI-121) label multiple sites with a pharmacological profile characteristic of the DA transporter in primate and human brain (59,67,77,81). Radioligand binding to COS cells transfected with the cloned cocaine-sensitive DA transporter demonstrates two sites for binding of [^{3}H]WIN 35,428 to the protein expressed from a single cDNA (*13*). Whether the multiple cocaine binding sites represent altered functional forms or states of the DA transporter, or discrete recognition sites on the DA transporter protein, remains unclear.

Pharmacological studies have demonstrated a lack of correspondence between DA transport function and ligand binding (*67*). These findings provide additional support for the incomplete correspondence of pharmacologically overlapping sites for [^{3}H]WIN 35,428, [^{3}H]GBR 12,935, and [^{3}H]mazindol labeling of the DA transporter in native membrane preparations from rat brain (*68,69*). Pharmacological heterogeneity of the cloned and native human DA transporter was suggested further by the dissociation of [^{3}H]WIN 35,428 and [^{3}H]GBR 12,935 binding sites (*67*). The proportion of observed high- and low-affinity [^{3}H]WIN 35,428 binding sites differs across studies using cloned (*13,21,67*) or native membranes (*59,68,69*). The binding of [^{3}H]WIN 35,428 to the cloned rat (*13*) and human (*67*) DA transporter demonstrates multiple recognition sites, and it has been suggested that only the high-affinity component is functionally correlated with that of the cloned DA uptake process (*67*). Using the same expression system, COS-7 cells, Eshleman et al. (*21*) detected a single high-affinity binding site for [^{3}H]WIN 35,428 on the cloned human DA transporter, but, with C6 glioma cells as the expression system, they observed labeling of both a high- and low-affinity binding site in 50% of their experiments (*21*).

Saturation binding of the cocaine congeners [^{3}H]WIN 35,428, (*43,79*), [^{125}I]RTI-55, (*54,77*) and [^{125}I]RTI-121 (*79*) is biphasic, indicating the presence of multiple cocaine recognition sites on the DA transporter. In contrast, the binding of [^{3}H]GBR 12935 (*61*) and [^{3}H]mazindol (Staley and Mash, unpublished observations) to the human striatum is monophasic, suggesting that these radioligands may interact differently with the DA transporter. The binding site densities in human striatum, estimated from saturation isotherms for the cocaine congeners ([^{3}H]WIN 35,428 (*80*), [^{125}I]RTI-55 (*77*), and [^{125}I]RTI-121 (*81*) (approx 150–200 pmol/g original wet weight tissue) are in agreement with that observed for the noncocaine-like transport inhibitors [^{3}H]mazindol (Fig. 1) and [^{3}H]GBR 12935 (*61*). The total binding densities corresponding to both the high- and low-affinity cocaine recognition sites were comparable to noncocaine-like transport inhibitors, which recognize a single class of sites associated with the DA transporter (Fig. 1).

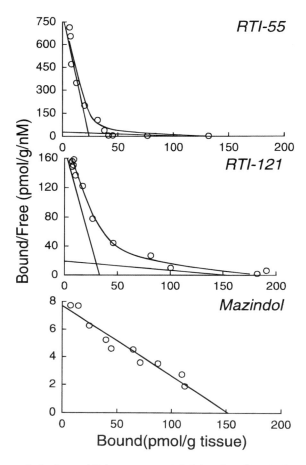

Fig. 1. Rosenthal plots of DA transport inhibitor binding in human striatum. Saturation binding studies of [^{125}I]RTI-55, [^{125}I]RTI-121, and [^{3}H]mazindol binding to human striatal membranes were conducted in 10 mM sodium phosphate buffer (pH 7.4) containing 0.32 M sucrose, as previously described by Staley et al. (77,81). Data were analyzed using the iterative nonlinear curve-fitting program EBDA/LIGAND (Elsevier, Amsterdam, The Netherlands, Biosoft). In these representative experiments, the cocaine congeners RTI-55 and RTI-121 recognized high- and low-affinity binding sites, with affinity values of 0.1 nM and 4.1 nM for RTI-55 and affinity values of 0.2 and 8.0 nM for RTI-121. The density values corresponding to the high- and low-affinity binding sites were 23.8 and 108.9 pmol/g for RTI-55 and 33.1 and 153.6 pmol/g tissue for RTI-121. In contrast, the noncocaine-like DA transport inhibitor [^{3}H]mazindol labeled a single binding site in the presence of paroxetine and desipramine with a K_d value of 19.2 nM and B_{max} value of 148.8 pmol/g tissue.

Multiple cocaine recognition sites associated with the DA transporter have not been consistently reported in human striatum (*55,67;* Kish, personal communication). The binding density corresponding to a single high-affinity site is significantly lower than that comprised by both high- and low-affinity cocaine recognition sites in human brain (*54,55,67,77,79,81*). In some instances, the existence of only a single component for WIN 35,428 (*55,66*) or RTI-121 (*78*) may result from different conditions of the binding assay. For example, in the human striatum the binding of RTI-121 is biphasic, depending on the assay buffer (*81*). RTI-121 saturation curves performed in sucrose-phosphate buffer reveal high- and low-affinity cocaine recognition sites, with a total density of approx 200 pmol/g tissue. When saturation binding assays are conducted in a high-salt–containing buffer, a significant decrease in the overall density of binding (50 pmol/g tissue) is observed (*81*). Similar total density values have been reported for [^{125}I]RTI-55 and [^{3}H]WIN 35,428 binding to human striatal membranes in Tris buffers (*54,55*). Rosenthal plots of RTI-121 binding, obtained in the presence of high-sodium–containing buffers, demonstrate a selective decrease in the density of the low-affinity binding component (*81*). These findings suggest that the low-affinity cocaine recognition site may overlap with sites on the transporter that confer ionic dependence of DA transport. Consonant with this observation, Little et al. (*56*) reported one binding site for [^{125}I]RTI-121 in human striatal membranes in high-salt buffer. Taken together, the heterogeneity of radioligand binding suggests that DA and cocaine interactions with the DA transporter are not mediated by a single class of recognition sites.

The functional significance of multiple cocaine recognition sites associated with the DA transporter remains unclear. The two cocaine recognition sites may reflect binding interactions with distinct domains of a single DA transporter polypeptide or with different conformations of the DA transporter, which are recognized with equal affinities by noncocaine-like DA transport inhibitors. The function of the DA transporter is to translocate DA together with Na^+ and Cl^- across the presynaptic nerve terminal into the cytoplasm. Re-orientation of the DA transporter from inside to outside, or structural folding of the protein that favors outward vs inward directed residues, may account for the pharmacological heterogeneity seen with different classes of radioligands that bind to the DA transporter.

The recent cloning and expression of the human DA transporter gene has provided extensive information on the pharmacological signature of the DA transporter protein (21,30,45). The cloned DA transporter cDNA encodes a single polypeptide strand of 620 amino acids, which corresponds to a protein of 68,517 Dalton (30). The cDNA encodes consensus sites—for glycosylation and phosphorylation, suggesting that secondary processing may contribute to the regulation of the transport protein. Like other neurotransmitter carriers, the predicted structure of the DA transporter based on hydropathicity analysis suggests the presence of 12 transmembrane domains with an intracellular N-terminus and C-terminus (30). Expression of the cloned DA transporter in COS-7, mouse fibroblast, or glioma cell lines (21,30,67) afforded biochemical characterization of saturable, Na^+-dependent DA transport, which was blocked by psychostimulants (cocaine, amphetamine, and phencyclidine) and DA transport inhibitors (GBR 12909, mazindol, nomifensine, amnfoleic acid) with potency values that correlate well with those observed for competition of radiolabeled cocaine congener binding. The pharmacological profile observed for inhibition of binding of the cocaine congeners RTI-55 and RTI-121 in human striatum agrees with the values observed for inhibition of DA uptake and [^{3}H]WIN 35,428 binding to the cloned human DA transporter (Table 1).

The molecular structure of the rat DA transporter has been modified, using site-directed mutagenesis to further characterize the regions of the transporter that mediate cocaine's interaction (44,45). In transmembrane (TM) 1, mutation of Asp 79 dramatically reduced uptake of [^{3}H]DA and decreased the binding affinity of the cocaine congener [^{3}H]WIN 35,428. Replacement of serine residues 356 and 359 in TM 7 decreased [^{3}H]DA uptake and had a minimal effect on [^{3}H]WIN 35,428 binding (44). These studies suggest that cocaine congeners and DA may interact with distinct, yet overlapping domains within the DA transporter complex. Discrete domains for cocaine, classic tricyclic antidepressant and substrate binding, ionic dependence, and substrate uptake have been delineated by the use of chimeric dopamine–norepinephrine transporters (15,31). Regions from the amino terminus through TM 5 are important for ionic dependence and DA uptake (15,31); regions within TM 6–8 confer tricyclic antidepressant and cocaine binding and cocaine interactions with DA transport (31). Transmembrane regions 4–8 are important for substrate translocation; TM 9 through the C-terminus may be responsible for stereoselectivity and high-affinity substrate interactions (15,31). Giros et al. (31) caution that the involvement of a particular region of the protein in a given function does not imply that other regions of the

Table 1

Pharmacological Characterization of Cloned and Native Human Brain DA Transporter[a]

	Cloned human DA transporter		Human brain DA transporter		
Inhibitor	[³H]DA Uptake K_i, nM[b,c]	[³H]WIN 35,428 K_i, nM[d,e]	[³H]WIN 35,428 K_i, nM[f]	[¹²⁵I]RTI-55 IC₅₀, nM[g]	[¹²⁵I]RTI-121 IC₅₀, nM[g]
Mazindol	11; 60	3; 24	15	8	7
GBR 12909	17; 14	nd; 4	30	15	1
(–) Cocaine	58; 743	39; 240	68	151	42
Pimozide	344; nd	nd	nd	141	nd
Buproprion	330; 784	121; 950	560	nd	nd
Nomifensine	17; 53	nd; 42	40	nd	18
Desipramine	13000; nd	3320; nd	nd	2014	1560

[a]nd; not determined.

[b]Giros et al. (30) and Giros and Caron (29): K_i values for inhibition of [³H]DA uptake into Ltk⁻ cells expressing human DA transporter were calculated from monophasic inhibition curves. There was only one [³H]DA uptake component.

[c]Pristupa et al. (67): K_i values for inhibition of [³H]DA uptake into COS-7 cells expressing human DA transporter were calculated from monophasic inhibition curves. There was only one [³H]DA uptake component.

[d]Eshleman et al. (21): K_i values for inhibition of [³H]WIN 35,428 binding to COS-7 cells expressing human DA transporter were calculated from monophasic inhibition curves. There was only one [³H]WIN 35,428 binding component with nonspecific binding defined by 5 μM mazindol.

[e]Pristupa et al. (67): K_i values for inhibition of [³H]WIN 35,428 binding to COS-7 cells expressing human DA transporter were calculated from inhibition curves that were monophasic for the particular compounds shown in this table. There were two [³H]WIN 35,428 binding components with at least 70% of the radioligand bound to high-affinity sites in the absence of inhibitor (nonspecific binding defined by 1 μM mazindol).)

[f]Pristupa et al. (67): K_i values for inhibition of [³H]WIN 35,428 binding to human native caudate membranes were calculated from monophasic inhibition curves. There was only one [³H]WIN 35,428 binding component with nonspecific binding defined by 1 μM mazindol.

[g]Staley et al. (77) and gStaley et al. (81): IC₅₀ values are shown for inhibition of [¹²⁵I]RTI-55/121 binding to human native caudate membranes. There were two [¹²⁵I]RTI-55/121 binding components with nonspecific binding defined by 50 μL cocaine. Because, in the absence of inhibitor, most of the radioligand was bound to the high-affinity component, 88 vs 12% to low-affinity sites, the IC₅₀ reflects primarily the K_i for the high-affinity sites.

protein are not implicated in that function, but it does suggest the possibility that certain properties of these functions are specified by modular structural entities (*31*). The discovery that in some chimeras the binding of cocaine can be virtually eliminated without interfering with the reuptake of DA suggests that a specific determinant for cocaine binding must exist independent of the binding of DA. Since the DA transporter is the endogenous target of cocaine action (*49,70*), these findings raise the important possibility that selective antagonists of cocaine's interaction with the DA transporter could be developed for clinical use in the treatment of drug abuse.

In Vitro and In Vivo Mapping of the DA Transporter in Human Brain

The DAergic systems in brain comprises three distinct pathways, including the nigrostriatal, mesocortical, and mesolimbic projections. The nigrostriatal pathway originates in the substantia nigra pars compacta and terminates in the striatum. The mesolimbic pathway originates in the ventral tegmental area (VTA) and projects to the limbic sectors of the striatum, amygdala, and olfactory tubercle. The mesocortical pathway originates in the VTA and terminates within particular sectors of the cerebral cortical mantle, including the prefrontal, cingulate, and entorhinal cortices (*12*). The human striatum is organized into distinct neurochemical compartments termed patch (striosome) and matrix (*32*). The DAergic terminals within the patch arise from cell bodies localized to the substantia nigra pars compacta; the DAergic projections to the matrix compartment originate from the VTA (rostrorubral area) and the substantia nigra pars compacta (*32,40*). Autoradiographic visualization of the distribution of DA transporters indicates that the topographic distribution of the DA transporter correlates well with DA innervation with high densities localized to nigrostriatal terminals, moderate densities within the mesolimbic terminals, and low densities within the mesocortical terminals (*33,57*).

The regional distribution of the DA transporter varies, depending on the probe and the target (message or protein). *In situ* hybridization histochemistry reveals high densities of DA transporter mRNAs localized to the ventral substantia nigra, VTA, and the retrorubral cell groups (*40*). Abundant DA transporter mRNA is found within the substantia nigra pars compacta, which contains the cell bodies that project primarily to the motor sectors of the striatum corresponding to the increased gradient in DA transporter protein. Matrix-directed neurons have the lowest level of DA transporter mRNA, but the DA terminals in the matrix of the striatum maintain the highest density of DA transporter binding. These results suggest that there may not be a precise correlation between mRNA and ligand binding to the DA transporter protein (*40*).

The regional distribution of the DA transporter in the human brain has been mapped in vitro, using ligand binding and autoradiography on postmortem brain sections, and visualized in vivo, using PET and SPECT. The first detailed regional maps of the distribution of the DA transporter in postmortem human brain were generated with [³H]mazindol (*20*). When binding to the norepinephrine transporter was occluded with desipramine, [³H]mazindol labeling was most evident in the striatum, with local gradients corresponding to the pattern of DAergic projections. Moderate to low [³H]mazindol labeling was visualized over DA cell body fields, including the substantia nigra compacta, VTA, and the cell group in the retrorubral field (*20*).

Autoradiographic mapping of the DA transporter in human brain using [³H]cocaine (*11*) and the cocaine congeners [³H]WIN 35,428 (*43,79*), [¹²⁵I]RTI-55 (*77*), and [¹²⁵I]RTI-121 (*81*) have demonstrated high densities of labeling over the striatum, with moderate labeling over DAergic cell body fields. Autoradiographic visualization of the labeling of the radiolabeled cocaine congeners demonstrates distinct regional distibution patterns (Fig. 2). Although these radioligands have been useful for determining the regional distribution of ligand binding sites associated with the DA transporter, the overlapping affinities for the serotonin and/or the norepinephrine transporter make studies aimed at mapping regulatory changes in the DA transporter by cocaine difficult (*11,14,22,54,77*). The distribution of [¹²⁵I]RTI-55 binding is very widespread, with binding sites prevalent throughout the cerebral cortex, striatum, thalamus, hypothalamus, and amygdala (Fig. 2A). This pattern of labeling correlates with the known distribution of monoaminergic nerve terminals and is consistent with binding of [¹²⁵I]RTI-55 to both 5-HT and DA transporters (*22,77*). Selective visualization of the DA transporter may be achieved by occluding the binding of [¹²⁵I]RTI-55 to the 5-HT transporter with the serotonin reuptake inhibitors paroxetine or citalopram (Fig. 2B; *22,77*). The DA transporter has been selectively labeled in vitro using the novel cocaine congener [¹²⁵I]RTI-121 (*81*). The anatomical distribution of [¹²⁵I]RTI-121 binding (Fig. 2C) is much more restricted and better correlates with the known distribution and density of DA pro-

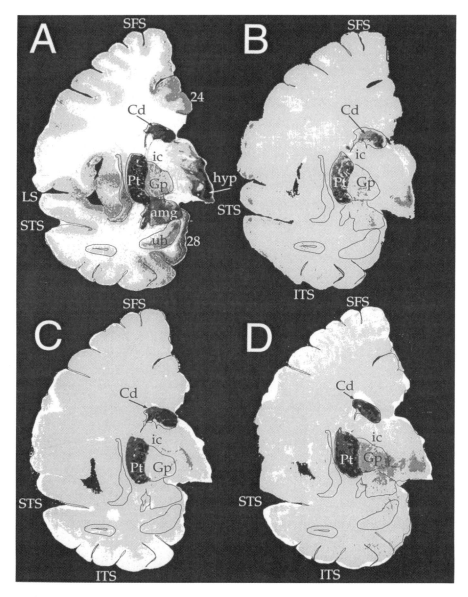

Fig. 2. In vitro autoradiography of radiolabeled cocaine congeners in human brain. (**A–D**) Gray-scale images of [^{125}I]RTI-55 (50 pM); [^{125}I]RTI-55 (50 pM) in the presence of 500 nM citalopram; [^{125}I]RTI-121 (20 pM); and [^{3}H]WIN 35,428 (2 nM), respectively. amg, amygdala; Cd, caudate; Gp, globus pallidus; hyp, hypothalamus; ic, internal capsule; ITS, inferior temporal sulcus; LS, lateral sulcus; Pt, putamen; sn, substantia nigra; SFS, superior frontal sulcus; STS, superior temporal sulcus; th, thalamus; uh, uncus.

jection systems than the distribution of either [^{125}I]RTI-55 or [^{3}H]WIN 35,428 (Fig. 2D). The anatomical distribution of [^{3}H]WIN 35,428 labeling is more highly correlated with the pattern of the [^{3}H]cocaine labeling than [^{125}I]RTI-55 (58).

The regional distribution of the DA transporter has been examined in vivo in human brain using ^{11}C-nomifensine (8,72), [^{11}C]dl-*threo*-methylphenidate (19), [^{11}C]cocaine (24,26), ^{11}C-WIN 35,428 (91), [^{11}C]β-CIT (also called RTI-55) (22), [^{123}I]β-CIT (63,66,75), [^{123}I]β-CIT-FE (51), and [^{123}I]β-CIT-FP (50). In the living human brain, the regional distribution of [^{11}C]cocaine and [^{11}C]dl-*threo*-methylphenidate is heterogenous, with high radiotracer labeling apparent in the striatum and low labeling seen throughout the cerebral cortex. The psychostimulants [^{11}C]cocaine and [^{11}C]dl-*threo*-methylphenidate bind to the DA transporter, with low in vivo occupancy of NE and 5-HT transporters (19,24). Administration of DA transport inhibitors significantly decreased striatal [^{11}C]cocaine and [^{11}C]dl-*threo*-methylphenidate uptake, further demonstrating that these radioligands primarily labeled the DA transporter. The cocaine congeners [^{11}C]WIN 35,428 (91, [^{11}C]β-CIT (22), and [^{123}I]β-CIT (63,66,75) also demonstrated marked radiotracer accumulation in the striatum with low levels of binding to the thalamus, hypothalamus, midbrain, and pons. Binding of the radiotracer to the extrastriatal regions was occluded by pretreatment with mazindol and citalopram, indicating that the labeling in these regions was primarily to the 5-HT and NE transporters and not to the DA transporter (22,66,75). The binding of [^{123}I] β-CIT to the thalamus, hypothalamus, midbrain, and pons was significantly reduced in depressed patients treated with the selective 5-HT reuptake inhibitor citalopram (66). Recently, cocaine congeners ([^{123}I]β-CIT-FP, [^{123}I]β-CIT-FE) demonstrating greater selectivity for binding to the DA transporter have been synthesized and radiolabeled (50,51). In vivo imaging of [^{123}I]β-CIT-FP or [^{123}I]β-CIT-FE was not detected in the thalamus, hypothalamus, or cerebral cortical areas, and the specific binding measured in the striatum was approx 10% less than that observed for [^{123}I]β-CIT. Considering that the ratio of 5-HT to DA terminals in the human striatum is approx 1:10, the 10% decrease probably corresponds to the decreased labeling of striatal serotonin transporters. The regional distribution for these radiotracers correlated well with the distribution of nigrostriatal and mesolimbic DAergic terminals and indicates that [^{123}I]β-CIT-FP and [^{123}I]β-CIT-FE (50,51) are highly promising imaging agents to assess the regulation of the DA transporter in vivo in human brain. In vitro and in vivo imaging techniques failed to detect DA transporters in neocortical regions known to receive DAergic projections, including the amygdala, hippocampus, frontal, cingulate, and entorhinal cortices. The lack of DA transporters in corticolimbic regions may be caused by the markedly lower densities of DA transporters in these brain areas, low sensitivity of the imaging agents, or, alternatively, may indicate the existence of a pharmacological subtype of DA transporter associated with mesocortical and mesolimbic projections. Understanding the effects of antidepressant drugs on corticolimbic DA transporters may be important for clarifying the role of the DA transporter in various neuropsychiatric disease states.

Regional Variability and the Effect of Age on the Human DA Transporter

Anatomical studies with different classes of radiolabeled DA transport inhibitors and cocaine congeners have demonstrated distinct subregional rostrocaudal, mediolateral, and dorsoventral gradients within the human striatum. For example, autoradiographic localization of [^{3}H]mazindol demonstrated the highest binding in ventral sectors of the striatum, with a decreasing rostral to caudal gradient in both the caudate and putamen (20). The gradient for [^{3}H]GBR 12935 binding has not been described in human brain. However, in the rat brain a decreasing rostral to caudal gradient was evident for striatal [^{3}H]GBR 12935 binding (90). Localization of [^{3}H]WIN 35,428 binding demonstrated an increasing medial to lateral and dorsal to ventral gradient, but binding was uniform throughout the anterior to posterior extent of the rat striatum (90). In the human brain, total [^{125}I]RTI-55 binding demonstrated a decreasing lateral to medial gradient and was uniform across the rostral to caudal boundaries of the human striatum. In contrast, when binding to the 5-HT transporter was occluded with citalopram, binding of [^{125}I]RTI-55 was high in the anterior sectors and lower in the posterior sectors of the striatum (77). A similar topographic pattern for the distribution of the DA transporter was visualized using [^{125}I]RTI-121 (81). The heterogeneity in topographic profiles obtained with different radioligands in the human striatum in vitro provides additional evidence to support the nonidentity of pharmacological sites associated with the DA transporter. One possibility is that DA transporters may be differentially regulated, depending upon their signaling rates within discrete anatomical target regions. Additional functional studies are needed to relate different patterns of radioligand binding to the DA transporter with parameters of DA neurotransmission and innervation from substantia nigra and ventral tegmental DAergic projection neurons.

Pharmacological heterogeneity for binding of the radiolabeled DA transport inhibitors may be caused by the labeling of binding sites that are not related to the DA transporter. A question has been raised regarding the DAergic nature of the diphenyl-substituted piperazine derivative ([³H]GBR 12935) binding in the human frontal cortex (3,5,6,37). Although DA is a potent inhibitor of [³H]GBR 12935 binding in the human striatum, it is inactive in inhibition assays conducted in the human frontal cortex (3,5,6). One possible explanation for these results is that DA and [³H]GBR 12935 binding reflects distinct, nonoverlapping binding domains on the DA transporter (34,35,35). However, this hypothesis fails to explain the ability of DA to compete for binding to DA transporters in the striatum, but not the frontal cortex. Pharmacological evidence suggests a profile for [³H]GBR 12935 binding to the frontal cortex consistent with that of the piperazine acceptor site on the cytochrome p450 complex (5,6). DA transport inhibitors exhibit significantly lower potencies for competition of [³H]GBR 12935 binding in the human frontal cortex and platelet membranes as compared to striatal membranes, however, piperazine analogs, including cis-flupentixol, proadifen, lobeline, budipine, and quinidine, inhibit [³H]GBR 12935 binding with potency values characteristic of the piperazine acceptor site in human frontal cortex. Ligand binding studies have shown that piperazine derivatives (GBR 12909 and GBR 12935) and antidepressants (buproprion and maprotiline) are substrates for cytochrome P450IID1 (debrisoquine 4-hydroxylase) (64). In the frontal cortex, the binding of [³H]GBR 12935 is biphasic, suggesting the involvement of multiple binding sites (35,36,37). The overall higher density of the piperazine acceptor sites in this brain region, and the high affinity of the GBR analogs for these sites, may render this radioligand unsuitable for assaying DA transporter regulation in the brain areas with low densities of DA transporter expression. The regional binding densities (B_{max}) reported for [³H]GBR 12935 binding do not correlate well with the distribution and overall densities of DA neuronal projections, providing additional evidence for the labeling of sites unrelated to the DA transporter. The distribution of cocaine congeners corresponds to the regional density of DA presynaptic markers, with the highest densities localized in the caudate and putamen, and significantly lower densities in the cerebral cortex. In contrast, the regional densities for [³H]GBR 12935 binding to the frontal cortex are equivalent to or higher than the density of DA transporters measured within the human striatum (*36*). Nonspecific binding of [³H]GBR 12935 in the frontal cortex, defined with different DA transport inhibitors, gives variable percentages of specific binding dependent on the choice of inhibitor (*5,6*). These results suggest that studies of [³H]GBR 12935 binding should be interpreted with caution, but may disclose some novel regional variability in specific properties of the transport carrier.

Little information about the effects of chronic cocaine exposure on the human brain DAergic system is currently available. Reductions in DA and DA-related synaptic markers in the striatum are known to contribute to the cognitive and motor deficits associated with normal aging. Although cocaine, unlike methamphetamine, does not appear to be neurotoxic in experimental animals (*47*), this question has not been fully resolved in the human. In the postmortem human striatum, a progressive decrease in DA transporter density with age has been demonstrated using [³H]GBR 12935 (*4,18,34,93*). Decreases in DA transporter density of 75 and 65% were reported for subjects ranging from 19–100 yr (*4*) and 18–88 yr (*18*), respectively. In vivo imaging of the DA transporter with cocaine and cocaine congeners ([¹¹C]cocaine [*86*] and [¹²³I]β-CIT [*84*] and the classical DA transport inhibitor [¹¹C]nomifensine [*82*]) also demonstrated a decline of DA transporters with increasing age. With [¹¹C]cocaine, a gradual decline in the density of cocaine recognition sites was detected over an age range of 21–63 yr (*86*). Using [¹²³I]β-CIT, a 51% decline in DA transporter density was observed over an age range of 18–83 yr (*84*). A decrease in the [¹¹C]nomifensine striatum/cerebellum ratios was observed over an age range of 24–81 yr (*82*). Taken together, in vivo imaging with a variety of radiotracers demonstrates age-related declines in DA transporter density that occur at a rate of approximately 10% per decade. It is unclear whether or not chronic cocaine abuse may lead to accelerated aging of DAergic neurons or that aging cocaine addicts may be at increased risk for neuroleptic-induced extrapyramidal disturbances. Neuropsychiatric sequelae of cocaine abuse are frequently treated with neuroleptic medications, and Parkinsonism and acute dystonia have been precipitated in cocaine addicts by DA receptor antagonists (*17,53,73*). One of the long-term consequences of psychostimulant abuse is withdrawal-emergent psychopathology, including depression and anhedonia, that could be related to a brain DA deficiency.

In keeping with the marked decline in DA transporters with normal aging, studies of the mRNA encoding the DA transporter demonstrated a profound loss of DA transporter gene expression in DA-containing substantia nigra neurons with increasing age (10). Although a precipitous age-related decline (>95% in subjects >57 old) was reported for DA transporter mRNA, the mRNA for tyrosine hydroxylase (another phenotypic marker of DA neurons) decreased linearly with age (62). The abrupt decline in the DA transporter at the end of the fifth decade was surprising, considering that the decrease in DA transporter density was linear over the lifespan. This difference may reflect differential regulation of DA transporter mRNA and protein with normal aging. However, additional studies with more subjects may disclose a decline in DA transporter message that more closely correlates with the decrease in DA transporter densities.

At present, it is not known if this decline in DA transporter density corresponds to a loss of DA nerve terminals or to a decrease in the number of DA transporters expressed by aging DAergic neurons. Comparable changes in DAergic pre- and postsynaptic markers and DA transporter densities suggest that the decline in DA transporter labeling may be caused by reduced integrity of DAergic projections (18). Age-related decreases have been shown for tyrosine hydroxylase (62), striatal DA content (2,38), and D1 and D2 receptors (18). This decrease in DA synaptic markers suggests that the observed decrease in DA transporter density with normal aging may be caused by actual decline of DA neurons. Alternatively, if the DA transporter is regulated by synaptic DA content, the decrease in DA transporter density may be a compensatory response to the age-related decline in neuronal DA content, with correspondingly abnormal rates of DA turnover. The marked decline in striatal DA transporter density with normal aging clearly demonstrates the importance of choosing well age-matched control subjects for assessing the effects of chronic cocaine abuse on the neuroadaptive regulation of synaptic DA transporters in cohorts of cocaine addicts.

Regulatory Changes in the Human DA Transporter by Cocaine Abuse

New tools from the neurosciences have led to proliferation of research approaches aimed at understanding the neurobiological consequences of chronic cocaine use on the human brain. The recent development of radioligands with high specific activity and selectivity for neurotransmitter carriers have provided the tools necessary to map and quantify neuroadaptations to cocaine exposure in postmortem brain from cocaine abusers. Since the DA transporter is a key regulator of DA neurotransmission, alterations in the number, affinity, or allosteric regulation of the DA transporter by cocaine may lead to marked alterations in DA-ergic signaling. Understanding the sites of cocaine actions in the brain, and the acute and long-term neurobiological effects, may help shed light on the clinical relevance of regulatory changes in DA transporter function to the behavioral effects of chronic cocaine use.

The cocaine congeners [^{3}H]WIN 35,428 and [^{125}I]RTI-55 have been used to visualize the regional density of DA transporters postmortem in the human brain from victims of fatal cocaine overdose and cocaine-related deaths caused by homicide and motor vehicle accidents. Postmortem radioligand binding and autoradiographic studies demonstrated significant increases in DA transporter densities, using the cocaine congeners [^{125}I]RTI-55 and [^{3}H]WIN 35,428 throughout the caudate, putamen, and nucleus accumbens from cocaine-related deaths (55) and fatal cocaine overdose victims (Figs. 3 and 4 [78,79]). Saturation binding analysis confirmed the increase in [^{3}H]WIN 35,428 binding to putamen membranes of cocaine overdose victims, as compared to drug-free and age-matched control subjects (78,79). Rosenthal plots of the saturation binding data demonstrated that the increase of [^{3}H]WIN 35,428 binding observed in the cocaine overdose victims was caused by an elevation in the apparent density of the high affinity cocaine recognition site on the DA transporter (78,79). The elevations in DA transporter densities demonstrated in the postmortem brain from human cocaine abusers have been confirmed by in vivo SPECT imaging in human cocaine-dependent subjects (60). The striatal uptake of [^{123}I]β-CIT (also called RTI-55) was significantly elevated (25%) in acutely abstinent (≥96 h) cocaine-dependent subjects (Fig. 5). These studies suggest that the high-affinity cocaine binding site may upregulate in the human striatum with chronic cocaine abuse as a compensatory response to elevated synaptic levels of DA. This compensatory effect on the DA transporter may result in an acute decrease in the intrasynaptic concentration of DA following cocaine challenge. If this regulatory change in high-affinity [^{3}H] WIN 35,428 binding sites on the human DA transporter actually reflects an increased ability of the protein to transport DA, it may help to explain the addictive liability of cocaine. As the transporter upregulates its apparent density in the nerve terminal to more effi-

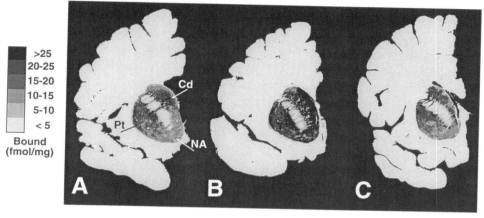

Fig. 3. Elevated densities of [³H]WIN 35,428 binding to the DA transporter in human cocaine overdose victims. (**A–C**) Gray scale images of [³H]WIN 35,428 labeling in coronal sections of a drug-free control subject; cocaine overdose victim; and excited delirium victim. A marked increase in the density of [³H]WIN 35,428 binding was observed throughout the ventral sectors of the anterior striatum in the cocaine overdose victim, as compared to a drug-free, age-matched control subject. The gray-scale bar at the left depicts the relationship between the [³H]WIN 35,428 binding site density (fmol/mg of tissue equivalent) and the gray scale intensity.

ciently transport DA, more cocaine will be needed to experience cocaine's reinforcing effects and euphoria. Once cocaine is no longer present to block reuptake, increased DA transport will result in a net DA deficit in the synapse, which may explain the reports of anhedonia associated with the post-cocaine crash.

In contrast to the elevated densities of DA transporters seen with radiolabeled cocaine congeners, [³H]mazindol binding was lower in the caudate and putamen from cocaine-related death victims, as compared to age-matched and drug-free controls (*39*). The different regulatory profile seen with [³H]mazindol binding provides additional evidence for the nonidentity of different classes of DA transporter radioligands. Consistent with this view, previous studies in rats have also failed to demonstrate significant changes with chronic administration of cocaine in the binding of noncocaine-like dopamine transport inhibitors, including [³H]nomifensine (*65*), [³H]GBR 12935 (*41,42,52,92*), and [³H]mazindol (Mash, unpublished observations). Many experimental cocaine treatment paradigms have been developed as animal models of human cocaine abuse and it has been reported that the dose, route, and frequency of administration influ-

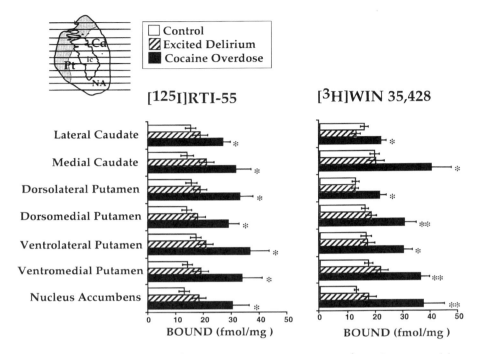

Fig. 4. Region-of-interest densitometric measurements of cocaine recognition sites in striatum of human cocaine overdose victims with and without pretermi-nal excited delirium and drug-free control subjects. The density of DA trans-porter in the striatum was assessed by using [^{125}I]RTI-55 (50 pM); 2 nM [^{3}H]WIN 35,428. Values (fmol/mg of tissue equivalent) representing the mean (±SE) for drug-free control subjects (white bars), cocaine overdose (black bars), and excited delirium victims (stripped bars) are shown. The drawing in the upper left hand corner illustrates in diagrammatic form the regional sites sampled from the autoradiograms at the anterior level of the striatum. The quantitative densitometric measurements demonstrate elevated [^{3}H]WIN 35,428 and [^{125}I] RTI-55 binding throughout the anterior sectors of the striatum in the cocaine overdose deaths (*$p < 0.01$; **$p < 0.001$). Cd, caudate; ic, internal capsule; na, nucleus accumbens; Pt, putamen. Part of the data reproduced with permission from ref. 78.)

ence the effects of chronic cocaine on DA transporter densities. Chronic treatment of rats with intermittent doses of cocaine demon-strated a two to five-fold increase in the apparent density of [^{3}H]cocaine and [^{3}H]BTCP binding in the striatum (1). Rats allowed to self-administer cocaine in a chronic unlimited access paradigm had significant increases in [^{3}H]WIN 35,428 binding observed when the

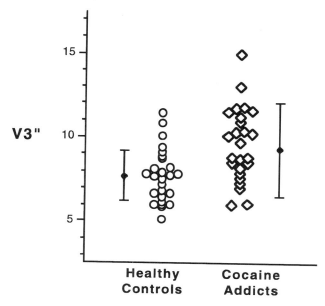

Fig. 5. Scatterplot illustrating the [^{123}I]β-CIT binding in cocaine abusers and drug-free control subjects. Subjects received a bolus injection of 9.5 ± 1.4 mCi [^{123}I]β-CIT followed by SPECT imaging on d 2. The ratio of specific to nonspecific activity [(striatal-occipital)/occipital], a measure known as the specific to nonspecific equilibrium partition coefficient (V3″) and proportional to the binding potential (B_{max}/K_d), was used to estimate differences in DA transporter levels between groups. Results showed significantly ($p = 0.02$; unpaired two-tailed t-test) increased V3″ values (mean ± SD) in cocaine addicts (9.6 ± 2.1) vs healthy controls (7.8 ± 1.6). Courtesy of Robert T. Malison (Yale University School of Medicine).

animals were sacrificed on the last day of cocaine access (*90*). Rabbits and mice treated chronically with cocaine show an elevation in the density of [^{3}H] WIN 35,428 binding sites in the caudate (*7,48*). Taken together, these results demonstrate that cocaine exposure leads to an apparent increase in the density of high-affinity cocaine binding sites on the DA transporter, but not the recognition sites for noncocaine-like DA transport inhibitors.

Regulatory changes in DA transporter densities have been visualized in parallel with different classes of DA transport inhibitors. In the brains of animals allowed to self-administer cocaine for 7 wk and sacrificed on the last day of access to cocaine, binding of [^{3}H]WIN 35,428 and [^{3}H]GBR 12935 to the DA transporter were elevated throughout the rostral sectors of the caudate-putamen and nucleus accumbens (90). In the cell body fields (substantia nigra and VTA), binding of both radioligands was elevated; however, only the density of [³H]GBR 12935 binding reached significance. After a 3 wk withdrawal period, [³H]WIN 35,428 binding to the DA transporter returned to baseline levels throughout the caudate, putamen, substantia nigra, and VTA, and was decreased significantly in the nucleus accumbens. In contrast, [³H]GBR 12935 binding was significantly decreased throughout all sectors of the striatum. Similar decreases were reported in previous studies of cocaine withdrawal models (23,76). The results demonstrate that different patterns of DA transporter regulation are observed with cocaine-like and nonocaine-like DA transport inhibitors with chronic cocaine adminstration. The time since the last cocaine administration has a marked effect on measurements of DA transporter density.

In keeping with these findings, in vivo SPECT measurements of DA transporter densities in cocaine abusers vary, depending on the time since the last cocaine administration. When the DA transporter was imaged in vivo after periods of drug abstinence, [¹²³I]β-CIT measures were still elevated, but decreased in their level of statistical significance (60). Initial imaging studies with [¹²³I]β-CIT in cocaine-dependent subjects abstinent for 3–18 mo demonstrated a significant trend toward a return to baseline densities measured in drug-free control subjects. In another study, chronic cocaine abusers had significantly lower [¹¹C]cocaine uptake in the basal ganglia and thalamus when screened 10–90 d after the last use of cocaine (85). The uptake of [¹¹C]cocaine was negatively correlated with cocaine craving and with depressive symptoms, suggesting an association between withdrawal symptoms and DA transporter densities. The results of human and rodent studies suggest that the DA transporter upregulates in response to acute binges of cocaine administration, but may gradually normalize or decrease with long periods of drug abstinence. The decrease in DA transporter densities in the striatal reward centers suggests that decreased DA transporter densities may reflect lower DAergic tone. A hypo-DAergic state may be one of the triggers of cocaine craving during abstinence that causes the addict to relapse to previous patterns of drug use.

A case series of cocaine overdose victims who died following a syndrome of excited delirium was first described in 1985 (89). We have compared the regulatory patterns of DA transporter in fatal cocaine overdose victims to the excited delirium subgroup, using ligand binding and in vitro autoradiography. Autoradiographic mapping with a single concentration of [³H]WIN 35,428 and [¹²⁵I]RTI-55 failed to demonstrate an elevation in the apparent density of the DA transporter in the striatum (Figs. 3c and 4; [78,80]) of excited delirium subjects, as compared to drug-free and age-matched control subjects. Rosenthal analysis of saturation binding curves for [³H]WIN 35,428 and [¹²⁵I]RTI-55 demonstrated a significant decrease in total binding sites for the excited delirium subgroup of cocaine overdose victims. Analysis of curvilinear Rosenthal plots demonstrated that there was no change in the apparent density of the high-affinity cocaine recognition site in the excited delirium victims, as compared to age-matched and drug-free control subjects. However, the density of the low-affinity cocaine recognition site was significantly decreased in the excited delirium victims (78,80). We have speculated that the differential regulation of cocaine recognition sites on the DA transporter in the excited delirium subgroup may indicate a diminished capacity for DA reuptake during a cocaine challenge or short-term binge use. Since the concentration of synaptic dopamine is controlled by the reuptake mechanism(s), the lack of a compensatory increase in cocaine recognition sites could be the molecular defect that explains the paranoia and agitation associated with this syndrome. Paranoia in the context of cocaine abuse is common and several lines of evidence suggest that this phenomenon may be related to the function of the DA transporter protein (28). Genetic differences in the makeup of individuals who abuse cocaine may underlie some of these differences in susceptibility to adverse neuropsychiatric effects of chronic cocaine abuse.

Clinical Relevance of DA Transporter Regulation for Understanding Cocaine Addiction

A unique advantage of in vivo imaging is that drug interactions within the brain can be assessed while simultaneously monitoring the behavioral effects and the plasma bioavailability of the drug (87). In vivo imaging with [¹¹C]cocaine has demonstrated that the time-course of cocaine binding to the striatum correlates with the onset of the euphoric experience (16,24). These studies support the hypothesis that the high or euphoria induced by psychostimulants is related to the rapid occupancy of DA transporter and the corresponding rise in the synaptic concentration of DA (87). Similar studies with [¹¹C]dl-*threo*-methylphenidate also demonstrated rapid uptake, which correlates with the onset of the behavioral effects. When compared to [^{11}C]cocaine, [^{11}C]dl-*threo*-methylphenidate exhibited slower clearance from the striatum. Since methylphenidate has lower abuse liability compared to cocaine, it is possible that kinetic differences in the rates of occupancy of the DA transporter by [^{11}C]dl-*threo*-methylphenidate may explain the lack of the euphoriant rush and lower arousal (*19*). Rothman (*71*) suggested that DA transport inhibitors with slow rates of entry into the brain and slow onset of action may be candidate drugs for treating cocaine dependence.

The investigation of compounds to reduce cocaine use by diminishing craving and reducing withdrawal symptoms have received the most attention in recent years (*46,88*). Although there is still controversy regarding the long-term sequelae of chronic cocaine abuse, pharmacological treatment strategies have been based on the assumption that chronic cocaine abuse leads to neuroadaptive changes in the sensitivity of DA pre- and postsynaptic markers, with increased DA turnover and a resultant DA depletion (*17,27*). The compensatory increase in high-affinity cocaine recognition sites on the human DA transporter may indicate an enhanced ability of cocaine to inhibit DA transport in chronic cocaine users. An elevation in [^{3}H]methylphenidate binding to the DA transporter has been shown to occur as early as 1 h after the acute administration of cocaine to drug-naive rats (*74*), indicating that DA transporters may undergo rapid regulatory changes in the membrane to regulate synaptic levels of neurotransmitter. Persistent increases in the apparent density of the DA transporter after cocaine levels have fallen in blood and brain may result in an acute decrease in the intrasynaptic concentration of DA and lower DAergic tone. If this regulatory change in high-affinity [^{3}H] WIN 35,428 binding sites on the human DA transporter reflects increased DA transporter function, it may help to explain the addictive liability of cocaine. As the transporter carrier upregulates its apparent density in the nerve terminal to more efficiently transport DA, more cocaine will be needed to experience the reinforcing effects and euphoria. During acute abstinence from cocaine, enhanced function of the DA transporter could lead to net depletion in synaptic DA. This depletion of DA may serve as a biological substrate for anhedonia, the cardinal feature of cocaine withdrawal symptomatology. Further studies are needed to define the relevance of cocaine-induced alterations in radioligand binding sites to the molecular mechanisms regulating DA transporter function. The newly developed tools to map and characterize the regulation and function of the DA transporter will clarify the definite role of the DA transporter in cocaine addiction.

Acknowledgments

This work was funded by grants from the National Institute on Drug Abuse (DA 06227 and DA 09484). We are grateful to Michael H. Baumann for his helpful discussion and editorial comments on this chapter.

References

1. Alburges, M. E., Narang, N., and Wamsley, J. K. Alterations in the dopaminergic receptor system after chronic administration of cocaine. *Synapse* **14** (1993) 314–323.

2. Adolfsson, R., Gottfries, C.-G., Roos, B.-E., and Winblad, B. Post-mortem distribution of dopamine and homovanillic acid in human brain, variations related to age, and a review of the literature. *J. Neural Transm.* **45** (1979) 81–105.

3. Allard P. Questions about the dopaminergic nature of [^{3}H]GBR 12935 binding in the human frontal cortex. *J. Neurochem.* **63** (1994) 1182,1183.

4. Allard, P. and Marcusson, J. O. Age-correlated loss of dopamine uptake sites with [^{3}H]GBR 12935 in human putamen. *Neurobiol. Aging* **10** (1989) 661–664.

5. Allard, P., Marcusson, J. O., and Ross, S. B. [^{3}H]GBR 12935 binding to cytochrome P450 in the human brain. *J. Neurochem.* **62** (1994) 342–348.

6. Allard, P., Danielsson, M., Papworth, K., and Marcusson, J. O. [^{3}H]GBR 12935 binding to human cerebral cortex is not to dopamine uptake sites. *J. Neurochem.* **62** (1994) 338–341.

7. Aloyo, V. J., Harvey, J. A., and Kirifides, A. L. Chronic cocaine increases WIN 35,428 binding in rabbit caudate. *Soc. Neurosci. Abstr.* **19** (1993) 1843.

8. Aquilonius, S. M., Bergstrom, K., Eckernas, S. A., Hartvig, P., Leenders, K. L., Lundquist, H., Antoni, G., Gee, A., Rimland, A., Uhlin, J., and Langstrom, B. In vivo evaluation of striatal dopamine reuptake sites using ^{11}C-nomifensine and positron emission tomography. *Acta Neurol. Scand.* **76** (1987) 283–287.

9. Baker S. P. *The Injury Fact Book.* 2nd ed. Oxford University Press, New York, 1992.

10. Bannon, M. J., Poosch, M. S., Xia, Y., Goebel, D. J., Cassin, B., and Kapatos, G. Dopamine transporter mRNA content in human substantia nigra decreases precipitously with age. *Proc. Natl. Acad. Sci.* USA **89** (1992) 7095–7099.

11. Biegon, A., Dillon, K., Volkow, N. D., Hitzemann, R. J., Fowler, J. S., and Wolf, A. P. Quantitative autoradiography of cocaine binding sites in human brain postmortem. *Synapse* **10** (1992) 126–130.

12. Bjorklund, A. and Lindvall, O. Dopamine-containing systems in the CNS. In Bjorklund, A. and Hokfelt , T. (eds.) *Handbook of Chemical Neuroanatomy, Vol. 2, Classical Transmitters in the CNS, Part I*, Elsevier, New York, 1994, pp. 55–122.

13. Boja, J. W., Markham, L., Patel, A., Uhl, G., and Kuhar, M. J. Expression of a single dopamine transporter cDNA can confer two cocaine binding sites. *Neuro. Rep.* **3** (1992) 247,248.

14. Boja, J. W. Vaughen, R., Patel A., Shaya, E. K., and Kuhar, M. J. The dopamine transporter. In Niznik, H. (ed.), *Dopamine Receptors and Transporters.* Dekker, New York (1994), pp. 611–644.
15. Buck, K. J. and Amara, S. G. Chimeric dopamine-norepinephrine transporters delineate structural domains influencing selectivity for catecholamines and 1-methyl-4-phenylpyridinium. *Proc. Natl. Acad. Sci. USA* **91** (1994) 12,584–12,588.
16. Cook, C. E., Jeffcoat, A. R., and Perez-Reyes, M. Pharmacokinetic studies of cocaine and phencyclidine in man. In Barnett, G. and Chiang, C. N. (eds) *Pharmacokinetics and Pharmacodynamics of Psychoactive Drugs*, Biomedical, Foster City, CA, 1985, pp. 48–74.
17. Dackis, C. A. and Gold, M. S. Bromocriptine as a treatment of cocaine abuse. *Lancet* **1** (1985) 1151,1152.
18. DeKeyser, J., Ebinger, G., and Vauquelin, G. Age-related changes in the human nigrostriatal dopaminergic system. *Ann. Neurol.* **27** (1990) 157–161.
19. Ding, Y.-S., Fowler, J. S., Volkow, N. D., Gatley, S. J., Logan, J., Dewey, S. L., Alexoff, D., Fazzini, E., and Wolf, A. P. Pharmacokinetics and in vivo specificity of [^{11}C]dl-threo-methylphenidate for the presynaptic dopaminergic neuron. *Synapse* **18** (1994) 152–160.
20. Donnan, G. A., Kaczmarczyk, S. J., Paxinos, G., Chilco, P. J., Kalnins, R. M., Woodhouse, D. G., and Mendelsohn, F. A. O. Distribution of catecholamine uptake sites in human brain as determined by quantitative [^{3}H]mazindol autoradiography. *J. Comp. Neurol.* **304** (1991) 419–434.
21. Eshleman, A. J., Neve, R. L., Janowsky, A., and Neve, K. A. Characterization of a recombinant human dopamine transporter in multiple cell lines. *J. Pharm. Exp. Therap.* **274** (1995) 276–283.
22. Farde, L., Halldin, C., Muller, L., Suhara, T., Karlsson, P., and Hall, H. PET Study of [^{11}C]β-CIT binding to monoamine transporters in the monkey and human brain. *Synapse* **16** (1994) 93–103.
23. Farfel, G. M., Kleven, M. S., Woolverton, W. L., Seiden, L. S., and Perry, B. D. Effects of repeated injections of cocaine on catecholamine receptor binding sites, dopamine transporter binding sites and behavior in rhesus monkey. *Brain Res.* **578** (1992) 235–243.
24. Fowler, J. S., Volkow, N. D., Wolf, A. P., Dewey, S. L., Schyler, D. J., Macgregor, R. R., Hitzemann, R., Logan, J., Bendrien, B., Gatley, S. J., and Christman, D. Mapping cocaine binding sites in human and baboon brain in vivo. *Synapse* **4** (1989) 371–377.
25. Galloway, M. P. Neurochemical interactions of cocaine with the dopaminergic system. *Trends Pharmacol. Sci.* **9** (1988) 451–454.
26. Gatley, S. J., Volkow, N. D., Fowler, J. S., Dewey, S. L., and Logan, J. Sensitivity of striatal [^{11}C]cocaine binding to decreases in synaptic dopamine. *Synapse* **20** (1995) 137–144.
27. Gawin, F. H. and Ellinwood, E. H. Cocaine and other stimulants. *N. Engl. J. Med.* **318** (1988) 1173–1182.
28. Gerlernter, J., Kranzler, H. R., Satel, S. L., and Rao, P. A. Genetic association between dopamine transporter protein alleles and cocaine-induced paranoia. *Neuropsychopharmacology* **11** (1994) 195–200.
29. Giros, B. and Caron, M. G. Molecular characterization of the dopamine transporter. *Trends Pharmacol. Sci.* **14** (1993) 43–49.

30. Giros, B., Mestikawy, S. E., Godinot, N., Zheng, K., Han, H., Yan-Feng, T., and Caron, M. G. Cloning, pharmacological characterization and chromosome assignment of the human dopamine transporter. *Mol. Pharm.* **42** (1992) 383–390.

31. Giros, B., Wang, Y. M., Suter, S., McLeskey, S. B., Pifl, C., and Caron, M. G. Delineation of discrete domains for substrate, cocaine, and tricyclic antidepressant interactions using chimeric dopamine-norepinephrine transporters. *J. Biol. Chem.* **269** (1994) 15,985–15,988.

32. Graybiel, A. M. and Moratalla, R. Dopamine uptake sites in the striatum are distributed differentially in striosome and matrix compartments. *Proc. Natl. Acad. Sci.* **86** (1989) 9020–9024.

33. Graybiel, A. M. and Ragsdale, C. W. Histochemically distinct compartments in the striatum of human, monkey and cat demonstrated by acetylcholinesterase staining. *Proc. Natl. Acad. Sci. USA* **75** (1978) 5723–5726.

34. Hitri, A., Casanove, M. F., Kleinman, J. E., Weinberger, D. R., and Wyatt, R. J. Age-related changes in [³H]GBR 12935 binding site density in the prefrontal cortex of controls and schizophrenics. *Biol. Psych.* **37** (1995) 175–182.

35. Hitri, A., Hurd, Y. L., Wyatt, R. J., and Deutsch, S. I. Molecular, functional, and biochemical characteristics of the dopamine transporter: regional differences and clinical relevance. *Clin. Neuropharm.* **17** (1994) 1–22.

36. Hitri, A., Venable, D., Nguyen, H. Q., Casanova, M. F., Kleinman, J. E., and Wyatt, R. J. Characteristics of [³H]GBR 12935 binding in the human and rat frontal cortex. *J. Neurochem.* **56** (1991) 1663–1672.

37. Hitri, A. and Wyatt, R. J. Questions about the dopaminergic nature of [³H]GBR 12935 binding in the human frontal cortex. *J. Neurochem.* **63** (1994) 1181–1182.

38. Hornykiewicz O. Dopamine changes in the aging human brain. In Agnoli, A., Grepaldi, G., Spano P. F., and Trabucchi, M. (eds.) *Aging Brain and Ergot Alkaloids*, Vol. 23, Raven, New York, 1983, pp. 9–14.

39. Hurd, Y. L. and Herkanham, M. Molecular alterations in the neostriatum of human cocaine addicts. *Synapse* **13** (1993) 357–369.

40. Hurd, Y. L., Pristupa, Z. B. Herman, M. M., Niznik, H. B., and Kleinman, J. E. The dopamine transporter and dopamine D2 receptor messenger RNAs are differentially expressed in limbic- and motor-related subpopulations of human mesencephalic neurons. *Neuroscience* **63** (1994) 357–362.

41. Izenwasser, S. and Cox, B. M. Daily cocaine treatment produces a persistent reduction of [³H]dopamine uptake in vitro in rat nucleus accumbens but not in the striatum. *Brain Res.* **531** (1990) 338–341.

42. Katz, J. L., Griffiths, J. W., Sharpe, L. G., De Souza, E. B., and Witkin, J. M. Cocaine tolerance and cross-tolerance. *J. Pharm. Exp. Ther.* **264** (1993) 183–192.

43. Kaufman, M. J. and Madras, B. K. Severe depletion of cocaine recognition sites associated with the dopamine transporter in Parkinson's diseased striatum. *Synapse* **9** (1991) 43–49.

44. Kitayama, S., Shimada, S., Xu, H., Markham, L., Donovan, D. M., and Uhl, G. R. Dopamine transporter site-directed mutations differentially alter substrate transport and cocaine binding. *Proc. Natl. Acad. Sci. USA* **89** (1992) 7782–7785.

45. Kitayama, S., Wang, J.-B., and Uhl, G. R. Dopamine transporter mutants selectively enhance MPP+ transport. *Synapse* **15** (1993) 58–62.

46. Kleber, H. D. Pharmacotherapy, current and potential, for the treatment of cocaine dependence. *Clin. Neuropharm.* **18** (1995) S96–S109.

47. Kleven, M. S., Woolverton, W. L., and Seiden, L. S. Lack of long-term monoamine depletions following repeated or continuous exposure to cocaine. *Brain. Res. Bull.* **21** (1988) 233–237.

48. Koff, J. M., Shuster, L., and Miller, L. G. Chronic cocaine administration is associated with behavioral sensitization and time-dependent changes in striatal dopamine transporter binding. *J. Pharm. Exp. Ther.* **268** (1994) 277–282.

49. Kuhar, M. J., Ritz, M. C., and Boja, J. W. The dopamine hypothesis of the reinforcing properties of cocaine. *TINS* **14** (1991) 299–302.

50. Kuikka, J. T., Akerman, K., Bergstrom, K. A., Karhu, J., Hiltunen, J., Haukka, J., Heikkinen, J., Tiihonen, J., Wang, S., and Neumeyer, J. L. Iodine-123 labelled N-(2-fluoroethyl)-2β-carbomethoxy-3β-(4-iodophenyl)nortropane for dopamine transporter imaging in the living human brain. *Eur. J. Nuc. Med.* **22** (1995) 682–686.

51. Kuikka, J. T., Bergstrom, K. A., Ahonen, A., Hiltunen, J., Haukka, J., Lansimies, E., Wang, S., and Neumeyer, J. L. Comparison of iodine-123 labelled 2β-carbomethoxy-3β-(4-iodophenyl)tropane and iodine-123 labelled 2β-carbomethoxy-3β-(4-iodophenyl)-N-(3-fluoropropyl)nortropane for imaging of the dopamine transporter in the living human brain. *Eur. J. Nuclear Med.* **22** (1995) 356–360.

52. Kula, N. S. and Baldessarini, R. J. Lack of increase in dopamine transporter binding or function in rat brain tissue after treatment with blockers of neuronal uptake of dopamine. *Neuropharmacology* **30** (1991) 89–92.

53. Kumor, K. Sherer M., and Jaffe, J. Haloperidol-induced dystonia in cocaine addicts. *Lancet* **ii** (1986) 1341, 1342.

54. Little, K. Y., Carroll, F. I., and Cassin, B. J. Characterization and localization of [125I]RTI-121 binding sites in human striatum and medial temporal lobe. *J. Pharmacol. Exp. Ther.* **274** (1995) 1474–1483.

55. Little, K. Y., Kirkman, J. A., Carroll, F. I., Breese, G. R., and Duncan, G. E. [125I]RTI-55 bindng to cocaine-sensitive dopaminergic and serotonergic uptake sites in the human brain. *J. Neurochem.* **61** (1993) 1996–2006.

56. Little, K. Y., Kirkman, J. A., Carroll, F. I., Clark, T. B., and Duncan, G. E. Cocaine use increases [3H]WIN 35,428 binding sites in human striatum. *Brain Res.* **628** (1993) 17–25.

57. Lowenstein, P. R., Joyce, J. N., Coyle, J. T., and Marshall, J. F. Striosomal organization of cholinerigic and dopaminergic uptake sites and cholinergic M1 receptors in the adult human striatum: a quantitative receptor autoradiographic study. *Brain Res.* **510** (1990) 122–126.

58. Madras, B. K. and Kaufman, M. J. Cocaine accumulates in dopamine-rich region of primate brain after i.v. administration: comparison with mazindol distribution. *Synapse* **18** (1994) 261–275.

59. Madras, B. K., Spealman, R. D., Fahey, M. A., Neumeyer, J. L., Saha, J. K., and Milius, R. A. Cocaine receptors labeled by [3H]2β-carbomethoxy-3β-(4-fluorophenyl)tropane. *Mol. Pharmacol.* **36** (1989) 518–524.

60. Malison, R. SPECT imaging of DA transporters in cocaine dependence with [123I]β-CIT. *NIDA Res. Monogr.* **152** (1995) 60.

61. Marcusson J. and Ericksson K. [3H]GBR 12935 binding to dopamine uptake sites in the human brain. *Brain Res.* **457** (1988) 122–129.

62. McGeer, P. L., McGeer, E. G., and Suzuki, J. S. Aging and extrapyramidal function. *Arch Neurol.* **34** (1977) 33–35.

63. Neumeyer, J. L., Wang, S., Gao, Y., Milius, R. A., Kula, N. S., Campbell, A., Baldessarini, R. J., Zea-Ponce, Y., Baldwin, R. M., and Innis, R. B. N-w-Fluoroalkyl analogs of (1R)-2β-carbomethoxy-3β-(4-iodophenyl)-tropane (β-CIT): radiotracers for positron emission tomography and single photon emission tomography and single photon emission computed tomography imaging of dopamine transporters. *J. Med Chem.* **37** (1994) 1558–1561.

64. Niznik, H. B., Tyndale, R. F., Sallee, F. R., Gonzalez, F. J., Hardwick, J. P., Inaba, T., and Kalow, W. The dopamine transporter and cytochrome p450IIDI (debrisoquine 4-hydroxylase) in brain: resolution and identification of two distinct [³H]GBR 12935 binding proteins. *Arch. Biochem. Biophys.* **276** (1990) 424–432.

65. Peris, J., Boyson, S. J., Cass, W. A., Curella, R., Dwoskin, L. P., Larson, G., Lin, L.-H., Yasuda, R. P., and Zahinser, N. R. Persistence of neurochemical changes in dopamine systems after repeated cocaine administration. *J. Pharmacol. Exp. Therap.* **253** (1990) 38–44.

66. Pirker, W., Asenbaum, S., Kasper, S., Walter, H., Angellberger, P., Koc, G., Pozzera, A., Deecke, L., Podreka, I., and Brucke, T. β-CIT SPECT demonstrates blockade of 5HT-uptake sites by citalopram in the human brain in vivo. *J. Neural Transm.* **100** (1995) 247–256.

67. Pristupa, Z. B., Wilson, J. M., Hoffman, B. J., Kish, S. J., and Niznik, H. B. Pharmacological heterogeneity of the cloned and native human dopamine transporter: dissociation of [³H]WIN 35,428 and [³H]GBR 12935 binding. *Mol. Pharm.* **45** (1994) 125–135.

68. Reith, M. E. A., De Cosata, B., Rice, K. C., and Jacobsen, A. E. Evidence for mutually exclusive binding of cocaine, BTCP, GBR 12935, and dopamine to the dopamine transporter. *Eur. J. Pharmacol.* **227** (1992) 417–425.

69. Reith, M. E. A. and Selmeci, G. Radiolabeling of dopamine uptake sites in mouse striatum—comparision of bindings sites for cocaine, mazindol, and GBR 12935. *Naunyn-Schmeidebergs Arch. Pharmacol.* **345** (1992) 309–318.

70. Ritz, M. C., Lamb, R. J., Goldberg, S. R., and Kuhar, M. J. Cocaine receptors of dopamine transporters are related to self-administration of cocaine. *Science* **237** (1987) 1219–1223.

71. Rothman, R. B. High affinity dopamine reuptake inhibitors as potential cocaine antagonists: a strategy for drug development. *Life Sci.* **46** (1990) PL17–PL21.

72. Salmon, E., Brooks, D. J., Leenders, K. L., Turton, D. R., Hume, S. P., Cremer, J. E., Jones, T., and Frackowiak, R. S. J. A two-compartment description and kinetic procedure for measuring regional cerebral [¹¹C]nomifensine uptake using positron emission tomography. *J. Cereb. Blood Flow Metab.* **10** (1990) 307–316.

73. Satel, S. L. and Swann, S. C. Extrapyramidal symptoms and cocaine abuse. *Am. J. Psychiat.* **150** (1993) 347.

74. Schweri, M. M. Rapid increase of stimulant binding to the dopamine transporter after acute cocaine administration: physiological basis of drug craving. *Soc. Neurosci. Abstr.* **19** (1993) 936.

75. Seibyl, J. P., Wallace, E., Smith, E. O., Stabin, M., Baldwin, R. M., Zoghbi, S., Zea-Ponce, Y., Gao, Y., Zhang, W. Y., Neumeyer, J. L., Zubal, G., Charney, D. S., Hoffer, P. B., and Innis, R. B. Whole-body biodistribution, radiation absorbed dose and brain SPECT imaging with iodine-123——CIT in healthy human subjects. *J. Nuclear Med.* **35** (1994) 764–770.

76. Sharpe, L. G., Pilotte, N. S., Mitchell, W. M., and De Souza, E. B. Withdrawal of repeated cocaine decreases autoradiographic [^{3}H]mazindol-labelling of dopamine transporter in rat nucleus accumbens. *Eur. J. Pharm.* **203** (1991) 141–144.

77. Staley, J. K., Basile, M., Flynn, D. D., and Mash, D. C. Visualizing dopamine and serotonin transporters in the human brain with the potent cocaine analogue [^{125}I]RTI-55: In vitro binding and autoradiographic characterization. *J. Neurochem.* **62** (1994) 549–556.

78. Staley, J. K., Basile, M., Wetli, C. V., Hearn, W. L., Flynn, D. D., Ruttenber, A. J., and Mash, D. C. Differential regulation of the dopamine transporter in cocaine overdose deaths. *NIDA Res. Monogr.* **141** (1994) 32.

79. Staley, J. K., Hearn, W. L., Ruttenber, A. J., Wetli, C. V., and Mash, D. C. High affinity cocaine recognition sites on the dopamine transporter are elevated in fatal cocaine overdose victims. *J. Pharm. Exp. Therap.* **271** (1995) 1678–1685.

80. Staley, J. K., Wetli, C. V., Ruttenber, A. J., Hearn, W. L., and Mash, D. C. Altered dopaminergic synaptic markers in cocaine psychosis and sudden death. *NIDA Res. Monogr.* 153:491 (1995).

81. Staley, J. K., Boja, J. W., Carroll, F. I., Seltzman, H. H., Wyrick, C. D., Lewin, A. H., Abraham, P., and Mash, D. C. Mapping dopamine transporters in the human brain with novel selective cocaine analog [^{125}I]RTI-121. *Synapse* **21** (1995) 364–372.

82. Tedroff, J., Aquilonius, S. M., Hartvig, P., Lundquist, H., Gee, A. G., Uhlin, J., and Langstrom, B. Monoamine reuptake sites in the human brain evaluated in vivo by means of [^{11}C]nomifensine and positron emission tomography: the effects of age and Parkinson's disease. *Acta Neurol. Scand.* **77** (1988) 192–201.

83. Vandenbergh, S. J., Persico, A. M., and Uhl, G. R. A human dopamine transporter cDNA predicts reduced glycosylation, displays a novel repetitive element and provides racially-dimorphic Taq I RFLPS. *Mol. Brain Res.* **15** (1992) 161–166.

84. Van Dyck, C. H., Seibyl, J. P., Malison, R. T., Laruelle, M., Wallace, E., Zoghbi, S. S., Zea-Ponse, Y., Baldwin, R. M., Charney, D. S., Hoffer, P. B., and Innis, R. B. Age-related decline in striatal dopamine transporter binding with iodine-123—CIT SPECT. *J. Nuclear Med.* **36** (1995) 1175–1181.

85. Volkow, N. D., Fowler, J. S., Logan, J., Wang, G.-J., Hitzemann, R., MacGregor, R., Dewey, S. L., and Wolf, A. P. Decreased binding of 11-C-cocaine in the brain of cocaine addicts. *J. Nuclear Med.* **33** (1992) 888.

86. Volkow, N. D., Fowler, J. S., Wang, G.-J., Logan, J., Schlyer, D., MacGregor, R. Hitzemann, R., and Wolf, A. P. Decreased dopamine transporters with age in healthy human subjects. *Ann. Neurol.* **36** (1994) 237–238.

87. Volkow, N. D., Ding, Y.-S., Fowler, J. S., Wang, G.-J., Logan, J., Gatley, J. S., Dewey, S., Ashby, C., Liebermann, J., Hitzemann, R., and Wolf, A. P. Is methylphenidate like cocaine? *Arch. Gen. Psychiatry* **52** (1995) 456–463.

88. Weiss, R. D. and Mirin, S. M. Psychological and pharmacological treatment strategies in cocaine dependence. *Ann. Clin. Psych.* **2** (1990) 239–243.

89. Wetli, C. V. and Fishbain, D. A. Cocaine-induced psychosis and sudden death in recreational cocaine users. *J. Foresci. Sci.* **30** (1985) 873–880.

90. Wilson, J. M., Nobrega, J. N., Carroll, M. E., Niznik, H. B., Shannak, K., Lac, S. T., Pristupa, Z. B., Dixon, L. M., and Kish, S. J. Heterogenous subregional bind-

ing patterns of ^{3}H-WIN 35,428 and ^{3}H-GBR 12,935 are differentially regulated by chronic cocaine self-adminstration. *J. Neurosci.* **14** (1994) 2966–2974.

91. Wong, D. F., Yung, B., Dannals, R. F., Shaya, E. K., Ravert, H. T., Chen, C. A., Chan, B., Folio, T., Scheffel, U., Ricaurte, G. A., Neumeyer, J. L., Wagner, H. N., and Kühar, M. J. In vivo imaging of baboon and human dopamine transporters by positron emission tomography using [11C]WIN 35,428. *Synapse* **15** (1993) 130–142.

92. Yi, S.-J. and Johnson, K. M. Effects of acute and chronic administration of cocaine on striatal uptake, compartmentalization and release of [3H]dopamine. *Neuropharmacology* **29** (1990) 475–486.

93. Zelnik, N., Angel, I., Paul, S. M., and Kleinman, J. E. Decreased density of human striatal dopamine uptake sites with age. *Eur. J. Pharmacol.* **126** (1986) 175, 176.

CHAPTER 12

Role of Axonal and Somatodendritic Monoamine Transporters in Action of Uptake Blockers

Nian-Hang Chen and Maarten E. A. Reith

Introduction

There is a large body of evidence indicating the presence of neuronal monoamine transport systems for dopamine (DA), norepinephrine (NE), and serotonin (5-HT) not only in axon terminals, but also in somatodendrites (6,38,44,61,67,82,100). Monoamine transporters are central to the actions of uptake blockers such as antidepressants and psychostimulants. This chapter focusses on recent findings obtained from in vitro and in vivo studies with uptake blockers at the level of both somatodendritic and axonal monoamine transporters, with particular attention to our findings on the monoamine effects of various uptake blockers in the axonal and somatodendritic areas of the DA pathway. These findings have provided new insights into the roles of both axonal and somatodendritic monoamine transporters in determining the potency, the selectivity, and the regulation of the action of uptake blockers. Further elucidation of these roles may assist in understanding the complex mechanisms responsible for various neuropathophysiological conditions, for the therapeutics of antidepressants, and for the reinforcement by abused drugs such as cocaine.

Distribution of Monoamine Transporters in Somatodendritic and Axonal Areas

Localization of monoamine transporters in the brain has been studied by quantitative autoradiographic techniques with various radioli-

Neurotransmitter Transporters: Structure, Function, and Regulation
Ed.: M. E. A. Reith Humana Press Inc., Totowa, NJ

gands (*13,25,38,44,57,61,82,100*). The distribution of monoamine transporters in DA axonal and somatodendritic areas is summarized in Table 1. These DA regions are also terminal regions of the NE and 5-HT system, and, with additional information on monoamine transporters in NE and 5-HT somatodendritic areas, it is possible to compare their distribution in all three monoamine systems. Three features appear prominent in the distribution of monoamine transporters in DA pathways. First, the highest density of DA transporters is found in DA terminal regions, such as striatum (STR) and nucleus accumbens (NAC), but a relative lower density is seen in the substantia nigra and the ventral tegmental area (VTA), which contain the DA cell bodies giving rise to the nigrostriatal and mesolimbocortical DA system. This distribution pattern is markedly different from that of NE and 5-HT transporters. In the latter cases, the highest density of NE or 5-HT transporters is observed over the locus coeruleus or dorsal raphe nucleus, regions rich in NE or 5-HT cell bodies. If the effect of an uptake blocker is only dependent on the occupancy of transporters, a DA uptake blocker would be expected to preferentially act in DA axonal regions; a NE or 5-HT uptake blocker would do so in NE or 5-HT somatodendritic regions. Second, DA transporters are predominant in DA pathways in comparison with NE and 5-HT transporters. If a higher transporter density would result in a relative higher occupancy of uptake sites by a given synaptic concentration of uptake blockers, the relative density of the three monoamine transporters in a single region would contribute to the apparent specificity of an uptake blocker in that region. Consequently, a nonselective uptake blocker may tend to preferentially enhance extracellular DA in DA transporter-rich regions, but some selective NE or 5-HT uptake blockers may not necessarily produce selective monoamine effect in these DA pathways, especially when present at higher concentrations. Third, NE and 5-HT transporters have a relatively higher proportion in DA somatodendritic regions than in DA axonal regions. In fact, the density of 5-HT transporters in the substantia nigra and the ventral tegmental area is only below that in the raphe nuclei. In addition, some studies suggest that the density of NE transporters is also higher in DA somatodendritic regions than in DA axonal regions (*39,44*). The higher population of NE and 5-HT transporters in the DA cell body areas may provide an anatomical substrate for DA uptake into non-dopaminergic terminals. If this really happens, the effect of NE or 5-HT uptake blockers on extracellular monoamines will be more complicated in DA cell body areas than in DA terminal regions.

Table 1
Distribution of Monoamine Transporters in Axonal and Somatodendritic Areas[a]

Transporter	Radioligand	Brain region[b]						Refs.
		STR	NAC	SN	VTA	LC	RN	
DA	Mazindol[c]	9.1	5.3	3.2	6.1	—	—	39
	Mazindol	12–16	12–16	4–7.20	4–7.20	1.60–4	1.60–4	61
	GBR12935	24.4	11.97	4.61	7.51	nd	nd	82
	GBR12935	340	159	54.4	nd	nd	nd	100
NE	Desipramine	0.20	0.21	0.15	nd	3.92	1.17	13
	Mazindol[c]	—	—	0.23	0.1	2.0	1.0	39
	Tomoxetine	<0.52	<0.52	0.52–1.16	0.52–1.16	1.16–1.55	0.52–1.16	44
	Mazindol	0.08–0.4	0.08–0.4	0.08–0.4	0.08–0.4	3–4	0.4–1	61
5-HT	Paroxetine[c]	0.99	1.26	2.64	2.57	3.33	6.64	25
	Paroxetine	0.48	nd	0.59	0.59	nd	0.73	38
	Paroxetine	0.47	nd	0.83	nd	0.80	1.27	57

[a]The transporter density is expressed as pmol/mg protein and approximated from autoradiographic ligand binding data by taking into account the K_d of the ligand and the ligand concentration used. Undetectable binding is shown as dashes (—).

[b]nd, not determined; LC, locus coeruleus; NAC, nucleus accumbens; RN, raphe nuclei; SN, substantia nigra; STR, striatum; VTA, ventral tegmental area.

[c]Normalized from mg tissue to mg protein by multiplying the value/mg tissue with 10.

It is necessary to emphasize that only few DA axon terminals have been documented in DA cell body areas (5,33,111). Thus, the possibility that the observed density of DA transporters in DA cell body areas includes those located on axon terminals is probably immaterial. In contrast, it is unclear whether NE transporters seen in the locus ceruleus are on the cell bodies of the locus ceruleus group (47) or on terminals of projections from the lateral tegmental system (83). In the raphe nuclei, although a large fraction of the 5-HT transporters are located on the somatodendritic portion of the 5-HT neurons, a small number of 5-HT transporters belong to 5-HT axon terminals from internuclear connections or from lower 5-HT cell groups (14,84,95).

Characteristics of Somatodendritic and Axonal DA Transporters

Although evidence that monoamine transporters exist not only in axonal terminals but also in cell bodies is compelling, it is not clear whether axonal and somatodendritic transporters have the same properties. The findings from several studies comparing DA uptake in axonal regions with that in somatodendritic regions are controversial. Thus, [^{3}H]DA uptake into slices of rat ventral tegmentum shows sensitivity to Na^+ and temperature, and is inhibited by various compounds, in a similar manner as uptake into NAC slices (6); however, caution is needed when interpreting these results, because other observations indicate the potential for [^{3}H]DA uptake into NE and 5-HT terminals (27,73,108). The binding of [^{3}H]WIN 35,428 in monkey substantia nigra, measured by autoradiography in coronal brain sections, is inhibited by various uptake blockers, with a rank order similar to that in slices from STR (70). However, there is no detailed comparative information, as far as the STR and the substantia nigra are concerned, about the potency of various uptake blockers.

Potential differences between axonal and somatodendritic DA transporters have recently been examined in our laboratory (31) by comparing the binding of [^{3}H]WIN 35,428 to membranes prepared from the rat NAC, STR, and ventral mesencephalon (VM) containing A_9 and A_{10} DA cell bodies (Table 2). These measurements are obtained in the presence of citalopram and desipramine to occlude 5-HT and NE transporters. Saturation of binding in all regions, conducted by varying either nonradioactive WIN 35,428 or [^{3}H]WIN 35,428, is best described by a one-site model. There are no statistically significant differences between the STR, NAC, and VM in the K_d for

Table 2
Binding of [³H]WIN 35,428 to Rat Axonal and Somatodendritic DA
Transporters[a]

Compound	STR	NAC	VM
[³H]WIN 35,428			
K_d (nM)	6.2 ± 1.3 (4)	5.2 ± 0.2 (8)	7.7 ± 1.2 (6)
B_{max} (pmol/mg)	8.8 ± 1.3 (4)[b]	3.46 ± 0.44 (8)[b]	0.53 ± 0.16 (6)[b]
Cocaine			
K_i (nM)		47.4 ± 0.98 (3)	66.4 ± 7.82 (3)
Hill number		0.96 ± 0.03 (3)	0.99 ± 0.08 (3)
GBR 12909			
K_i (nM)		2.8 ± 0.36 (3)	1.9 ± 0.54 (2)
Hill number		1.3 ± 0.29 (3)	1.2 ± 0.12 (2)

[a]Membranes were prepared from the STR, NAC, and the VM containing A_9 and A_{10} dopamine cell bodies. The binding of [³H] WIN 35,428 was determined in the presence of citalopram (90 nM) and desipramine (90 nM) to occlude serotonin and norepinephrine transporters. Values are mean ± SEM of data collected for the number of independent membrane preparations indicated between parentheses.
[b]$p < 0.01$ compared with the B_{max} value from any other brain region (Tukey's multiple comparisons test following significant one-way analysis of variance).

[³H]WIN 35,428 binding and the inhibitory potency of cocaine and GBR 12909. The lack of difference between the VM and the NAC suggests that axonal and somatodendritic DA transporters have comparable affinities for cocaine- and GBR-related compounds. In addition, the affinity of the transport complex for WIN 35,428 is similar in the two terminal areas of the mesolimbic (NAC) and the nigrostriatal (STR) pathways. Other reports have described generally similar properties of DA transporters in the STR and the NAC (12,15). These results suggest that the DA transporter is similar in DA axonal and somatodendritic areas, except for the density of transporters. In parallel with the autoradiographic data, the rank order for the B_{max} of [³H]WIN 35,428 binding sites is STR > NAC > VM (Table 2).

These results do not rule out the possibility that there are regionally dependent differences in DA transporter functioning beyond the level of blocker and Na⁺recognition. In fact, the [³H]DA uptake into somatodendritic preparations in the presence of desipramine and citalopram is substantially lower than expected from the DA transporter density as measured with [³H]WIN 35,428 binding in comparison with NAC preparations (*31*). Under similar conditions, the GBR 12909-sensitive dopamine accumulation in the substantia nigra slices is also quite low (*108*). These facts indicate slower dynamics of DA uptake in somatodendrites than in axon terminals. It remains unknown whether the somatodendritic DA transporter density indicated by autoradiographic and binding techniques includes immature uptake sites at the rough endoplasmic reticulum of the cell body prior to their transport to cell membranes. Transmitters may be better taken up by mature DA transporters on terminals.

Methodological Considerations in Investigating the Monoamine Effect of Uptake Blockers in Somatodendritic Areas

Brain slices labeled with radioactive monoamines represent the in vitro preparation most widely used for investigating the direct effect of uptake blockers on monoamine transmission. In this preparation, the neuronal connections between cell body and terminal regions are severed, allowing us to pinpoint the effects of uptake blockers locally. It should be recalled that labeled and endogenous monoamine release does not always occur in parallel. The major causes for this include the potential presence of a large newly-synthesized component in endogenous release and the uneven distribution of labeled monoamines within the endogenous releasable pool (*53*). For investigation of the effect of uptake blockers in DA somatodendritic areas, two additional points should be considered: the vesicular storage of DA, and the specificity of the labeling process.

The relative lack of a vesicular storage pool in DA cell body areas received much attention more than a decade ago (for refs., *see 32*). The low vesicular representation would make ongoing DA synthesis more important in maintaining a releasable pool, but ongoing DA synthesis may not be available for the pool of labeled DA when radioactive DA is used for labeling the slices. In addition, lack of sequestration of cytosolic [^{3}H]DA into vesicles may result in a relative larger cytoplasmic compartmentation of [^{3}H]DA, especially when a monoamine oxidase inhibitor has been added to the slice system. Under conditions of cytoplasmic compartmentation, DA can be released through DA transporters (*58,90*). This release process probably does not operate under an exocytosis-like mechanism (*79*), compromising the capacity of the DA cell body areas to release [^{3}H]DA in an impulse-dependent manner and thereby diminishing the effect of uptake blockers on depolarization-induced release. In a Na^+-containing medium, this transporter-mediated DA release may be less sensitive to uptake blockers inhibiting both transporter-mediated uptake and transporter-mediated release. It should be pointed out here that the widely assumed lack of vesicles in DA cell body areas has been questioned recently by investigations with a polyclonal antiserum against the vesicular monoamine transporter VMAT2 localized by electron microscopy (23). In both the substantia nigra and VTA, VMAT2 is found in dendrites, frequently the same ones that contain tyrosine hydroxylase; VMAT2-containing vesicles are often near dendritic membranes apposed to glial processes or unlabeled dendrites (substantia nigra) or other VMAT2-containing dendrites (VTA) (23). These new findings, along with recent dialysis data (*see* Regional Differences Following Focal Application of Uptake Blockers), should reopen the debate on the classically held view that somatodendritic DA release does not involve vesicles and does not depend on impulse flow-mediated depolarizations blockable by tetrodotoxin (TTX).

DA cell body areas are brain regions in which NE and 5-HT terminals coexist with DA somatodendrites (*89*). A potential limitation with slices prepared from such a region is that radioactive DA can enter other nondopaminergic terminals, confounding the effect of DA uptake blockers (*25*). This problem may not be satisfactorily circumvented by using low concentrations of labeled DA or by adding specific uptake blockers during the labeling phase. One reason is that some monoamines, for instance DA and NE, have similar affinities for the NE transporter (*47,91,101*), which makes it impossible to prevent labeled DA uptake into NE terminals only by decreasing the concentration of labeled DA. The other reason is that the specificity of an uptake blocker depends on the concentration used. Practically, an uptake blocker cannot fully inhibit one category of transporters without affecting another. Our work with VM slices (*27*) provides a good example. A concentration of 10 nM of [³H]DA, which presumably is close to the extracellular level of endogenous DA, still labels the 5-HT terminals to a significant extent. The presence of up to 1 µM fluoxetine in the loading phase does not seem to completely prevent the labeling of 5-HT terminals by [³H]DA. A further increase in the concentration of fluoxetine during the preloading period partly prevents labeling of DA somatodendrites by [³H]DA, causing the somatodendritic [³H]DA release itself to be too small to be detected reliably. This unavoidable drawback probably plays a significant role in the unexpectedly small somatodendritic effect of DA uptake blockers observed in the in vitro studies with VM slices preloaded with 1 μM fluoxetine (27).

The debate on the lack of vesicles and the cross-labeling of nontarget monoamine terminals, in the context of the monoamine effects of uptake blockers, does not apply only to DA cell body regions. A lack of vesicles has also been proposed to exist in raphe nuclei (24,95). In addition, appreciable density of DA/5-HT or DA/NE transporters has been found in the locus coeruleus or dorsal raphe (see Table 1).

Determination of endogenous transmitters offers the possibility of studying monoamine transmission without any previous manipulation of the transmitter pools. However, the in vitro effect of uptake blockers on endogenous DA in DA somatodendritic areas has seldom been measured, because of the technical difficulties in determining low concentrations of endogenous monoamines in superfusion fluid. Intracerebral dialysis has the advantage, but also the complexity, of investigating effects of uptake blockers on endogenous monoamine transmission in an intact nervous system. Although focal application of a compound into a brain region via dialysis probes can circumvent pharmacokinetical factors and minimize the effect of the compound on other brain structures that could indirectly influence the monoamine transmission in the target region, it cannot occlude the impact normally exerted by other brain structures, through numerous neuronal circuits, on the target region. When dialyis studies are undertaken in DA cell body areas without imposed blockade of NE and 5-HT transporters, it is not impossible that a portion of the dialysate DA, in fact, has originated from NE and 5-HT terminals, which contribute to the in vivo DA effect of uptake blockers. For comparing the axonal and somatodentritic monoamine effects of uptake blockers in vivo, it is important to carry out the experiments in conscious animals. Inherent in dialysis studies using anesthetized animals is the concern that the anesthetic itself may compromise the activity of monoamine neurons in somatodendritic regions (19,71,72). The axonal and somatodendritic monoamine effects of uptake blockers may be differentially contingent upon the activity of monoamine neurons. Despite some disadvantages, the mentioned in vitro and in vivo approaches constitute important research tools at this time. Undoubtedly, the combination of both is helpful for a rational evaluation of the monoamine effects of uptake blockers.

Effects of Uptake Blockers on Monoamine Transmission in Axonal and Somatodendritic Areas

Both in vitro and in vivo approaches can be used to identify the axonal and somatodendritic monoamine effect of uptake blockers. To date, little knowledge about the in vitro effect of uptake blockers in NE or 5-HT somatodendritic areas has been obtained. The DA system is the only monoamine system in which the effect of uptake blockers on axonal and somatodendritic DA transmission has been investigated with both in vitro and in vivo approaches.

DA Uptake Blockers

Electrically induced [^{3}H]DA release from VM slices appears to be, for the most part, of somatodendritic origin, provided uptake of [^{3}H]DA into NE and 5-HT terminals is inhibited by labeling the slices with [^{3}H]DA in the presence of selective NE and 5-HT uptake blockers (27). Under these conditions, the electrically induced [^{3}H]DA release from the VM is enhanced by selective and nonselective DA uptake blockers. The DA effect of cocaine is abolished by preperfusion of the VM slices with the selective DA uptake blocker GBR 12909, confirming that the cocaine-induced increase in the [^{3}H]DA release is caused by inhibition of DA uptake into somatodendrites. However, all tested uptake blockers are much less effective in augmenting electrically induced [^{3}H]DA release in VM than in NAC and STR (27). Compared with the STR and NAC, the spontaneous release of [^{3}H]DA in the VM is much higher, but the electrically induced release is less responsive to uptake blockers, supporting a potential role for cytoplasmic compartmentation of [^{3}H]DA (Table 3).

When various uptake blockers are applied directly to the NAC or VTA via dialysis probes, in line with in vitro studies, three DA uptake blockers, cocaine (Fig. 1), GBR 12935 (29,80), and nomifensine (66), show significantly more potent effects on extracellular DA levels in the NAC than in the VTA. The threshold concentrations for a significant DA response to these uptake blockers are almost 10-fold higher in VTA than in NAC. At 1–100 µM perfusate concentrations, the fractional or absolute DA response in the NAC to focally applied cocaine is approx 3- or 15-fold as high as that in the VTA (Fig. 1, Table 4). A similar trend is also observed for the DA response to focally applied GBR 12935 (Table 4).

In our studies with dual dialysis probes, the extracellular DA levels after systemic administration of uptake blockers are investigated

Table 3
Effects of DA Uptake Blockers on Electrically Induced and Spontaneous
[³H]DA Release from Superfused Slices of DA Axonal and Somatodendritic
Areas in Rats[a]

[³H]DA	Brain region		
release and treatment	STR	NAC	VM
Electrically induced [³H]DA release			
S_1	0.61 ± 0.04 (6)	0.94 ± 0.07 (6)[b]	0.98 ± 0.06 (6)[b]
S_2/S_1			
Control	0.92 ± 0.04 (5)	0.98 ± 0.05 (7)	0.97 ± 0.04 (7)
GBR 12909 1 μM	4.05 ± 0.85 (3)	2.65 ± 0.38 (3)[b]	1.53 ± 0.25 (4)[b]
Nomifensine 10 μM	4.10 ± 0.17 (3)	2.84 ± 0.10 (3)[b]	1.50 ± 0.10 (4)[b]
Cocaine 10 μM	2.54 ± 0.31 (3)	2.50 ± 0.38 (3)	1.28 ± 0.10 (7)[b]
Spontaneous [³H] DA release			
B_1	0.40 ± 0.01 (6)	0.38 ± 0.02 (6)	2.36 ± 0.07 (6)[b]
B_2/B_1			
Control	0.81 ± 0.02 (5)	0.90 ± 0.06 (7)	0.75 ± 0.02 (7)
GBR 12909 1 μM	2.61 ± 0.28 (3)	2.65 ± 0.37 (3)	0.96 ± 0.04 (4)[b]
Nomifensine 10 μM	1.68 ± 0.03 (3)	1.57 ± 0.06 (3)	0.86 ± 0.04 (4)[b]
Cocaine 10 μM	1.96 ± 0.10 (3)	1.88 ± 0.10 (3)	0.84 ± 0.02 (7)[b]

[a]Slices were prepared from the STR, NAC, and the VM, containing A_9 and A_{10} dopamine cell bodies. The slices were labeled with [³H]DA (0.1 μM) in the presence of 0.5 μM desipramine (for all slices), and 1 μM fluoxetine (only for VM slices) to prevent [³H]DA from labeling norepinephrine and serotonin terminals. S_1 or S_2 correspond to the sum of increased fractional release above the baseline in three 5-min samples after the start of the first or the second electrical stimulation. S_2/S_1 corresponds to the ratio of fractional release for electrically induced release. B_1 or B_2 correspond to the percentage of the tissue radioactivity released spontaneously in one 5-min sample just before the first or the second stimulations. B_2/B_1 corresponds to the ratio of fractional release for spontaneous release. Drugs were added 20 min before the second stimulation and maintained throughout the rest of the experiment. Values are mean ± SEM of data for the number of independent experiments indicated between parentheses.

[b]$p < 0.05$ compared with the value from STR (one-way ANOVA followed by the Newman Keul's test).

simultaneously in both the NAC and VTA of awake animals. Intraperitoneal injection of cocaine (20 mg/kg) or GBR 12935 (15 mg/kg) enhances the dialysate DA output simultaneously in both regions. However, the regional difference in the magnitude of the DA

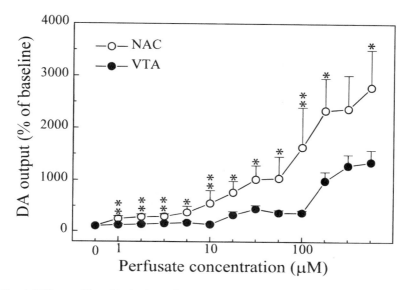

Fig. 1. Effects of local infusion of cocaine on dialysate DA levels from rat NAC and VTA. Progressively higher concentrations of cocaine (1, 10, and 100 μM) were perfused into the tested brain regions via the probe and each concentration was perfused for 80 min (4 samples). Values are mean ± SEM (n = 5–9). All data were evaluated by a two-way ANOVA with repeated measures over time: time, $F_{(12,144)}$ = 152, $p < 0.0001$; region, $F_{(1,16)}$ = 22, $p = 0.0002$; interaction, $F_{(12,144)}$ = 3.7, $p = 0.0001$. *$p < 0.05$, *$p < 0.01$ compared with VTA at each time point (unpaired Student's t test).

effect is diminished as compared with focal administration. When the DA levels are expressed as percent change from baseline, both cocaine and GBR 12935 produce a similar magnitude of DA increase in the NAC and VTA (Fig. 2, Table 4). It is noted that the maximal effects of systemic cocaine and GBR 12935 on extracellular DA levels in the VTA, at the doses tested, are close to those of local cocaine and GBR 12935 when applied through the probe at 10 μM. In contrast, the maximal DA effects of both compounds are markedly smaller in the NAC upon systemic administration than upon focal administration (Table 4). In addition, the time-course of the blocker-induced DA output differs between the NAC and the VTA. Thus, the stimulatory effect of cocaine or GBR 12935 on somatodendritic DA output is relatively persistent, lasting more than 3–6 h postinjection, while that on axonal DA output is significantly shorter, lasting less than 2–3 h and then declining to levels below baseline (Fig. 2). All data taken

Table 4
Comparison of Effects of Uptake Blockers on Dialysate DA Levels in the
NAC and the VTA of Freely Moving Rats[a]

| | Dialysate DA levels | | | |
| | Fractional increase, % | | Absolute increase, fmol/20 min | |
Compound	NAC	VTA	NAC	VTA
Cocaine				
10 µM	710 ± 244	241 ± 46[b]	377 ± 129	25.3 ± 4.9[b]
20 mg/kg	359 ± 40	256 ± 21	190 ± 33	24.7 ± 2.2[b]
GBR12935				
10 µM	611 ± 170	288 ± 48[b]	324 ± 90	30.3 ± 5.0[b]
15 mg/kg	172 ± 51	227 ± 15	55 ± 9	13.6 ± 1.8
Desipramin				
10 µM	84 ± 16	66 ± 21	47 ± 9	6.8 ± 2.2
10 mg/kg	20 ± 11	99 ± 20	5.7 ± 3.3	5.8 ± 0.8

[a]The uptake blockers were either focally infused into the NAC or VTA via the dialysis probe for 80 min, or intraperitoneally injected. The local uptake blocker-induced DA output is the average of four 20-min samples collected during infusion of the compound. The systemic uptake blocker induced DA output is the maximal output following administration of the compound. Values are mean ± SEM of 4–9 animals. The basal levels (fmol/20 min) of dialysate DA were 50.3 ± 4 ($n = 49$) in the NAC and 10.5 ± 1.1 in the VTA ($n = 39$) for the experiments with local application of uptake blockers, and 39 ± 3 ($n = 25$) in the NAC and 6.9 ± 0.4 ($n = 27$) in the VTA for the experiments with systemic application of uptake blockers.

[b]$p < 0.05$ compared with the value from NAC (one-way ANOVA followed by Least Significant Difference Multiple-Range Test).

together suggest that extracellular DA in the NAC is affected less by systemic than by focal administration of uptake blockers. As mentioned, systemic administration of cocaine (or GBR 12935) causes a similar percent increase in DA output in the NAC and VTA (Table 4), and the same observation has been reported by other investigators for cocaine administered systemically to conscious animals (68,70,91). In anesthetized animals, the results are contradictory. One dialysis study shows that the DA response to intravenous cocaine is greater in magnitude and persists longer in the NAC than in the VTA (17). However, an electrochemical study claims that subcutaneous application of cocaine concurrently decreases DA in both NAC and VTA,

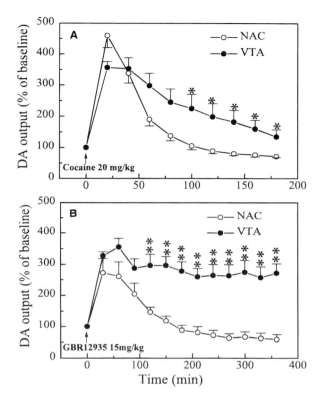

Fig. 2. Effects of systemic administration of cocaine (**A**) and GBR 12935 (**B**) on dialysate DA levels from rat NAC and VTA. Cocaine (20 mg/kg, ip) or GBR 12935 (15 mg/kg, ip) was injected at time zero. Values are mean ± SEM ($n = 6$–7). All data were evaluated by a two-way ANOVA with repeated measures over time. For cocaine: time, $P_{(9,99)} = 542$, $p < 0.0001$; region, $F_{(1,12)} = 3.73$, $p = 0.07$; interaction, $F_{(9,99)} = 6$, $p < 0.0001$. For GBR 12,935; time, $F_{(12,132)} = 15$, $p < 0.0001$; region, $F_{(1,12)} = 23$, $p = 0.0005$; interaction, $F_{(12,132)} = 5$, $p < 0.0001$. *$p < 0.05$ compared with NAC at each time point (unpaired Student's t test).

with the VTA more vulnerable to this effect than the NAC (*18*). These findings taken together demonstrate that methodological factors (anesthetized animals vs conscious animals, dialysis vs voltammetry, i-v vs s-c) affect the DA response to cocaine.

The data also indicate that uptake blockers exert a significantly greater somatodendritic effect in vivo than in vitro. For example, cocaine concentrations of 10 and 100 µ*M* increase DA release from superfused VM slices only by about 28% (*27*); similar concentrations in perfusates increase dialysate DA from the VTA by 240 and 900%

(29). If we consider that only a small fraction of the perfused cocaine can pass through the dialysis membrane (about 10%), the in vivo somatodendritic effect of cocaine is even more impressive. This fact argues against our earlier speculation drawn from the in vitro studies that the local effect of cocaine on somatodendritic DA release is not appreciable (27). There are various methodological differences that play a significant role in the discrepancy between the in vitro and in vivo results (see section on Methodical Considerations).

NE and 5-HT Uptake Blockers

To our knowledge, only one study has compared NE axonal and somatodendritic areas in the effects of uptake blockers on NE transmission. It reports that focal application of cocaine produces a greater percent increase in the extracellular level of NE in the locus ceruleus than in the hippocampus and frontal cortex, but systemic application of cocaine (20 mg/kg) elevates extracellular NE only in the locus ceruleus, but not in the hippocampus and prefrontal cortex (109). Similar results have been found following administration of desipramine in the same lab. Thus, the predominant NE effect of uptake blockers has been suggested to occur in the NE cell body area. However, other studies have shown a significant stimulatory effect of systemic cocaine (again 20 mg/kg) or desipramine on the extracellular NE in the hippocampus and the prefrontal cortex (37,42,81), arguing against a negligible effect of NE uptake blockers in the terminal regions. Probably, the most important difference between these studies is that the former experiments were conducted in anesthetized rats and the latter in freely moving rats. Uptake blockers have been found less effective in inhibiting NE neurons in unanesthetized animals than in anesthetized animals (35), which can account for the appreciable terminal effects of NE uptake blockers in awake animals. Even so, it is still possible that, in awake animals, NE uptake blockers have a greater effect in the NE cell body area than in the axon terminal regions. This possibility requires further experimental validation.

The effects of several 5-HT uptake blockers in 5-HT axonal and somatodendritic areas have been compared primarily in the frontal cortex and the dorsal raphe (2,9,59). Systemic application of citalopram, or fluvoxamine, produces a markedly greater increase in dialysate 5-HT in the dorsal raphe than in the frontal cortex. In the former region, the effect is also long lasting. Some investigators have found no increase at all in the frontal cortex following systemic application of clomipramine, although local application of this compound appears to increase dialysate 5-HT in the two regions to a similar degree. It is not clear whether such regional differences also exist between the raphe nuclei and other 5-HT terminal regions. In other 5-HT terminal regions, 5-HT uptake blockers do cause two- to five-fold increases in extracellular levels of 5-HT (21,29,96,105).

Factors Contributing to the Difference Between the Axonal and Somatodendritic Monoamine Effects of Uptake Blockers

Regional Differences Following Focal Application of Uptake Blockers

One reason for studying direct effects of uptake blockers on axonal and somatodendritic monoamine transmission is to address the question whether the mechanisms governing monoamine release in both regions are similar. Some earlier in vivo and in vitro investigations, as well as studies based on postmortem tissue analysis, conclude that somatodendritic DA release is not comparable to axonal DA release, because it is dependent neither on neuronal impulse-activity, nor on DA autoreceptor occupancy (32,86,87). A similar conclusion has been advanced also for somatodendritic 5-HT release (3,54). Such differences could account for the different ability of uptake blockers to increase monoamines in axonal and somatodendritic regions (85,94). However, multiple dialysis studies have shown not only that DA release from the VTA or substantia nigra (66,103,106), but also 5-HT release from raphe nuclei (8,16), is sensitive to TTX, dependent on Ca^{2+}, and regulated by autoreceptors. Our in vitro and in vivo release studies also support the involvement of impulse flow and autoregulation in somatodendritic DA release (27,29). Thus, somatodendritic monoamine release shares the same properties with axonal release, even if part of the former might not be of vesicular origin (*see* section on Methodological Considerations). The DA effect of nomifensine in the substantia nigra is sensitive to TTX (103). The monoamine effects of cocaine in the VTA are virtually abolished by infusion of TTX (Fig. 3), are substantially enhanced by DA autoreceptor antagonist (*see* section on DA Transporter), and are independent of cocaine's local anesthetic activity (29). These facts strongly suggest that, as their effects in terminal regions (21,88), the DA effects of uptake blockers in the DA somatodendritic areas are also dependent on the impulse activity of DA neurons.

Important factors contributing to the regional difference of uptake blockers may be the different characteristics of axonal and somatodendritic transporters. As mentioned earlier, our binding data indicate a comparable potency for cocaine and GBR 12909 in

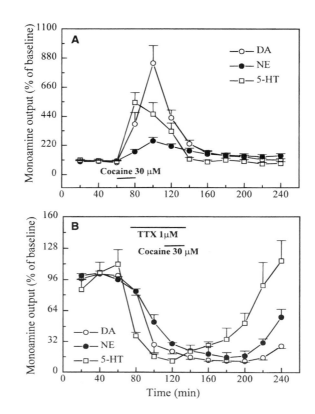

Fig. 3. Effects of local infusion of TTX into the rat VTA on local cocaine-induced changes in VTA dialysate levels of DA, NE, and 5-HT (**A**) in the absence of TTX (adapted with permission from ref. *28*) and (**B**) in the presence of TTX (adapted with permission from ref. *29*). The short horizontal bar denotes the 20-min period of cocaine infusion. The long horizontal bar denotes the 80-min period of TTX infusion. The dialysate levels of the three monoamines were measured simultaneously. Values are mean ± SEM (*n* = 3–7). All data were evaluated by a one-way ANOVA with repeated measures over time. For cocaine alone, $F_{(11, 24)}$ = 19, 7.4, and 17 for DA, NE, and 5-HT, respectively, $p < 0.0001$. For cocaine plus TTX, $F_{(11, 24)}$ = 159, 45, and 11 for DA, NE, and 5-HT, respectively, $p < 0.001$.

inhibiting [³H]WIN 35,428 binding in DA cell body and terminal regions (*31*). Thus, the findings showing that the local DA effects of uptake blockers are smaller in DA cell body areas than in terminal regions are probably not the result of a lower affinity of uptake blockers for somatodendritic as compared with axonal DA transporters. However, if the somatodendrites transport DA slowly, as indicated by the in vitro uptake assays, the blockade of somatodendritic transporters by uptake blockers would be expected to cause less accumulation of endogenous DA in the extracellular fluid. Of course, the lower density of DA transporters in the somatodendritic areas may be the most important factor. Because of the lower density, the number of sites occupied by a given concentration of blockers will be relatively smaller in the cell body areas, causing a smaller DA output.

The differential effects of focally applied uptake blockers probably also depend on the rate of ongoing monoamine release in the two regions. The basal levels of DA in dialysates from the NAC are almost fourfold higher than those from the VTA (*see* Table 4 footnote). This seems related to a smaller reserve capacity in DA cell body areas. Indeed, the tissue levels of DA in the cell body areas are approximately 10% of those in the NAC (our unpublished data). Two pharmacological treatments used to release DA, amphetamine and high potassium, display much smaller release ability in the cell body areas than in the NAC (*65,69*). Since uptake blocker-induced increase in extracellular DA is dependent on impulse-generated transmitter release, the region with a higher basal release would be expected to show the larger absolute increase in DA output in the presence of uptake blockers.

Taken together, the two- to fourfold higher DA transporter density combined with the fourfold higher basal DA release in the NAC, as compared with the VTA, and the potentially slower DA uptake dynamics in the VTA, could be thought to underlie the 10- to 14-fold regional difference in the absolute DA change induced by focal application of uptake blockers.

Regional Differences Following Systemic Application of Uptake Blockers

Unlike the in vitro and in vivo local perfusion approaches, in which effects of uptake blockers are limited to a discrete brain region, uptake blockers, when administered systemically, will affect both axon terminal and somatodendritic events. Because of the various regulating loops impinging on the monoamine circuits, it is not surprising that, upon systemic application of an uptake blocker, the change in the extracellular level of monoamines in a given brain region is not completely in line with that predicted, based on its transporter density and its basal release. In this context, the diminished regional difference in the maximal DA response between NAC and VTA, as well as the augmented regional difference in the NE/5-HT response between some terminal regions and the locus oeruleus/raphe nuclei, upon systemic application of uptake blockers, may reflect an inhibitory effect exerted by various regulating mechanisms on the monoamine release in the monoamine axon terminal regions.

The regional differences in the DA effects of three different uptake blockers, GBR 12935, cocaine, and desipramine, have been compared in the mesolimbic DA system (Table 4). We use the NAC/VTA ratio for the percent increase of dialysate DA output as a quantitative index reflecting the regional difference. The mechanisms underlying the direct DA stimulatory effects of these uptake blockers are not exactly the same: for desipramine, mostly because of blockade of NE transporters (*see* Involvement of Monoamine Interaction section); for GBR 12935, mostly blockade of DA transporters; and for cocaine, mostly blockade of both DA and NE transporters. However, the regional difference in their systemic DA effects varies following a common regulation that is positively associated with the regional difference in their direct DA effects (Fig. 4). The regression equation is $NAC_{sys}/VTA_{sys} = -0.75 + 0.74 \times NAC_{loc}/VTA_{loc}$. Thus, the systemic application of a blocker will produce a stimulatory effect on the extracellular DA in the NAC only when the NAC_{loc}/VTA_{loc} ratio for its direct DA effects is more than 1 (cocaine and GBR 12935), almost no effect when the ratio is close to 1 (desipramine), and an inhibitory effect when the ratio is less than 1. This regression equation can be expressed as $NAC_{sys} = 0.74 \times NAC_{loc} \times (VTA_{sys}/VTA_{loc}) - 0.75 \times VTA_{sys}$. The latter equation indicates that, when the uptake blocker is given systemically, its NAC DA effect is proportional to its direct NAC DA effect, but partly counteracted by its VTA DA effect. Moreover, this correlation analysis implies that the regulating mechanism underlying the regional differences in the systemic DA effect is similar for the three uptake blockers in the mesolimbic DA pathway. A similar relationship is also revealed by correlation analysis of the absolute values ($p = 0.02$, figure not shown).

There may be an alternative interpretation to explain the regional differences after systemic uptake blockers. For example, it has been reported that extracellular cocaine is higher in the VTA than in the medial prefrontal cortex following systemic administration (*92*). However, it is unlikely that the diminished DA effects observed here are caused by lower extracellular concentration of systemic uptake blockers in the NAC, because the NE and 5-HT effects of both cocaine and GBR 12935, determined simultaneously with their DA effects, do not show a consistent trend of reduced output or shortened time-

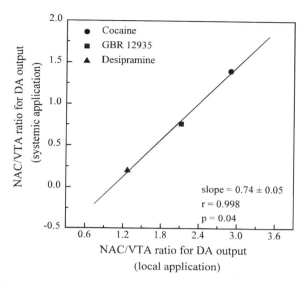

Fig. 4. Relationship between the regional difference caused by local application and that caused by systemic application in the effect of uptake blockers on dialysate DA levels from rat NAC and VTA. The NAC/VTA ratio is defined as the ratio of the % increase in the dialysate DA level from the NAC over the % increase in the dialysate DA level from the VTA. The data for the plot are from Table 4. For other details, *see* Table 4.

course in the NAC in response to systemic administration (manuscript in preparation). In addition, the transient regional difference in the extracellular concentration of cocaine observed in the first 40 min cannot explain the persistently higher DA effect of cocaine in the VTA. Likewise, the differential effect of clomipramine cannot be attributed to pharmacokinetic reasons, because systemic application causes similar clomipramine concentrations in the cortex and the midbrain (43).

Selectivity of Uptake Blockers in DA Somatodendritic and Axonal Areas

The specificities of monoamine uptake blockers for DA, NE, and 5-HT transporters in in vitro uptake and binding assays have been widely documented (73,98,99,101,102,104). However, to what extent the in vitro specificities of these compounds can be extrapolated to their in vivo specificities is not clear. The simultaneous measurement of extracellular levels of DA, NE, and 5-HT by intracerebral dialysis makes it possible to evaluate the in vivo profiles of uptake blockers in raising extracellular monoamines in the brain. With this paradigm, important trends about how uptake blockers act in mesolimbic DA pathway where the three monoamine systems coexist have been revealed in experiments in our laboratory (*30,31,82*). The apparent in vivo selectivity of uptake blockers is compared with their in vitro selectivity in Table 5.

The results show that the apparent in vivo selectivity of an uptake blocker is not completely comparable with its in vitro selectivity in a number of ways. First, although the selective DA uptake blocker GBR 12935 and the selective 5-HT uptake blocker fluoxetine show prominent effects on the level of their target extracellular monoamine, the apparent selectivity for increasing extracellular monoamine levels in vivo is less than expected from the in vitro studies. Second, desipramine and nisoxetine, both of which have been demonstrated to be potent and selective NE uptake blockers in vitro do not show a strong preference for increasing extracellular NE in vivo. In fact, both of them are as potent in enhancing 5-HT output as in enhancing NE output, and both show an appreciable DA effect. Third, the in vivo selectivity varies with the tested brain region. For instance, the NE/DA ratio for the EC_{100} (concentration required for a onefold increase) of desipramine or the 5-HT/DA ratio for the EC_{100} of fluoxetine is 13- or 49-fold lower in the NAC than in the VTA, but the DA/NE ratio for the EC_{100} of cocaine is 12-fold lower in the NAC than in the VTA (Table 5).

The possibility should be considered that the focal perfusion protocol produces a high concentration of the selective uptake blockers in the tested brain region that may not be obtained with systemic administration of the drugs, thus diminishing their selectivity. However, there are two lines of reasoning arguing against this. First, if we take into account the limited in vitro recoveries of dialysis probes for uptake blockers, most of the perfusate concentrations used are expected to give extracellular concentrations no higher than the peak total brain concentrations reported by others following pharmacologically relevant systemic doses (*29*). Moreover, the stimulatory effects of desipramine and nisoxetine on dialysate DA and 5-HT start at low perfusate concentrations (1–10 µM, resulting in at least 10-fold lower extracellular concentrations because of the probe recovery), and hence are not likely to be the consequence of accumulation of high concentrations of these drugs. Second, systemic administration

Table 5
The In Vivo Apparent Selectivity (EC$_{100}$) of Uptake Blockers on Dialysate Monoamine Output: Comparison with the In Vitro Selectivity (K_i) of Uptake Blockers on Synaptosomal Monoamine Uptake

| Compound | EC$_{100}$ (μM)^a | | | | | | K_i (nM)^b | | | Refs. |
| | NAC | | | VTA | | | | | | |
	DA	NE	5-HT	DA	NE	5-HT	DA	NE	5-HT	
Cocaine	0.28	5.59	0.08	2.45	3.58	2.34	270	155	180	99
GBR 12935	0.28	1.24	128.30	1.65	19.20	21.80	3.7^c	1261^{c,d}	289^c	104
Desipramine	164.00	5.56	4.82	23.90	10.20	6.90	5200	0.9	340	99
Nisoxetine	1.82	2.95	2.79	1.01	1.48	1.60	510	1.3	310	99
Fluoxetine	857.60	192.10	1.57	12.20	37.60	1.12	1600	280	12	99
Citalopram	—	—	—	99.40	233.80	0.14	28,000	4000	1.3	99

^{a}The EC$_{100}$ is defined as the perfusate concentration of a compound required for a onefold increase in the monoamine output from rat NAC or VTA, as estimated by standard linear or nonlinear regression analysis ($r > 0.96$) of the mean dialysis monoamine output as a function of the perfusate concentration of a compound. Dialysate levels of DA, NE, and 5-HT were measured simultaneously in one run. For the determination of the dose–response relationship, progressively higher concentrations (0.1–1000 μM) of compounds were perfused through the probe and each concentration was perfused for 80 min (four samples). The dialysate monoamine output was summed over the 80-min sampling period after infusion of each concentration of a compound (AUC) and expressed as the percentage of the baseline AUC. Each value was obtained from 4–9 animals.

^{b}The K_i is the inhibition constant for blockade of [^{3}H] monoamine uptake into rat brain synaptosomes.

^{c}IC$_{50}$ (nM).

^{d}For inhibiting [^{3}H] nisoxetine binding.

of the selective NE uptake blockers desipramine (20 mg/kg) or oxaproptiline (10 mg/kg) do increase the extracellular DA in the prefrontal cortex (22). We also find that systemic desipramine produces a significant DA and 5-HT effect in the VTA, and systemic GBR 12935 or citalopram can influence extracellular levels of monoamines other than their target monoamine (80). Taken together, these facts support the notion that selective uptake blockers can produce "nonselective" effects, even when they are given systemically. Thus, caution should be exercised in the interpretation of results from in vivo studies using "selective" uptake blockers.

An important issue for consideration of the discrepancy between the in vivo profile of uptake blockers on extracellular monoamine levels and their in vitro blocking effects is the regional difference in the distribution of monoamine systems. The in vitro uptake or binding assays are carried out routinely in a brain region predominantly containing the target transporters; the in vivo dialysis technique tests effects of various uptake blockers in DA axon terminal and somatodendritic areas that are mildly innervated by NE terminals, but moderately or highly innervated by 5-HT terminals when compared with other brain regions. As summarized in Table 1, in both NAC and VTA, the NE transporter has the lowest density, followed by that of the 5-HT transporter, and, at the far end of the spectrum, the DA transporter. This anatomical feature may permit a NE uptake blocker to occupy DA or 5-HT transporters to some extent, particularly at higher concentrations, and hence can partly account for the unexpectedly high DA and 5-HT responses to selective NE uptake blockers. However, the relative density of monoamine transporters cannot account for the nonselective DA effect of NE uptake blockers observed at their low perfusate concentrations (29,80), or observed in a region relatively poor in DA transporters, such as the prefrontal cortex (22). Certainly, other factors are involved. In this context, in addition to the autoregulation of monoamine release (*see* Autoregulation of Action of Uptake Blockers section) and the activation of other adaptive cellular responses, there are many other possible ways that NE, DA, and 5-HT could interact to change each other's output (*see* Involvement of Monoamine Interaction section).

It should be pointed out that the absolute levels of synaptic transmitters, rather than fractional levels, determine the transmission. When we evaluate the in vivo local monoamine effect of an uptake blocker, we should discuss not only the in vivo selectivity derived from the fractional change, but also consider the impact of basal release. In the NAC, DA release is much higher than NE and 5-HT release. The basal levels of dialysate DA, NE and 5-HT are 53, 2.5, and 6.4 fmol/20 min, respectively (*80*). A small fractional change in the DA output by uptake blockers actually results in a great absolute change in the DA output, but a great fractional change in the NE or 5-HT output only produces a small absolute change in the NE or 5-HT output. In terms of the absolute change, one finds that the nonselective uptake blocker, cocaine, very much like the selective uptake blocker, GBR 12935, predominantly enhances the extracellular level of DA, rather than that of NE and 5-HT (*80*; manuscript in preparation). Likewise, the DA effects of NE uptake blockers prevail over their other monoamine effects in the NAC. In contrast, the basal levels of dialysate DA, NE, and 5-HT in the VTA are all close together: 10.5, 9.8, and 6.2 fmol/20 min, respectively (*29*). In this region, unlike GBR 12935, cocaine and NE uptake blockers, at 10 μ*M* or pharmacologically relevant systemic doses, enhance the absolute levels of the three monoamines to a similar degree (*29*; manuscript in preparation). Therefore, their monoamine profiles are really nonselective in the VTA.

In a recent study by Jordan et al. (*63*), fractional changes are reported for extracellular levels of DA, NE, and 5-HT in the medial prefrontal cortex of freely moving rats on focal or intraperitoneal application of uptake blockers. In agreement with our results, Jordan et al. concluded that the so-called 'selective serotonin reuptake inhibitors,' such as fluoxetine and fluvoxamine, are not entirely selective for serotonin. In fact, focal application of fluoxetine enhances not only prefrontal 5-HT, but also DA and NE appreciably. Although a 5-HT/DA interaction has been suggested (*see* Role of 5-HT in the DA Effect of Uptake Blockers), this is not likely to be an underlying factor, because focal fluvoxamine is as potent as fluoxetine in enhancing prefrontal 5-HT, but much less effective in increasing DA (and NE), and intraperitoneal administration of fluvoxamine produces less DA (and NE) output than intraperitoneal fluoxetine; DA output following focal or systemic imipramine is also much lower than that after fluoxetine by the respective route, even though the 5-HT effect by local imipramine is the same as that of fluoxetine and fluvoxamine (*63*). Of course, in interpreting the systemic effects of blockers, one needs to take into account also the impact of autoregulatory events (*see* section on Regional Differences Following Systematic Application and section on Autoregulation of Action of Uptake Blockers) and monoamine interactions (section on Involvement of Monoamine Interactions in the DA response) in monoamine cell body areas.

Autoregulation of Action of Uptake Blockers in Axonal and Somatodendritic Areas

Both axonal and somatodendritic monoamine transporters are involved in regulating the levels of monoamines in synaptic clefts. However, the end points may be different. Generally, the axonal transporters, by terminating the effect of monoamine on postsynaptic receptors, can play a decisive role in regulating monoamine-mediated behaviors. The somatodendritic transporters, by terminating the effect of monoamines on somatodendritic autoreceptors, play a primary role in regulating the activity of monoamine neurons. What, then, is the relative importance of the axon terminal transporters vs the somatodendritic transporters in determining the action of an uptake blocker? This issue can be considered in light of the monoamine autoregulation and monoamine transporter density.

DA Transporter

A prominent feature of the DA system is that the density of DA transporters is higher in axon terminal regions than in somatodendritic regions. Correspondingly, local application of DA uptake blockers preferentially increases extracellular DA level in terminal regions. Also, there is extensive evidence that the behavioral effects of DA uptake blockers are caused by the action of increased concentrations of DA on postsynaptic target neurons in various axon terminal regions (36,41,51). On the other hand, it is well established that DA uptake blockers inhibit the firing of DA neurons (40). This ability of DA uptake blockers is mediated by increased DA available for interaction with somatodendritic autoreceptors, as a consequence of the blockade of somatodendritic DA uptake processes (40,76). Local infusion of sulpiride (a D_2/D_3 DA autoreceptor antagonist) into the VTA strikingly enhances both local and systemic cocaine-induced DA output in this region (Fig. 5). Thus, the VTA DA effect of cocaine is self-limiting, because of the concomitant blockade of the somatodendritic DA transporters and the activation of somatodendritic DA autoreceptors. In contrast, despite this self-limiting property, the VTA DA response to systemic uptake blockers lasts much longer than the NAC DA response (Fig. 2 and *see* Role of NE in the DA Effect of Uptake Blockers). A slower dynamics of DA uptake into somatodendrites might partly account for this feature (*see* Characteristics of Somatodendric and Axonal DA Transporters). Such a long VTA DA response could play an important role in determining the impulse activity of DA neurons.

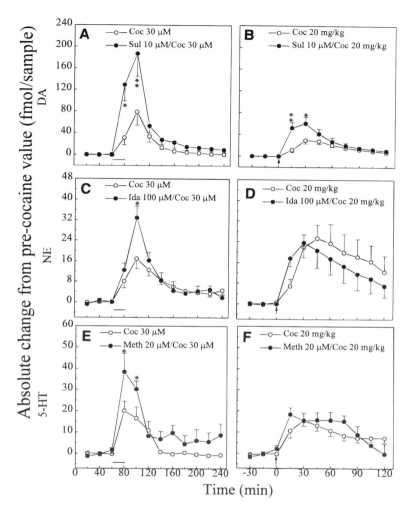

Fig. 5. Effects of local infusion of the monoamine auroreceptor antagonists sulpiride (Sul, D_2/D_3), idazoxan (Ida, α_2), and methiothepin (Meth, 5-HT_1/5-HT_2) into the VTA on local and systemic cocaine (Coc)-induced changes in VTA dialysate levels of DA, NE, and 5-HT. Horizontal bars denote the 20-min period of cocaine infusion. Arrows denote the time of cocaine injection. Values are means ± SEM (n = 5–7). *p < 0.05, **p < 0.01 compared with the corresponding cocaine alone group (Neuman Keul's test). (Adapted with permission from ref. *28*.)

Because of the functional and anatomic links between axonal and somatodendritic areas, the blockade of somatodendritic DA transporters and subsequent inhibition of DA neurons is also important in determining the availability of DA in axonal terminal regions and thus the behavioral activity after systemic cocaine. In the section on Effects of Uptake Blockers, we mentioned that systemic administration of cocaine and GBR 12935 increases extracellular DA in the NAC to a smaller degree (% change) with a shorter time-course than expected. This cannot be attributed to a relatively stronger autoregulation by terminal DA autoreceptors if we consider the equal DA responses to D_2 agonist and antagonists in the NAC and the DA cell body regions (27,66), as well as the greater DA effect in the NAC than in the VTA by local cocaine and GBR 12935. Therefore, an inhibitory effect, mediated by activation of somatodendritic autoreceptors after systemic application of DA uptake blockers, on terminal DA response is strongly suggested. Indeed, blockade of somatodendritic DA autoreceptors locally in the VTA by sulpiride dramatically enhances the systemic cocaine-induced motor activity (28). As the extracellular DA level in the VTA is not only a consequence of excitation of DA cells, but also a cause of inhibition of DA cells, it is to be expected that no certain correlation exists between the dialysate DA output from the VTA and the locomotion after systemic cocaine administration. However, with simultaneous local infusion of sulpiride into the VTA, a positive correlation is observed after cocaine challenge (Fig. 6). It is possible that, after blockade of somatodendritic DA autoreceptors, the extracellular DA level in the VTA is unable to mediate autoinhibition, and thus becomes a better indicator of the excitation of DA cells. In this situation, the higher the impulse activity is of DA neurons in the VTA, the greater the cocaine-induced DA output is in the NAC, and thus the more active the animal becomes. Recently, unilateral administration of D_2 DA receptor antisense oligodeoxynucleotides into the substantia nigra has been reported to decrease nigral D_2 autoreceptor binding site density, and to markedly stimulate contralateral rotation in response to systemic cocaine (107). Both observations demonstrate that somatodendritic DA autoreceptors play an essential role in reducing the motor response to cocaine. Clearly, cocaine can also limit its own axon terminal action by enhancing somatodendritic autoregulation through its blocking somatodendritic DA transporters.

The unresolved issue is to what extent the terminal effect of DA uptake blockers reflects changes at the cell body level. Surprisingly,

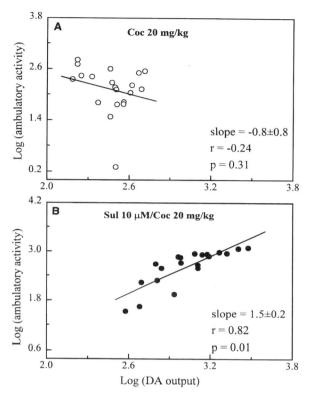

Fig. 6. Effects of local infusion of sulpiride (Sul) into the rat VTA on the relationship between dialysate DA levels from the VTA and ambulatory activity of animals after cocaine (Coc) challenge. (**A**) In the absence of sulpiride. (**B**) In the presence of sulpiride. Data are shown in a double logarithmic plot of monoamine levels in VTA dialysate vs ambulatory activity of animals. Data for either regression line were obtained from the first four samples after ip injection of cocaine in five rats. Adapted with permission from ref. *28*.

two labs have reported that administration of cocaine or nomifensine into the substantia nigra does not change DA release in the ipsilateral striatum (*58,103*). However, such results were obtained either from animals anesthetized by halothane, which is known to increase the firing of DA neurons in substantia nigra (*19*), or by a short time of nomifensine infusion (20 min) (*103*). Recently, with an 80-min infusion paradigm in awake animals, we found that infusion of cocaine into the VTA reduces the dialysate DA output in the ipsilateral NAC. In addition, by comparing the % change of dialysate DA output between focal and systemic application of uptake blockers, we estimate that somatodendritic autoregulation reduces the NAC DA effect of systemic uptake blockers by approx 50% or more (Table 4).

NE and 5-HT Transporter

In the NE system, the locus ceruleus has the highest density of NE transporters. It is possible that NE transporters in NE somatodendritic areas play a pivotal role in determining the overall effect of NE uptake blockers. Indeed, extracellular NE levels in the locus ceruleus are more responsive to the focal application and intraperitoneal injection of cocaine than the hippocampus and the frontal cortex (*109*). Moreover, the blockade of both axonal and somatodendritic NE autoreceptors by systemic application of idazoxan potentiates the terminal NE response to systemic desipramine to a much greater extent (approx 3500%) than the blockade of axonal NE autoreceptors alone by local application of idazoxan (approx 600%) (*36*). This is consonant with a predominant action of uptake blockers in the somatodendritic regions and a predominant role of somatodendritic autoreceptors in regulating the terminal NE effect of uptake blockers.

In this context, the 5-HT system has been examined more than the other two monoamine systems. It has been suggested that the 5-HT transporters in the raphe nuclei play a crucial role in determining the net effect of uptake blockers on 5-HT transmission in the brain. This conclusion is drawn from the following observations. First, systemic 5-HT uptake blockers preferentially enhance extracellular 5-HT levels in raphe nuclei (*2,9,59*). Second, an increase in the extracellular level of 5-HT in raphe nuclei by focal infusion with a 5-HT uptake blocker reduces the extracellular 5-HT level in the terminal region frontal cortex (*2*). Third, when uptake is first blocked by infusing a 5-HT uptake blocker into terminal regions, peripheral 5-HT uptake blockers, which should preferentially block uptake in the raphe nuclei, result in a reduction in terminal 5-HT output (*55,105*). Fourth, blockade of 5-HT$_{1A}$ autoreceptors by systemic administration of the selective 5-HT$_{1A}$ receptor antagonist UH-301, or by intra-raphe application of the nonselective 5-HT receptor antagonist methiothepin, potentiates or uncovers the 5-HT stimulatory effect of a systemic 5-HT uptake blocker in terminal regions (*56,59*) Fifth, blockade of 5-HT$_{1B}$ autoreceptors by focal infusion of autoreceptor antagonists into terminal regions increases 5-HT output only when a 5-HT uptake blocker is focally applied, but not when it is systemically applied (*56*). These observations demonstrate that 5-HT somatodendritic transporters are the major targets of 5-HT uptake blockers. The elevation

ity of extracellular NE itself to enhance the DA effect of cocaine (28). Instead, a NE transporter-mediated mechanism seems more plausible. DA is synthesized as a precursor of NE in NE neurons (20,112), and has a higher affinity, even higher than NE itself, for NE transporters (49,91,101). DA uptake into NE terminals by the NE transporter has been shown to exist in DA cell body regions in in vitro studies (73,108). It may be one of the mechanisms potentially involved in keeping extracellular DA levels low in somatodendritic areas. Thus, NE uptake blockers may increase DA output partly by blocking NE transporters on NE terminals, thereby preventing DA uptake into NE terminals. This mechanism may offer a partial explanation for the significantly better effect of cocaine on the DA release in in vivo dialysis studies than in in vitro superfusion experiments. In the latter situation, the presence of desipramine during the labeling phase allows pinpointing of the interaction between DA and 5-HT, while excluding the contribution of NE terminals to the DA output in the presence of cocaine.

This NE transporter-mediated mechanism may play a greater role in areas with a higher ratio of NE over DA transporters. Following NE uptake inhibition, Carboni et al. (22) described a profound increase in extracellular DA of prefrontal cortex as opposed to that of striatum, and Kihara and Masuto (74) reported a greater increment in dialysate DA of prefrontal cortex than that of NAC. In the mesolimbic DA pathway, the NAC has a lower ratio of NE over DA transporters as compared with the VTA. Thus, the positive association between DA and NE output, following the focal application of various uptake blockers, is weaker in the NAC than in the VTA (Fig. 7).

Systemic administration of desipramine (10 mg/kg) enhances the dialysate DA level in the VTA by more than onefold, but it gradually reduces the dialysate DA level in the NAC. The increase in dialysate DA in the VTA is parallel with the reduction in dialysate DA in the NAC for several hours, suggesting a functional link between the two events (Fig. 8). Probably, the sustained increase in VTA DA by desipramine inhibits the activity of DA neurons, and thus causes a reduced DA release in NAC. This reduced DA release may exceed the enhanced DA output by blockade of NE transporters, resulting in a net reduction in the DA output in the NAC. Although electrophysiological measurements in anesthetized animals do not show the expected reduction in firing of DA neurons upon intravenous application of desipramine (40), our finding that intraperitoneal application of NE uptake blockers persistently increases extracellular DA in

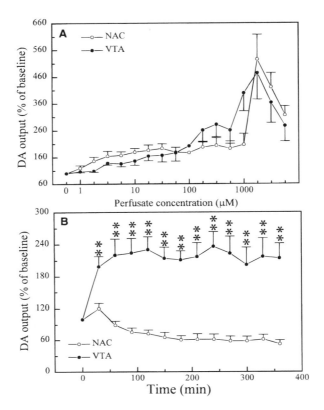

Fig. 8. Effects of local (**A**) and systemic (**B**) administration of desipramine on the dialysate DA levels from rat NAC and VTA. For local administration, progressively higher concentrations of desipramine (1, 10, 100, and 1000 μM) were perfused into the tested brain regions via the probe and each concentration was perfused for 80 min (4 samples). For systemic administration, desipramine (10 mg/kg, ip) was injected at time zero. Values are means ± SEM (n = 6–7). All data were evaluated by a two-way ANOVA with repeated measures over time. For local administration: time $F_{(16, 171)} = 30$, $p < 0.0001$; region, $F_{(1, 12)} = 0.04$, $p = 0.85$; interaction, $F_{(16, 171)} = 2.8$, $p = 0.0004$. For systemic administration: time, $F_{(12, 144)} = 2.3$, $p = 0.009$; region, $F_{(1, 12)} = 37$, $p = 0.0001$; interaction, $F_{(12, 144)} = 6$, $p < 0.0001$. **$p < 0.01$ compared with NAC at each time point (unpaired Student's t test).

the VTA of awake animals argues for their ability to depress the firing of DA neurons, provided the animals are conscious and freely moving. Since the A_{10} group of DA neurons in the VTA is also the origin of most dopaminergic fibers that innervate the prefrontal cortex, the DA effect of NE uptake blockers in the prefrontal cortex (22,74) is probably also under the impact of its DA effect in the VTA. This interpretation is supported by the relative short time-course of the DA effect of desipramine in the prefrontal cortex (1 h), compared with its long lasting NE effect in the cortex (>5 h) (37) and its long lasting DA effect in the VTA (>6 h) (Fig. 8). A sustained enhancement of extracellular DA in the VTA by NE uptake blockers would tend to partly counteract the NE uptake blocker-induced DA increase in the terminal regions by inhibiting the impulse activity of DA neurons, thus shortening the time-course of their DA effects in the prefrontal cortex. Blockade of somatodendritic DA autoreceptors will remove such autoinhibitory tone, allowing the DA effect of NE uptake blockers in the prefrontal cortex to become more appreciable and longer, which could account for the greater DA response in the prefrontal cortex observed following NE uptake blockers with systemically administered haloperidol than without (22).

Role of 5-HT in the DA Effect of Uptake Blockers

Numerous studies have been carried out to investigate the interaction between DA and 5-HT. Some earlier in vitro studies describe a stimulatory effect of exogenous 5-HT on [^{3}H]DA release from the midbrain slices (7,113). A number of in vivo studies report a stimulatory effect of 5-HT on terminal DA release, such as an increase in extracellular DA in NAC following central administration of a 5-HT$_3$ receptor agonist (26,62), an increase in extracellular DA in NAC following focal infusion of 5-HT involving both 5-HT$_3$ and 5-HT$_4$ receptors (93), a similar increase in the STR involving 5-HT$_{1-4}$ receptor subtypes (10), and an enhancing effect of endogenous striatal 5-HT following a high concentration of a 5-HT uptake blocker (114). The interpretation of these results is confounded by many factors, such as cross-labeling of the 5-HT terminals by [^{3}H]DA (27,73,108), the known activity of exogenous 5-HT and 5-HT$_3$ receptor agonist as DA transporter substrates (11,60,115), and nonspecific effects of 5-HT receptor agents, especially at their higher concentrations (45).

In our in vitro studies with STR, NAC, and VM slices (11,25), exogenous 5-HT and 5HT$_{1,2,3}$ receptor agonists fail to enhance electrically induced [^{3}H]DA release. In contrast, exogenous 5-HT increases spontaneous [^{3}H]DA release, which is most evident in fluoxetine-unpretreated VM slices. Our results with Ca^{2+}-free buffers, receptor antagonists, and uptake blockers indicate that the stimulatory effect of exogenous 5-HT on spontaneous [^{3}H]DA release is not mediated by 5-HT receptors, but by exchange diffusion via both DA and 5-HT transporters, mostly DA transporters in STR, NAC, and fluoxetine-pretreated VM slices, and mostly 5-HT transporters in fluoxetine-unpretreated VM slices.

Since 5-HT terminals can accumulate [³H]DA in vitro, one may ask whether the blockade of [³H]DA uptake into 5-HT terminals by cocaine could augment its stimulatory effect on impulse-dependent DA output. The existing experimental evidence is negative. In NAC and STR slices, DA transporters are predominant, and no evidence for a role of 5-HT transporters is observed in the effect of cocaine on electrically induced [³H]DA release. When the VM slices are labeled in the absence a 5-HT uptake blocker, to allow [³H]DA to enter 5-HT terminals, electrically induced [³H]DA release from the VM slices is mostly of 5-HT terminal origin, functionally modulated by 5-HT autoreceptors, rather than DA autoreceptors (Table 6). Under these conditions, uptake blockers that preferentially block DA transporters, such as GBR 12909 and nomifensine, are ineffective in increasing electrically induced [³H]DA release from the VM slices. Unexpectedly, cocaine significantly reduces electrically induced [³H]DA release. This inhibitory effect of cocaine on [³H]DA release may be a result of activation of terminal 5-HT autoregulation by blocking 5-HT re-uptake and enhancing synaptic 5-HT levels with a subsequent reduction in [³H]DA release from 5-HT terminals. This possibility is supported by the following observations. First, blockade of 5-HT transporters by preperfusion with fluoxetine, or blockade of terminal 5-HT$_{1B}$ autoreceptors by preperfusion with methiothepin, prevents the suppression of electrically induced [³H]DA release by cocaine. Second, under the same condition, the selective 5-HT uptake blocker fluoxetine and 5-HT itself also decrease [³H]DA release. Third, in the 5-HT release experiments, cocaine indeed impedes its own 5-HT stimulatory effect by indirectly activating 5-HT autoreceptors (Table 6). Thus, although 5-HT terminals can uptake and release [³H]DA, selective and nonselective 5-HT uptake blockers are unable to enhance electrically induced [³H] DA release by blocking 5-HT transporters.

Consonant with the in vitro studies, an increase in extracellular 5-HT levels in vivo by focal infusion of exogenous 5-HT (up to 0.4 µM) fails to increase VTA dialysate DA levels in awake animals (our unpublished data). Likewise, an increase in synaptic 5-HT levels by focal infusion of the selective 5-HT uptake blocker citalopram into the VTA (29) or fluoxetine into the NAC (80), does not produce an appreciable increase in dialysate DA levels. In addition, systemic administration of fluoxetine does not increase extracellular DA in the STR (96). These results indicate that both 5-HT itself, either exogenous or

Table 6
The Role of 5-HT Axonal Transporters in the In Vitro Effect of Cocaine on
Electrically Induced [³H]DA Release from Superfused Ventral
Mesencephalon Slices in Rats[a]

Pretreatment (labeling and/or $S_1 + S_2$)	Treatment, S_2	n	[³H]DA release, S_2/S_1
	Control	7	1.03 ± 0.04
	5-HT (0.1 μM)	4	0.76 ± 0.12^c
	Fluoxetine (10 μM)	3	0.81 ± 0.03^c
	Cocaine (10 μM)	7	0.62 ± 0.06^c
	Cocaine (100 μM)	5	0.47 ± 0.08^c
	Nomifensine (10 μM)	5	1.07 ± 0.03
	GBR 12909 (1 μM)	5	1.17 ± 0.05
	5-Methoxytryptamine (5 μM)	6	0.38 ± 0.06^c
	Methiothepin (1 μM)	3	1.34 ± 0.05^c
	Quinpirole (1 μM)	3	1.10 ± 0.10
	Sulpiride (10 μM)	3	1.14 ± 0.14
GBR 12909 1 μM ($S_1 + S_2$)	Cocaine (100 μM)[b]	3	0.43 ± 0.04^c
Fluoxetine 1 μM ($S_1 + S_2$)	Cocaine (100 μM)[b]	3	0.91 ± 0.01
Methiothepin 1 μM ($S_1 + S_2$)	Cocaine (10 μM)[b]	3	1.12 ± 0.06
Methiothepin 1 μM ($S_1 + S_2$)	Cocaine (100 μM)[b]	3	1.14 ± 0.16
Fluoxetine 1 μM (labeling)	Cocaine (100 μM)[b]	5	1.28 ± 0.07^c
Fluoxetine 1 μM	Cocaine (100 μM)[b]	3	1.61 ± 0.16^c

[a]Slices were labeled with [³H]DA (0.1 μM) in the presence of 0.5 μM desipramine. In some cases, fluoxetine was present during labeling period (labeling) to prevent [³H]DA from labeling serotonin terminals. Drugs were added at the start of the superfusion (S_1+S_2), or 20 min before the second stimulation (S_2) and maintained throughout the rest of the experiment. Values are mean ±SEM of n independent experiments. For other explanations, see Table 3.

[b]Control values in the absence of treatment are not shown here because pretreatment did not cause significant changes in S_2/S_1.

[c]$p < 0.05$ vs the control value (one-way ANOVA followed by the Newman Keul's test).

endogenous, and blockade of DA uptake into 5-HT terminals, are not capable of increasing the impulse-dependent DA output. To further investigate this issue, we have examined the effect of methiothepin on cocaine-induced DA output in the VTA. If the blockade of 5-HT$_{1B}$ receptors with methiothepin would reduce cocaine-induced DA output, it would be in favor of the notion that cocaine-induced 5-HT output stimulates DA release from the DA somatodendrites by activating 5-HT$_{1B}$ receptors located on accumbens-tegmental afferents to remove the GABA-mediated feedback inhibition to DA neurons (20,66). If this procedure would enhance the cocaine-induced DA output, it would be consistent with our in vitro findings that cocaine-induced 5-HT output inhibits DA release from the 5-HT terminals by activating terminal 5-HT$_{1B}$ autoreceptors (27). However, we have found no effect of methiothepin on either local or systemic cocaine-induced DA output in the VTA (28). Thus, it is questionable whether cocaine could modify its own in vivo DA effect through its 5-HT transporter blocking activity.

These in vivo studies do not exclude the possibility that endogenous DA could be taken up into, and released from, the 5-HT terminals in the VTA. Selective 5-HT uptake blockers, at moderate concentrations, may not be able to block DA and NE transporters, and endogenous DA released from the 5-HT terminals could still be removed effectively by DA somatodendrites and NE terminals. If 5-HT terminals indeed take up endogenous DA in vivo, one may ask why cocaine increases in vivo extracellular DA levels in DA cell body regions, rather than reduces them, as suggested by the in vitro studies with fluoxetine-unpretreated VM slices (Table 6). One explanation is that endogenous DA has much less chance to be taken up by 5-HT terminals than exogenous DA, and thus the impact of DA released from 5-HT terminals on the net DA output could be much less in vivo than in vitro. Under in vivo conditions, the somatodendritic DA effect of cocaine is predominant. Also, the above studies do not exclude the possibility that extracellular DA levels are modified by 5-HT in multiple or opposite ways (29).

Significance of Modulation of DA Transmission by NE and 5-HT System in the VTA

In the model with monoamine autoreceptor antagonists, one major finding is that, in the VTA, idazoxan or methiothepin appreciably elevate the basal DA level, in addition to increasing the basal NE or 5-HT levels (28), suggesting both NE and 5-HT systems may be involved, by receptor-mediated mechanisms, in the maintenance of a normal function of DA neurons under basal conditions. A low extracellular monoamine level in the DA cell body areas kept by ongoing uptake may be necessary for maintenance of the sensitivity of DA neurons to heteroregulating factors and physiological stimuli. DA uptake into NE and 5-HT terminals may be compensatory for the slower dynamics of DA uptake into somatodendrites. However, it is doubtful that heteroreceptor-mediated mechanisms can contribute to the DA effect of cocaine. On cocaine administration, nondopaminergic receptor-mediated modulation of DA neuron activity may be compromised because of the excessive levels of monoamine in the synaptic clefts or cocaine-induced depression of DA neuronal activity. If it is true that cocaine can increase extracellular DA by blocking NE transporters, it is not clear why it cannot do so by blocking 5-HT transporters. Perhaps the dynamic process for DA uptake into NE terminals and 5-HT terminals is different, because DA is a natural substrate for NE transporter, but it is not for 5-HT transporters, and because the affinity of DA for the NE transporter is much higher than that for the 5-HT transporter. In contrast to the above deduced lack of involvement of nondopaminergic receptor-mediated modulation of DA neuron activity in the effect of cocaine, NE transporter-mediated mechanism may well contribute to the DA effect of cocaine. Since systemic application of NE uptake blockers modifies the DA transmission in the NAC and VTA in an opposite way (enhancing extracellular DA levels in the VTA, and reducing extracellular DA levels in the NAC), the NE transporter-mediated mechanism might also play an role in triggering the autoinhibition of DA neurons and thus in limiting the terminal DA effect of systemic cocaine. Based on this, it would be of interest to investigate whether NE uptake blockers could alleviate the NAC DA effect of cocaine, and thus act as pharmacological adjuncts in the treatment of cocaine addiction.

Acknowledgments

The authors thank the National Institute on Drug Abuse for support (DA 03025 and 08379) of much of the work discussed in this chapter. We also thank Bob Burger for expert assistance in the HPLC aspects of the dialysis experiments, Lori L. Coffey for help in analyzing the experimental results, and Ming-Ya Li for collecting the most recent dialysis data presented in the chapter.

References

1. Ackerman, J. M. and White, F. J. A_{10} somatodendritic dopamine autoreceptor sensitivity following withdrawal from repeated cocaine treatment. *Neurosci. Lett.* **117** (1990) 181–187.

2. Adell, A. and Artigas, F. Differential effects of clomipramine given locally or systemically on extracellular 5-hydroxytryptamine in raphe nuclei and frontal cortex. *Naunyn-Schmiedebergs Arch. Pharmacol.* **343** (1991) 237–244.

3. Adell, A., Carceller, A., and Artigas, F. In vivo brain dialysis study of the somatodendritic release of serotonin in the raphe nuclei of the rat: Effect of 8-hydroxy-2-(di-n-propylamino)tetralin. *J. Neurochem.* **60** (1993) 1673–1681.

4. Arborelius, L., Chergui, K., Mruase, S., Nomikos, G. G., Höök, B. B., Chouvet, G., Hacksell, U., and Svensson, T. H. The 5-HT$_{1A}$ receptor selective ligands, (R)-8-OH-DPAT and (S)-UH-301, differentially affect the activity of midbrain dopamine neurons. *Naunyn-Schmiedebergs Arch. Pharmacol.* **347** (1993) 353–562.

5. Bayer, V. E. and Pickel, V. M. Somatic and dendritic basis for dopaminergic modulation in the ventral tegmental area. *Soc. Neurosci. Abstr.* **15** (1989) 483.4.

6. Beart, P. M. and McDonald, D. Neurochemical studies of the mesolimbic dopaminergic pathway: Somatodendritic mechanisms and GABAergic neurons in the rat ventral tegmentum. *J. Neurochem.* **34** (1980) 1622–1689.

7. Beart, P. M. and McDonald, D. 5-Hydroxytryptamine and 5-hydroxytryptaminergic–dopaminergic interactions in the ventral tegmental area of rat brain. *J. Pharm. Pharmacol.* **34** (1982) 591–593.

8. Becquet, D., Faudon, M., and Héry, F. The role of serotonin release and autoreceptors in the dorsalis raphe nucleus in the control of serotonin release in the cat caudate nucleus. *Neuroscience* **39** (1990) 639–647.

9. Bel, N. and Artigas, F. Fluvoxamine preferentially increase extracellular 5-hydroxytryptamine in the raphe nuclei: an in vivo microdialysis study. *Eur. J. Pharmacol.* **229** (1992) 101–103.

10. Benloucif, S., Keegan, M. J., and Galloway, M. P. Serotonin-facilitated dopamine release in vivo: Pharmacological characterization. *J. Pharmacol. Exp. Ther.* **265** (1993) 373–377.

11. Benuck, M. and Reith, M. E. A. Dopamine releasing effect of phenylbiguanide in tat striatal slices. *Naunyn-Schmiedebergs Arch. Pharmacol.* **345** (1992) 666–672.

12. Berger, P., Elsworth, J. D., Arroyo, J., and Roth, R. H. Interaction of [^{3}H]GBR12935 and GBR12909 with the dopamine uptake complex in nucleus accumbens. *Eur. J. Pharmacol.* **177** (1990) 91–94.

13. Biegon, A. and Rainbow, T. C. Localization and characterization of [^{3}H]desmethylimipramine binding sites in rat brain by quantitative autoradiography. *J. Neurosci.* **3** (1983) 1069–1076.

14. Bobillier, P., Seguin, S., Deguelurce, A., Lewis, B. D., and Pujol, J. F. The efferent connections of the nucleus raphe centralis superior in the rat as revealed by radioautography. *Brain Res.* **166** (1979) 1–8.

15. Boja, J. W. and Kuhar, M. J. [^{3}H]Cocaine binding and inhibition of [^{3}H]dopamine uptake is similar in both the rat striatum and nucleus accumbens. *Eur. J. Pharmacol.* **173** (1989) 215–217.

16. Bosker, F., Klompmakers, A., and Westenberg, H. Extracellular 5-hydroxytryptamine in median raphe nucleus of the conscious rat is decreased by nanomolar concentrations of 8-hydroxy-2-(di-n-propylamino)tetralin and is sensitive to tetrodotoxin. *J. Neurochem.* **63** (1994) 2165–2171.

17. Bradberry, C. W. and Roth, R. H. Cocaine increases extracellular dopamine in rat nucleus accumbens and ventral tegmental area as shown by in vivo microdialysis. *Neurosci. Lett.* **103** (1989) 97–102.

18. Broderick, P. A. Distinguishing effects of cocaine IV and SC on mesoaccumbens dopamine and serotonin release with chloral hydrate anesthesia. *Pharmacol. Biochem. Behav.* **43** (1992) 929–937.

19. Bunney, B. S., Walters, J. R., Roth, R. H., and Aghajanian, G. K. Dopaminergic neurons: effect of antipsychotic drugs and amphetamine on single cell activity. *J. Pharmacol. Exp. Ther.* **185** (1973) 560–571.

20. Cameron, D. L. and Williams, J. T. Cocaine inhibit GABA release in the VTA through endogenous 5-HT. *J. Neurosci.* **14** (1994) 6763–6767.

21. Carboni, E. and Chiara, G. Di. Serotonin release estimated by transcortical dialysis in freely-moving rats. *Neuroscience* **32** (1989) 637–645.

22. Carboni, E., Tanda, G. L., Frau, R., and Di Chiara, G. Blockade of the noradrenaline carrier increases extracellular dopamine concentrations in the prefrontal cortex: evidence that dopamine is taken up in vivo by noradrenergic terminals. *J. Neurochem.* **55** (1990) 1067–1070.

23. Chan, J., Nirenberg, M. J., Peter, D., Liu, Y., Edwards, R. H., and Pickel, V. M. Localization of the vesicular monoamine transporter-2 in dendrites of dopaminergic neurons: Comparison of rat substantia nigra and ventral tegmental area. *Soc. Neurosci. Abstr.* **21** (1995) 373.

24. Chan-Palay, V. Serotonin neurons and their axons in the raphe dorsalis of the rat and rhesus monkey: demonstration by high resolution autoradiography with ^{3}H-serotonin. In Chan-Palay V. and Palay S. L. (eds.), *Cytochemical Method is Neuroanatomy*, Liss, New York, 1982, pp. 357–386.

25. Chen, H.-T., Clark, M., and Goldman, D. Quantitative autoradiography of ^{3}H-paroxetine binding sites in rat brain. *J. Pharmacol. Toxicol. Meth.* **27** (1992) 209–216.

26. Chen, J., van Praag, H. M., and Gardner, E. L. Activation of 5-HT$_3$ receptor by 1-phenylbiguanide increases dopamine release in the rat nucleus accumbens. *Brain Res.* **543** (1991) 354–357.

27. Chen, N.-H. and Reith, M. E. A. [^{3}H]Dopamine and [^{3}H]serotonin release in vitro induced by electrical stimulation in A$_9$ and A$_{10}$ dopamine regions of rat brain: characterization and responsiveness to cocaine. *J. Pharmacol. Exp. Ther.* **267** (1993) 379–389.

28. Chen, N.-H. and Reith, M. E. A. Autoregulation and monoamine interactions in the ventral tegmental area in the absence and presence of cocaine: A microdialysis study in freely moving rats. *J. Pharmacol. Exp. Ther.* **271** (1994) 1597–1610.

29. Chen, N.-H. and Reith, M. E. A. Effects of locally applied cocaine, lidocaine, and various uptake blockers on monoamine transmission in the ventral tegmental area of freely moving rats: a microdialysis study on monoamine interrelationships. *J. Neurochem.* **63** (1994) 1701–1713.

30. Chen, N.-H. and Reith, M. E. A. Monoamine interaction measured by microdialysis in the ventral tegmental area of rats treated systemically with (±)-8-hydroxy-2-(Di-N-propylamino)tetralin. *J. Neurochem.* **64** (1995) 1585–1597.

31. Chen, N.-H., Xu, C., Coffey, L. L., and Reith, M. E. A. [^{3}H]WIN35,428(2b-carbomethoxy-3b-(4-fluorophenyl)tropane)binding to rat brain membranes: Comparing dopamine cell body areas with nerve terminal regions. *Biochem. Pharmacol.* **51** (1996) 563–566.

32. Cheramy, A., Leviel, V., and Glowinski, J. Dendritic release of dopamine in the substantia nigra. *Nature* **289** (1981) 537–542.

33. Cunningham, K. A. and Lakoski, J. M. The interaction of cocaine with serotonin dorsal raphe neurons. *Neuropsychopharmacology* **3** (1990) 41–50.
34. Cunningham, K. A., Paris, J. M., and Goeders, N. E. Chronic cocaine enhances serotonin autoregulation and serotonin uptake binding. *Synapse* **11** (1992) 112–123.
35. Curtis, A. L., Conti, E., and Valentimo, R. J. Cocaine effects on brain noradrenergic neurons of anaesthetized and unanesthetized rats. *Neurophamacology* **32** (1993) 419–428.
36. Delfs, J. M., Schreiber, L., and Kelley, A. E. Microinjection of cocaine into the nucleus accumbens elicits locomotor activation in the rat. *J. Neurosci.* **10** (1990) 303–310.
37. Dennis, T., L'heureux, R., Carter, C., and Scatton, B. Presynaptic alpha-2 adrenoceptors play a major role in the effects of idazoxan on cortical noradrenaline release (as measured by in vivo dialysis) in the rat. *J. Pharmacol. Exp. Ther.* **241** (1987) 642–649.
38. Dewar, K. M., Reader, T. A., Grondin, L., and Descarries, L. [^{3}H]Paroxetine binding and serotonin content of rat and rabbit cortical areas, hippocampus, neostriatum ventral mesencephalic tegmentum, and midbrain raphe nuclei region. *Synapse* **9** (1991) 14–26.
39. Donnan, G. A., Kaczmarczyk, S. J., McKenzie, J. S., Kalnins, R. M., Chilco, P. J., and Mendelsohn, F. A. O. Catecholamine uptake sites in mouse brain: distribution determined by quantitative [^{3}H]mazindol autoradiography. *Brain Res.* **504** (1989) 64–71.
40. Einhorn, L. C., Johansen, P. A., and White, F. J. Electrophysiological effects of cocaine in the mesoaccumbens dopamine system: studies in the ventral tegmental area. *J. Neurosci.* **8** (1988) 100–112.
41. Fibiger, H. C., Phillips, A. G., and Brown, E. E. The neurobiology of cocaine-induced reinforcement. *Ciba Found. Symp* **166** (1992) 96–124.
42. Florin, S. M., Kuczenski, R., and Segal, D. S. Regional extracellular norepinephrine responses to amphetamine and cocaine and effects of clonidine pretreatment. *Brain Res.* **654** (1994) 53–62.
43. Friedman, E. and Cooper, T. B. Pharmacokinetics of chlorimipramine and its demethylated metabolite in blood and brain regions of rats treated acutely and chronically with chlorimipramine. *J. Pharmacol. Exp. Ther.* **225** (1983) 387–390.
44. Gehlert, D. R., Gackenheimer, S. L., and Robertson, D. W. Localization of rat brain binding sites for [^{3}H]tomoxetine, an enantiomerically pure ligand for norepinephrine reuptake sites. *Neurosci. Lett.* **157** (1993) 203–206.
45. Glennon, R. A. and Dukat, M. Serotonin receptors and their ligands: a lack of selective agents. *Pharmacol. Biochem. Behav.* **40** (1991) 1009–1017.
46. Gonon, F. G. Nonlinear relationship between impulse flow and dopamine released by rat midbrain dopaminergic neurons as studied by in vivo electrochemistry. *Neuroscience* **24** (1988) 19–28.
47. Graznna, R. and Molliver, M. The locus coeruleus in the rat. *Neuroscience* **5** (1980) 21–40.
48. Grenholff, J. and Svensson, T. H. Prazosin modulates the firing pattern of dopamine neurons in rat ventral tegmental area. *Eur. J. Pharmacol.* **233** (1993) 79–84.

49. Gu, H., Wall, S. C., and Rudnick, G. Stable expression of biogenic amine transporters reveals differences in inhibitor sensitivity, kinetics, and ion dependence. *J. Biol. Chem.* **269** (1994) 7124–7130.

50. Harris, G. C. and Williams, J. T. Sensitization of locus ceruleus neurons during withdrawal from chronic stimulants and antipressants. *J. Pharmacol. Exp. Ther.* **261** (1992) 476–483.

51. Hemby, S. E., Jones, G. H., Justice, J. B., and Neill, D. B. Conditioned locomotor activity but not conditioned place preference following intra-accumbens infusions of cocaine. *Psychopharmacology* **106** (1992) 330–336.

52. Henry, D. J., Greene, M. A., and White, F. J. Electrophysiological effects of cocaine in the mesoaccumbens dopamine system: repeated administration. *J. Pharmacol. Exp. Ther.* **251** (1989) 833–839.

53. Herdon, H., Strupish, J., and Nahorski, S. R. Differences between the release of radiolabelled and endogenous dopamine from superfused rat brain slices: effects of depolarizing stimuli, amphetamine and synthesis inhibition. *Brain Res.* **348** (1985) 309–320.

54. Hery, F., Faudon, M., and Fueri, C. Release of serotonin in structures containing serotoninergic nerve cell bodies: Dorsalis raphe nucleus and nodose ganglia of the cat. *Ann. NY Acad. Sci.* **473** (1986) 239–255.

55. Hjorth, S. and Auerbach, S. B. Further evidence for the importance of 5-HT$_{1A}$ autoreceptors in the action of selective serotonin reuptake inhibitors. *Eur. J. Pharmacol* **260** (1994) 251–255.

56. Hjorth, S. Serotonin 5-HT$_{1A}$ autoreceptor blockade potentiates the ability of the 5-HT reuptake inhibitor citalopram to increase nerve terminal output of 5-HT in vivo: a microdialysis study. *J. Neurochem.* **60** (1993) 776–779.

57. Hrdina, P. D., Foy, B., Hepner, A., and Summers, R. J. Antidepressant binding sites in brain: autoradiographic comparison of [^{3}H]paroxetine and [^{3}H]imipramine localization and relationship to serotonin transporter. *J. Pharmacol. Exp. Ther.* **252** (1990) 410–418.

58. Hurd, Y. and Ungerstedt, U. Cocaine: an in vivo microdialysis evaluation of its acute action on dopamine transmission in rat striatum. *Synapse* **3** (1989) 48–54.

59. Invernizzi, R., Belli, S., and Samanin, R. Citalopram's ability to increase the extracellular concentrations of serotonin in the dorsal raphe prevents the drug's effect in the frontal cortex. *Brain Res.* **584** (1992) 322–324.

60. Jacocks III, H. M. and Cox, B. M. Serotonin-stimulated release of [^{3}H]dopamine via reversal of the dopamine transporter in rat striatum and nucleus accumbens: a comparison with release elicited by potassium, N-methyl-D-aspartic acid, glutamic acid and D-amphetamine. *J. Pharmacol. Exp. Ther.* **262** (1992) 356–364.

61. Javitch, J. A., Strittmatter, S. M., and Snyder, S. H. Differential visualization of dopamine and norepinephrine uptake sites in rat brain using [^{3}H]mazindol autoradiography. *J. Neurosci.* **5** (1985) 1513–1521.

62. Jiang, L. H., Ashby Jr., C. R., Kasser, R. J., and Wang, R. Y. The effect of intraventricular administration of the 5-HT$_3$ receptor agonist 2-methylserotonin on the release of dopamine in the nucleus accumbens: An in vivo chronocoulometric study. *Brain Res.* **513** (1990) 156–160.

63. Jordan, S., Kramer, G. L., Zukas, P. K., Moeller, M., and Petty, F. In vivo biogenic amine efflux in medial prefrontal cortex with imipramine, fluoxetine, and fluvoxamine. *Synapse* **18** (1994) 294–297.

64. Kalivas, P. W. Neurotransmitter regulation of dopamine neurons in the ventral tegmental area. *Brain Res. Rev.* **18** (1993) 75–113.

65. Kalivas, P. W., Bourdelais, A., Abhold, R., and Abbott, L. Somatodendritic release of endogenous dopamine: in vivo dialysis in the A_{10} dopamine region. *Neurosci. Lett.* **100** (1989) 215–220.

66. Kalivas, P. W. and Duffy, P. A comparison of axonal and somatodendritic dopamine release using in vivo dialysis. *J. Neurochem.* **56** (1991) 961–967.

67. Kalivas, P. W. and Duffy, P. Time course of extracellular dopamine and behavioral sensitization to cocaine. I. Dopamine axon terminals. *J. Neurosci.* **13** (1933) 265–275.

68. Kalivas, P. W. and Duffy, P. Time course of extracellular dopamine and behavioral sensitization to cocaine. I. Dopamine perikarya. *J. Neurosci.* **13** (1933) 276–284.

69. Kalivas, P. W. and Weber, B. Effects of daily cocaine and morphine treatment on somatodendritic and terminal field dopamine release. *J. Neurochem.* **50** (1988) 1498–1504.

70. Kaufman, M., Spealman, R. D., and Madras, B. K. Distribution of cocaine recognition sites in monkey brain: I. In vitro autoradiography with [^{3}H]CFT. *Synpase* **9** (1991) 177–187.

71. Kelland, M. D., Chiodo, L. A., and Freeman, A. S. Anesthetic influences on the basal activity and pharmacological responsiveness of nigrostriatal dopamine neurons. *Synapse* **6** (1990) 207–209.

72. Kelland, M. D., Freeman, A. S., and Chiodo, L. A. Chloral hydrate anesthesia alters the responsiveness of identified midbrain dopamine neurons to dopamine agonist administration. *Synapse* **3** (1989) 30–37.

73. Kelly, E., Jenner, P., and Marsden, C. D. Evidence that [^{3}H]dopamine is taken up and released from nondopaminergic nerve terminals in the rat substantia nigra in vitro. *J. Neurochem.* **45** (1985) 137–144.

74. Kihara, T. and Masato, I. Effects of duloxetine, a new serotonin and norepinephrine uptake inhibitor, on extracellular monoamine levels in rat frontal cortex. *J. Pharmacol. Exp. Ther.* **272** (1995) 177–183.

75. Koe, B. K. Molecular geometry of inhibitors of the uptake of catecholamines and serotonin in synaptosomal preparations of rat brain. *J. Pharmacol. Exp. Ther.* **199** (1976) 649–661.

76. Lacey, M. G., Mercuri, N. B., and North, R. A. Action of cocaine on rat dopaminergic neurones in vitro. *Br. J. Pharmacol.* **99** (1990) 731–735.

77. Lategan, A. J., Marien, M. R., and Colpaert, F. C. Effects of locus coeruleus lesions on the release of endogenous dopamine in the rat nucleus accumbens and caudate nucleus as determined by intracerebral microdialysis. *Brain Res.* **523** (1990) 134–138.

78. Lategan, A. J., Marien, M. R., and Colpaert, F. C. Suppression of nigrostriatal and mesolimbic dopamine release in vivo following noradrenaline depletion by DSP-4: a microdialysis study. *Life Sci.* **50** (1992) 995–999.

79. Levi, G. and Raiteri, M. Carrier-mediated release of neurotransmitters. *Trends Neurosci.* **16** (1993) 415–419.

80. Li, M-Y., Yan, Q-S., Coffey, L. L., and Reith, M. E. A. Extracellular dopamine, norepinephrine, and serotonin in the nucleus accumbens of freely moving rats

following focal cocaine and other monoamine uptake blockers. *J. Neurochem.* **66** (1996) 559–568.

81. Matsumoto, M., Yoshioka, M., Togashi, H., Hirokami, M., Tochihara, M., Ikeda, T., Smith, C. B., and Saito, H. Mu-opioid receptors modulate noradrenaline release from the rat hippocampus as measured by brain microdialysis. *Brain Res.* **636** (1994) 1–8.

82. Mennicken, F., Savasta, M., Peretti-Renucci, R., and Feuerstein C. Autoradiographic localization of dopamine uptake sites in the rat brain with ^{3}H-GBR 12935. *J. Neural. Transm.* **87** (1992) 1–14.

83. Moore, R. Y. and Card, J. P. Noradrenaline containing neuron systems. In Böjorklund, A. and Hökfelt T. (eds.), *Handbook of Chemical Neuroanatomy*, Elsevier, Amsterdam, 1984, pp. 123–153.

84. Mosko, S. S., Haubrich, D., and Jacobs, B. L. Serotonin afferents to the dorsal raphe nucleus: Evidence from HRP and synaptosomal uptake studies. *Brain Res.* **119** (1977) 269–290.

85. Nissbrandt, H., Engberg, G., and Pileblad, E. The effect of GBR12909, a dopamine re-uptake inhibitor, on monoaminergic neurotransmission in rat striatum, limbic forebrain, cortical hemispheres and substantia nigra. *Naunyn-Schmiedebergs Arch. Pharmacol.* **344** (1991) 16–28.

86. Nissbrandt, H., Pileblad, E., and Carlsson, A. Evidence for dopamine release and metabolism beyond the control of nerve impulses and dopamine receptors in rat substantia nigra. *J. Pharm. Pharmacol.* **37** (1985) 884–889.

87. Nissbrandt, H., Sundström, E., Jonsson, G., Hjorth, S., and Carlsson, A. Synthesis and release of dopamine in rat brain: comparison between substantia nigra pars compacta, pars reticulata, and striatum. *J. Neurochem.* **52** (1989) 1170–1182.

88. Nomikos, G. G., Damsma, G., Wenkstern, D., and Fibiger, H. C. In vivo characterization of locally applied dopamine uptake inhibitors by striatal microdialysis. *Synapse* **6** (1990) 106–112.

89. Oades, R. D. and Halliday, G. M. Ventral tegmental (A$_{10}$) system: 1. anatomy and connectivity. *Brain Res.* **434** (1987) 117–165.

90. Okuma, Y. and Osumi, Y. KCl-induced calcium-independent release of dopamine from rat brain slices. *Brain Res.* **363** (1986) 47–52.

91. Pacholczyk, T., Blakely, R. D., and Amara, S. G. Expression cloning of a cocaine- and antidepressant-sensitive human noradrenaline transporter. *Nature* **350** (1991) 350–354.

92. Pan, WH. T., Lim, L.-H., and Shiau, M-R. Difference in extracellular cocaine concentration between the ventral tegmental area and the medial prefrontal cortex following intravenous administration as revealed by quantitative microdialysis coupled with in vivo calibration. *J. Neurosci. Meth.* **53** (1994) 65–71.

93. Parsons, L. H. and Justice, Jr. J. B. Perfusate serotonin increases extracellular dopamine in the nucleus accumbens as measured by in vivo microdialysis. *Brain Res.* **606** (1993) 195–199.

94. Parsons, L. H. and Justice, J. B., Jr. Serotonin and dopamine sensitization in the nucleus accumbens, ventral tegmental area, and dorsal raphe nucleus following repeated cocaine administration. *J. Neurochem.* **61** (1993) 1611–1619.

95. Pecci Saavedra, J., Brusco, A., Peressini, S., and Oliva, D. A new case for a presynaptic role of dendrites: an immunocytochemical study of the N. raphe dorsalis. *Neurochem. Res.* **11** (1986) 997–1009.

96. Perry, K. and Fuller, R. W. Effect of fluoxetine on serotonin and dopamine concentration in microdialysis fluid from rat stratum. *Life Sci.* **50** (1992) 1683–1690.

97. Pitts, D. K. and Marwah, J. Electrophysiological actions of cocaine on noradrenergic neurons in rat locus coeruleus. *J. Pharmacol. Exp. Ther.* **240** (1987) 345–341.

98. Reith, M. E. A., Meisler, B. E., Sershen, H., and Lajtha, A. Structural requirements for cocaine congeners to interact with dopamine and serotonin uptake sites in mouse brain and to induce stereotyped behavior. *Biochem. Pharmacol.* **35** (1986) 1123–1129.

99. Richelson, E. and Pfenning, M. Blockade by antidepressants and related compounds of biogenic amine uptake into rat brain synaptosomes: most antidepressants selectively block norepinephrine uptake. *Eur. J. Pharmacol.* **104** (1984) 277–286.

100. Richfield, E. K. Quantitative autoradiography of the dopamine uptake complex in rat brain using [^{3}H]GBR 12935: Binding characteristics. *Brain Res.* **540** (1991) 1–13.

101. Ritz, M. C., Cone, E. J., and Kuhar, M. J. Cocaine inhibition of ligand binding at dopamine, norepinephrine and serotonin transporters: a structure-activity study. *Life Sci.* **46** (1990) 635–645.

102. Ritz, M. C., Lamb, R. J., Goldberg, S. R., and Kuhar, M. J. Cocaine receptors on dopamine transporters are related to self-administration of cocaine. *Science* **237** (1987) 1219–1223.

103. Robertson, G. S., Damsma, G., and Fibiger, H. C. Characterization of dopamine release in the substantia nigra by in vivo microdialysis in freely moving rats. *J. Neurosci.* **11** (1991) 2209–2216

104. Rothman, R. B., Lewis, B., Dersch, C., Xu, H., Radesca, L., de Costa, B. R., Rice, K. C., Kilburn, R. B., Akunne, H. C., and Pert, A. Identification of a GBR12935 homolog, LR1111, which is over 4,000-fold selective for the dopamine transporter, relative to serotonin and norepinephrine transporters. *Synapse* **14** (1993) 34–39.

105. Rutter, J. J. and Auerbach, S. B. Acute uptake inhibition increase extracellular serotonin in the rat forebrain. *J. Pharmacol. Exp. Ther.* **265** (1993) 1319–1324.

106. Santiago, M. and Westerink, B. H. C. Characterization and pharmacological responsiveness of dopamine release recorded by microdialysis in the substantia nigra of conscious rats. *J. Neurochem.* **57** (1991) 738–747.

107. Silvia, C. P., King, G. R., Lee, T. H., Xue, Z-Y., Caron, M. G., and Ellinwood, E. H. Intranigra administration of D_2 dopamine receptor antisense oligodeoxynucleotides establishes a role for nigrastriatal D_2 autoreceptors in the motor actions of cocaine. *J. Pharmacol. Exp. Ther.* **46** (1994) 51–57.

108. Simon, J. R. and Ghetti, B. Is there a significant somatodendritic uptake of dopamine in the substantia nigra? Evidence from the weaver mutant mouse. *Neurochem. Int.* **22** (1993) 471–477.

109. Thomas, D. N., Post, R. M., and Pert, A. Focal and systemic cocaine differentially affect extracellular norepinephrine in the locus coeruleus, frontal cortex and hippocampus of the anaesthetized rat. *Brain Res.* **645** (1994) 135–142.

110. Ugedo, L., Grenhoff, J., and Svensson, T. H. Ritanserin, a 5-HT receptor antagonist, activates midbrain dopamine neurons by blocking serotonergic inhibition. *Psychopharmacology* **98** (1989) 45–50.

111. Wassef, M., Berod, A., and Sotelo, C. Dopaminergic dendrites in the pars reticulata of the rat substantia nigra and their striatal input. Combined immunocytochemical localization of tyrosine hydroxylase and anterograde degeneration. *Neuroscience* **6** (1981) 2125–2139.

112. Westerink, B. C. and Devries, J. B. On the origin of dopamine and its metabolite in predominantly noradrenergic innervated brain areas. *Brain Res.* **330** (1985) 164–166.

113. Williams, J. and Davies, J. A. The involvement of 5-hydroxytryptamine in the release of dendritic dopamine from slices of rat substantia nigra. *J. Pharm. Pharmacol.* **35** (1983) 734–737.

114. Yadid, G., Pacak, K., Kopin, I. J., and Goldstein, D. S. Endogenous serotonin stimulates striatal dopamine release in conscious rats. *J. Pharmacol. Exp. Ther.* **270** (1994) 1158–1165.

115. Yi, S. J., Gifford, A. N., and Johnson, K. M. Effect of cocaine and 5-HT$_3$ receptor antagonists on 5-HT-induced [^{3}H] dopamine release from rat striatal synaptosomes. *Eur. J Pharmacol.* **199** (1991) 185–189.

Index